What a professor says about this book

Scientifically-based health professionals recognize that current approaches to weight-loss need to change. Extreme and often unpleasant diets do lead to some initial weight-loss. But, almost inevitably, hunger and dissatisfaction with the entire process lead back to old habits and the regain of most, if not all, of the lost weight. This chain of events is frustrating and unhealthy. Further attempts to lose weight with the same extreme approaches just repeat the process and the same dismal outcomes.

Many health professionals have also realized that there must be a healthful way to lose weight effectively and permanently. With its careful blending of science and practice, **WEIGHT-LOSS SALVATION** offers that way. This is a terrific approach for people who want to prevent additional weight-gain, for people who are overweight and need to lose some weight, and for people who are obese and need to lose a lot of weight.

There are no gimmicks, fad diets, or ridiculous exercise programs here. Rather, the key revolves around lifestyle and energy balance through developing a healthful, enjoyable, and sustainable eating pattern. This pattern can custom-fit each individual, and include the foods people prefer. Likewise, simple walking provides a base for physical activity and exercise. Walking and other exercise can be done in a way that's enjoyable and satisfying so that it becomes part of a more active lifestyle.

Rather than rigorous and inflexible procedures, **WEIGHT-LOSS SALVATION** provides many different strategies so that people can best shape a program that will fit into their lives. Numerous real-life examples of effective strategies, including those that helped one of the authors maintain a large weight-loss after years of turmoil and struggle, provide a rich base for people to develop their own effective programs.

But make no mistake about it, **WEIGHT-LOSS SALVATION** is not about yet another horrible diet to be followed for a few weeks and then abandoned. This wonderful book is all about doable, *sustainable* changes that will enable you to lose weight and then *maintain* that weight-loss, and make your entire lifestyle healthful and enjoyable.

– Richard A. Winett, Ph.D., Professor of Psychology,
Virginia Tech, Blacksburg, VA 24061, USA

Also by Stuart McRobert

Build Muscle, Lose Fat, Look Great

The Insider's Tell-All Handbook on Weight-Training Technique

Brawn

Beyond Brawn

Further Brawn

WEIGHT-LOSS SALVATION

HOW REAL PEOPLE LOSE WEIGHT AND KEEP IT OFF

First Edition

Stuart McRobert & Bradley Cailor

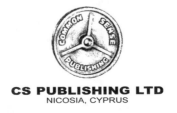

CS PUBLISHING LTD
NICOSIA, CYPRUS

Cover production and photo retouching by Phil Velikan: www.findphil.com
Cover copyright © 2010 by Stuart McRobert
Cover photographs courtesy of Jupiterimages®

CS Publishing Ltd., P.O. Box 20390, CY-2151 Nicosia, Cyprus
tel + 357-2233-3069   cspubltd@spidernet.com.cy
www.weightlosssalvation.com
www.hardgainer.com

Printed in the United States of America

Cataloging-in-Publication Data

McRobert, Stuart, 1958–
    Weight-loss salvation : how real people lose weight and keep it off /
    by Stuart McRobert and Bradley Cailor. -- 1st ed.
        p. : photos. ; cm.
    Includes index.
    ISBN: 978-9963-9163-7-5 (hardcover)
    1. Weight loss. 2. Nutrition   I. Cailor, Bradley, 1965– II. Title
RM222.2.M37 2010   613.2

Dedications

This book is for everyone who has a weight problem. And it's especially for people who are tired of failure from restrictive diets, fad diets, gimmicky pills, and exercise gadgets.

Once you follow this book's proven guidance you *will* lose weight and then *keep it off*.

  – Stuart McRobert and Bradley Cailor

To my late father, LaVerne, my late mother-in-law, Evelyn, and my late father-in-law, Sonny.

To my lovely wife, Lisa, who loved me just as much when I was fat as when I was slim; and to my mother, Lucy, whose belief in me never wavered.

To William Chill, whose steadfast support helped to make this project possible.

And to Stuart McRobert, who gave an unknown author a chance.

  – Bradley Cailor

To my wife, Maro, the rock of my life. Over many years she has sacrificed a great deal so that I could realize my dream of being a writer and a publisher. Without her love and support this book would never have happened.

  – Stuart McRobert

CONTENTS

PART IV
THE WHOLE-SCOOP SUMMARY OF WHAT
YOU MUST DO FOR WEIGHT-LOSS SUCCESS

Disclaimer

Trademarks

There's much more to this book than the account of how Brad achieved his terrific weight-loss success story.

WEIGHT-LOSS SALVATION incorporates much additional information and guidance that Brad wasn't aware of during his transformation, *to provide you with the definitive model for how to lose weight and keep it off.*

MISSION STATEMENT

How much weight do you want to lose?

Out of the hundreds of successful real-life dieters who were researched for this book, the average weight-loss was 25 to 45 pounds for women, and 40 to 60 for men. There were some 80-, 100-, and 150-pound triumphs, and there were also many 15- to 20-pound triumphs (which is a lot of weight for a five-foot tall woman to lose, for example).

But no matter how much weight the real-life dieters lost, *they all did essentially the same thing*. This means that the people who lost 20 or 30 pounds—and kept it off—followed basically the same approach that helped the much heavier people, like Brad, to lose their weight.

This book will teach you *precisely* how these people lost their weight and then *kept it off*.

How much weight do *you* want to lose—10 pounds, 25, 50, 100, or more than 100? Whether you want to lose a few pounds, or a few hundred pounds, this book has the proven guidance that's specific to *your* individual needs.

WEIGHT-LOSS SALVATION is for *everyone* who wants to lose weight, *regardless of how much*. And it's also for people who may already be content with their current weight *but who don't want to add weight as they age*.

Because the guidance promoted in this book worked for Brad and hundreds of real-life dieters, it's *proven*, and will work for you, too.

Introduction

WEIGHT-LOSS SALVATION is for everyone who has a weight problem. And it's especially for people who are tired of failure from restrictive diets, fad diets, gimmicky pills, and exercise gadgets.

The book explains what real people did to lose weight and then *keep it off*. By drawing on real-life success stories, the book takes the best elements from many weight-loss plans and presents them in an easy-to-follow guide.

And it covers the psychological and physiological issues that are at the root of many people's weight problems and weight-loss difficulties. Only after having addressed these issues will even a sensible weight-loss plan have a chance of success.

But aren't anorexics weighing under 70 pounds, and 400-plus pound people, the only ones who have eating disorders? *No.*

And isn't weight-loss simply about discipline and willpower? *No.*

Learn from real people who succeeded with weight-loss, and gain the confidence and know-how required to produce your own success story.

Ads that claim fast weight-loss results are usually snake-oil pitches, and are misleading and manipulative. People are duped by a multi-billion-dollar industry that preys on the gullible.

Co-author Brad Cailor has experienced all the trials and tribulations that come with trying to lose weight. Throughout his adult life he has regained well over 600 pounds of fat from yo-yo dieting. He lost it in different intervals, but kept putting it back on. It included more than a dozen 40- and 50-pound weight-losses. He was called "the human guinea pig for failed diets" by his friends.

But Brad's experiences with dieting aren't exceptional. They are common. And many people have lost far more weight than Brad. These people are among the real-life dieters Brad learned from, and who inspired him to research this topic thoroughly.

Chronic yo-yo dieting is a major reason why weight-related issues have become the second leading cause of preventable death in the United States—second only to smoking. And they may soon become the *leading* cause of preventable death, according to projections by the Centers for Disease Control and Prevention.

Brad needed to find a weight-loss plan that worked. It had to be one that wouldn't make him miserable. And it had to be one he could comfortably *sustain* while still enjoying life.

After experimenting with almost every pill and plan, Brad found a blueprint that works, based on a model of success that has worked for countless real-life people who lost weight and then *kept it off*.

Brad's final, continuous stretch of weight-loss yielded a 114-pound net fat-loss.

By this time Brad had a wealth of weight-loss knowledge—from his 30 years of trial-and-error experiences, and his 25 years of research that included interviewing hundreds of people who have been successful with long-term weight-loss.

He wondered if this knowledge could be the basis of a book. So he discussed the raw concept, and his research, with Stuart McRobert from CS Publishing in Cyprus. Stuart immediately saw the potential for a co-authored book. His research acumen, knowledge of exercise and nutrition, and experience of writing how-to instructional books, *in combination with Brad's unique, powerful contribution*, resulted in **WEIGHT-LOSS SALVATION**.

Stuart has long been the doyen of trustworthy guidance on exercise and related topics. He has authored several books, and he published and edited an exercise instruction magazine for 15 years. Here's what Dr. Gregory Steiner, a chiropractor from Texas, has said:

> *"In the field of physical training—where hyperbole, drugs, dishonesty, inappropriate training routines, insufficient attention to safety, and excessive commercialization are rampant—Stuart McRobert's books are unique. They are honest, safety-minded, health-conscious, inspirational, free of hype and drugs, and packed with instruction that works for all trainees."*

Although the worlds of weight-loss and physical training are different, they share common problems. Both are loaded with nonsense and dishonesty, and information that's highly commercialized because its purpose is to exploit gullible people.

Starting with Brad's concept, Brad and Stuart worked to bring to weight-loss the same no-nonsense, practical and thorough approach that Stuart used when he wrote his books on exercise instruction.

Brad was a personal trainer for seven years, a trainer of national- and world-caliber powerlifters, the president of Kent State University's Weightlifting and Exercise Association, and a competitive powerlifter. He also has a college degree in health education, post-graduate schooling in nutrition, and was a certified health teacher for almost a decade.

Brad has tremendous experience of dieting because he struggled with his weight for 30 years. Most so-called experts on weight-loss have never had such a struggle. Brad went through this agonizing struggle and eventually solved the problem.

Furthermore, Brad's father, mother-in-law, and father-in-law died prematurely as a consequence of excessive weight and the inability to be successful with weight-loss. This book presents the information that could have prevented those deaths, and will prevent similar deaths.

Part I is a brief analysis of some of Brad's weight-loss attempts, and what you can learn from his mistakes. It also explains why Brad got fat in the first place.

Part II details the psychological and physiological issues that are at the root of many people's weight problems and weight-loss difficulties, and explains how they should be addressed.

As weight-loss obsessed as Brad was, it wasn't until after 30 years of struggle that he acknowledged the contribution of psychological issues to his weight problem and the difficulties he had with applying weight-loss plans.

Of course, a sensible, practical and healthy lifestyle is essential for successful weight-loss—a regimen that's unlike most diets. But for many people, even a sensible regimen will work *only* if the related psychological and possibly physiological issues are understood and properly addressed.

Part III is the unique weight-loss guide written from the perspective of real-life experiences. It will teach you how to lose weight *and* keep it off.

WEIGHT-LOSS SALVATION isn't a diet book. Diets usually mean deprivation, discipline and dictates, and they invariably fail.

This isn't just another book on weight-loss.

As of late 2009—just prior to the publication of this book—Brad has maintained his ideal weight for just three-and-a-half years because that's the period since he completed his transformation. But many of the real-life dieters Brad researched—who followed *the same basic approach as he did*—made their transformations much earlier, and thus have maintained their ideal weights for much longer. *And the approach they all used—explained in this book—will work for you, too, if you apply it as they did. Be confident!*

The basic formula for weight-loss is common to all effective plans—*reduced caloric intake*, and *increased caloric output.*

But precisely *how* those two components are implemented makes the difference between a plan that can be carried out comfortably and enjoyably over the long-term, and a plan that can be carried out *only* over the short-term because it's *restrictive, unpleasant,* and *impractical.*

The lifestyle-reform, weight-loss and health model promoted in WEIGHT-LOSS SALVATION *is* comfortable and enjoyable to implement, and thus sustainable over the long-term, to produce the required weight-loss and then *keep it off*.

And not only will it transform your appearance, it will also transform your health, which will add life to your years, and probably add years to your life.

Read - Grasp - Apply - Persist . . . *Achieve*

Five critical preliminaries

1. "Diet" and "dieting" have bad connotations

"Going *on* a diet means someday you're going to go *off* a diet.
 You can't be on a diet your whole life."

This quote is from a man billed as the "world's greatest dieter" by
the *Guinness Book of World Records*, for losing the most weight in the
least time. He went from 1,100 pounds to 198 pounds, but then
regained all of his weight. So, he may also hold the unofficial
world record for *regaining* the most weight in the least time. He's a
prime example of how *fast* weight-loss from restrictive diets nearly
always leads to long-term failure.

"Diet" and "dieting" are usually associated with bouts of
suffering, sacrifice, and deprivation. And they usually result in
mere temporary change.

According to the Federal Trade Commission (FTC), restrictive
diets and fad diets have a 95% failure rate. They fail because the
dieters can't wait to get back to their comfort zone—the lifestyle
and habits that got them heavy in the first place.

New diet concepts or books are commonly based on supposedly
"new and revolutionary principles" that try to present quick and
easy paths to weight-loss. But these "revolutionary principles"
don't work *long-term* in at least 95% of the cases.

**Successful weight-loss plans that keep the weight off must
be based on behavior that you're already comfortable
with. Many dieters have said, "The best diet is the one
you don't know you're on." This makes sense, and is the
principle behind the guidance in this book.**

How many times have you seen someone embark on a diet only
to end up frustrated and heavier over the long-term? Has this
ever happened to you?

Deprivation diets usually don't work over the long-term.

Our bodies and minds naturally repel deprivation diets. And our
everyday lives make those diets impractical to follow.

No wonder the great majority of diets end up in failure. Brad's
deprivation diets failed every time.

If you can't see yourself exercising and eating in the new way for the rest of your life, don't bother starting, because you'll most likely fail.

There are no quick fixes for long-term weight-loss. Your changes must be small, gradual, enjoyable, and *sustainable* if they are to be permanent.

Restrictive or fad diets usually dictate that you strictly follow their rules and ways of eating. But people usually don't like being told what they can or can't eat.

WEIGHT-LOSS SALVATION teaches you how to modify your eating habits so that—within reason—you can continue to eat what you want. If a diet's rules take you too far from your normal routine, you'll sooner or later fail to follow it.

When *you* call the shots, and without the thought of having to experience the misery and frustration of a diet, you'll have a terrific chance of succeeding at weight-loss.

The words "diet" and "dieting" are usually reminders of memories of deprivation and failure.

You will, however, see the words "diet," "dieting" and "dieter" in this book because they are so commonly used. But be aware of their limitations, and have the positive, upbeat attitude that you're *not* on a diet, but that you have adopted a fresh outlook on life, nutrition, and health.

2. This book is for men and women

Although this book was written by two men, a majority of the hundreds of successful real-life dieters researched for this book were women. The principles learned from all of these dieters are what Brad applied to yield his own transformation.

This book's subtitle, "How real people lose weight and keep it off" is derived from the research amassed from these hundreds of real men and women. The research is highlighted in the dozens of sidebars, stories, and illustrative tie-ins presented in this book.

While some gender-specific issues affect weight and weight-loss—such as menopause, and hormones in general—the fundamental ways in which men and women lose weight and keep it off *are the same*.

Although the central character of this book is male, what you'll learn from his success and vast research will apply to you *regardless* of your gender.

Apply the guidance of this book to your own situation—whether you're male or female—and adjust your caloric intake based on your size, activity levels, and goals.

3. America is fat . . . *what's the skinny?*

Nearly two out of every three Americans are obese or overweight. What the heck's going on?

Restaurant portion-sizes are much bigger than they used to be. Large fast-food sizes have become the norm. Most people greatly underestimate the number of calories they consume.

And it's not just a calorie issue. Most people consume large quantities of sodium, sugar, and the wrong types of fats; and high-fructose corn syrup seems to be in just about everything.

Much of America is gorging on food with little nutritional value. Although oversupplied with calories, most Americans are deficient in some nutrients.

Fast-food restaurants and high-fructose corn syrup didn't exist 50 years ago. And obesity wasn't really a problem back then, either.

Average Americans are ingesting 300 more calories a day than they did 25 years ago. Those extra daily calories equate to 109,500 extra *annual* calories.

Furthermore, generally speaking, people are less active than they used to be. Approximately 80% of Americans are sedentary, and don't exercise at all.

So, because most people are doing nothing to use up the extra calories, it's no wonder that nearly two out of every three Americans are obese or overweight.

And the same problem also affects other countries—the UK, for example.

The consequences are grave—not just for the health and well-being of individuals, but in terms of the huge increase in the demands on national medical services.

4. Get a physical checkup before you begin

Your doctor should be an expert on weight-loss and nutrition. According to a study by New York University, only 3% of medical students take elective courses in nutrition.

If your doctor isn't an expert on weight-loss and nutrition, you may be referred to a bariatrician—a doctor who deals with the causes, prevention, and treatment of obesity.

5. This book is thorough

The greater your understanding of the practicalities of effective weight-loss, the more readily you're likely to lose weight and keep it off. And that's why this book is thorough.

WEIGHT-LOSS SALVATION has three categories of information:

>Information you're probably already familiar with because it's accurate material that's often promoted by other people.

>Subjects you're probably familiar with but not the specific information that this book presents.

>Information on topics unique to our research that you've probably never heard about.

The weight-loss model presented in this book has already worked for countless real-life people. Brad is but one example.

If you apply what this book teaches, you *will* lose weight *and keep it off.*

Part I

AN ANALYSIS OF SOME OF BRAD'S REAL-LIFE DIETS

Important terminology

Food processing can be something as simple as removing the skin from peaches, dicing carrots, or any form of cooking. But by "processed foods" we're referring to products that have undergone physical or chemical treatment that results in substantial change in the state of the food. Typically, nutrients are removed, taste and texture are altered, and sugar, fat, salt, emulsifiers, colorings, flavorings, and other additives are mixed in.

The two main categories of this type of processed food are "junk food" and "fast food." But some people use those terms interchangeably.

Junk food refers to items such as candy, that are high in calories but with no significant nutritional value; and products with nutritional value but that are made unhealthy by the processing method and added ingredients—for example, potato chips.

And fast food specifically refers to items such as hamburgers, pizza, or fried chicken, which are prepared by a standardized method and can be dispensed quickly and inexpensively.

Junk food is always unhealthy. But provided that natural ingredients are used, without harmful processing, meals can be fast yet healthy. But the fast food we refer to in this book, unless otherwise specified, is the unhealthy type.

Be informed and discerning—read nutrition labels.

"The ad claimed anyone could lose up to 100 pounds in as little as 12 weeks."

The "magical" weight-loss program

Many people who struggle with their weight have been lured into buying weight-loss pills and potions. They were deceived by unscrupulous claims for miraculous results from the use of scam products. It happened to Brad.

Brad has been a chronic yo-yo dieter for decades. He would eat healthily until summer, then balloon up by autumn and winter. By the time he was 25 he had lost and regained almost 300 pounds.

January was always the start of a new diet, which included the latest program or pill. In late 1991, with a new diet looming, Brad saw an ad for a mega-hype, mass-advertised program.

The ad claimed anyone could lose up to 100 pounds in as little as 12 weeks. Dramatic before-and-after pictures supported the claim.

Convinced that the program would work, Brad ponied up the $125. He now had the inspiration for his New Year's diet.

The program involved severe exercise, restricted eating, large quantities of water, and an array of pills. It mirrored the discipline required of a bodybuilder preparing for a competition. It was the most demanding plan Brad had ever seen, let alone attempted.

Brad ate frequent small meals with skinless chicken breasts, egg whites, tuna, and lots of fruits and vegetables. The daily gallon of water was claimed to "flush the fat out."

He ran wind sprints, and climbed bleacher stairs—he pushed himself so hard that he often vomited.

And he lifted weights ruthlessly.

He didn't know what the pills were, but they were part of the program. Brad followed the program without questioning it.

After 12 weeks he got down to 156 pounds—a loss of 52 pounds. This was the fourth time Brad had lost more than 50 pounds in a continuous stretch.

The program was brutal, but the results were dramatic. Brad's face was chiseled, he had visible veins in his limbs, and he finally had abs. His confidence soared.

Ironically, the basis for the mega-hype program's success was also the basis for its failure. Overwhelmed by its severity, Brad crossed the finish line and was *done*.

Deprived of burgers, chips, and pizza, he craved them more than ever. After returning to his normal eating routine it wasn't long before his abs were gone, and his belly was back.

ANALYSIS
Why this program worked, and failed

Brad ate small portions at frequent intervals, with a total daily intake of 1,000 to 1,200 calories. Coupled with lifting weights rigorously, and intensive running, he shedded body fat readily. The combination of severe exercise and dietary control was the "secret" of the program.

Besides the calories he burned during the workouts, the ultra-intensive exercise may have elevated his metabolism for a period after each workout, and further increased his caloric output.

Brad probably added a few pounds of muscle during this program, which further helped his efforts to lose fat.

The diet pills probably contributed a placebo effect and increased water loss, but they helped to justify the high cost of the program.

Most weight-loss pills—whether they claim to burn fat, control appetite, or help you lose weight in another way—have accompanying fine print that states: "results achieved are in conjunction with diet and exercise." The pills can, however, provide a placebo effect. If you believe that the pills burn fat, for example, you may be more likely to train and diet harder. Brad's experience exemplified this.

Ultra-restrictive plans don't work over the long-term because that degree of sacrifice can't be maintained for extended periods. Because partying, junk food, and fast food were important to Brad at the time, the mega-hype program had no chance of longevity.

And there were psychological issues behind Brad's weight and weight-loss problems. These needed to be addressed if he was to lose weight and *keep it off*.

"Because he was so mentally deprived from the tortuous dieting and exercising, each weekend usually resulted in some sort of late-night binge session."

The wedding diet

Have you ever tried a crash diet in an effort to lose weight quickly for a wedding, vacation, or class reunion, for example? It may have yielded short-term results, but it probably ended in long-term failure. This has happened to Brad many times.

Because Brad was so deprived from the restrictions of the mega-hype program outlined in the first chapter, food became an obsession. He had already regained 25 pounds when he began a relationship with his new girlfriend in the autumn of 1992, at the age of 27.

Although the relationship was going well, a dilemma was unfolding. Brad's girlfriend loved to dine out at restaurants, and eat fast food. Unknowingly, she was enabling the temptations that triggered Brad's underlying problems with overeating.

He now had a fixation for all-you-can-eat buffets, and fine dining, and a renewed interest in fast food. And because of this his weight climbed to 225 pounds—12 heavier than he'd ever been before.

He knew he was becoming unhealthy, but didn't care. He was finally content with his life, and fell into an unhealthy comfort zone.

If diets didn't work, why bother trying? Eating made Brad feel good, dieting didn't. He enjoyed eating too much to stop.

After a two-year courtship, Brad proposed to his girlfriend, and she accepted.

Although the relationship had Brad living in a state of elation, he was also living in denial.

While he was initially oblivious to how heavy he was becoming—because he was so fixated on enjoying his life—some people were now poking fun at his rotund appearance. The blunt comments made Brad realize that he was fat.

Brad promised his new fiancée that he would try not to embarrass them with his appearance for their once-in-a-lifetime day. He vowed to get in shape for the wedding, and had four months to do it. The wedding was set for February 24, 1995, one day before his 30th birthday.

He had a resurgence of motivation. Although he vowed to lose weight for his fiancée, Brad also needed to it for himself.

He really did look like "a potato on two toothpicks." The effects of his profound weight-gain finally hit home.

To lose the weight, Brad again turned to the principles learned from the mega-hype program—severe running and rigorous lifting of weights, coupled with six ultra-restrictive mini-meals a day. If it worked once, it should work again.

But because he was so mentally deprived from the tortuous dieting and exercising, each weekend usually resulted in some sort of late-night binge session. Whether it was an entire pizza, a bag of tacos, *two* late-night breakfasts at a local 24/7 restaurant, or a dozen mini-hamburgers, Brad couldn't control his binging.

Needless to say, the diet wasn't working and the weight wasn't coming off. Brad panicked. He lost composure and began to all but starve himself. By consuming nothing but skim milk, protein bars, peanut butter, and water for six weeks, he got down to 184 pounds for the wedding. He lost a lot of muscle, but he met his goal.

And now he had to lose even more weight, for their honeymoon in Los Angeles, California. They were going to beaches renowned for beautiful bodies. Brad had four more weeks to get in top shape.

He was now obsessed with weight-loss. It dominated his every thought and action.

Needing to lose weight even quicker, he was won over by the claims of "fast results" from a notorious fat-burning pill.

The pills (which were essentially "speed") created a nightmare. They made Brad moody, irritable, and nauseous. And he was often soaked in a cold sweat while his hands trembled. He even experienced frightening heart palpitations.

He further limited his food intake, to just 500 to 750 calories a day, from tiny rations of skim milk and peanut butter.

And despite that he had little energy due to the lack of calories, and he was so light-headed he could barely drive a car, Brad still exercised hard.

While the borderline-starvation plan produced fast weight-loss, Brad was now fat *and* skinny.

Although he was down to 168 pounds for his honeymoon, Brad still had a belly, and his arms and chest had shriveled to nothing.

He appeared emaciated because he had lost so much muscle mass. His face was gaunt. Prior to his departure, a friend asked, "Brad, are you on a hunger strike or something? You look like you're dying."

After arriving at the beach and watching athletic bodies frolic for a day, Brad's confidence sunk. Despite that he trained as hard as possible in an attempt to have a beach-worthy physique, his emaciated build—along with his ever-present belly—didn't measure up to the required standard.

He was so intimidated by the perfect bodies that he mentally surrendered. He abandoned all thoughts of health, and decided to enjoy the rest of his honeymoon without reservation. He became obsessed with food and couldn't control himself.

He ate so much that he was up to 183 pounds by the time he got home a week later, whereas his wife gained nothing. This was because Brad ate most of her meals as well his own.

He soon ballooned back to 225 pounds, by resorting to the comfort zone he thrived in—fast-food, partying, and all-you-can-eat binging.

Commenting that Brad was always starting a diet but never finishing one, his friends now began calling him "the human guinea pig for failed diets."

ANALYSIS
Why this diet worked, and failed

Brad's initial reason for weight-gain is common. "Dieting" was such a source of deep-rooted misery that he rebelled against it. He fell into an unhealthy comfort zone that allowed him to eat what he wanted, when he wanted. And he became content because he was freed from the source of frustration and unhappiness that had blighted his life for the last decade.

Brad was demonstrating many symptoms of binge-eating disorder. And his wife became an unknowing enabler who inadvertently put him into situations that triggered his underlying problems (which, at the time, neither of them realized he had).

Although Brad's wife enjoyed fast food and eating at restaurants, she always kept her portions in check. And she kept herself fit due to a lifelong commitment to exercise. As a result, she stayed slim.

Anyone who lives on fat burners, and small quantities of peanut butter and skim milk, will lose weight. But 500 to 750 calories a day is nowhere near sufficient to provide the nutrition necessary for proper sustenance.

Borderline starvation is dangerous. It can deplete your body of essential nutrients and electrolytes, and can cause stomach ulcers.

When you severely reduce your caloric intake, your body slows its basal metabolic rate as a means of self-preservation. Furthermore, your body is innately programmed to *store* fat if you starve yourself, and crash diets are a major trigger for this.

Brad's initial progress was negated by his over-indulgent weekends. By starving, then binging, over and over, he was training his body to physically preserve its fat stores.

And once he began his borderline-starvation diet full-time, his body actively stored every ounce of fat it could. This is why he had such a hard time losing his belly and fat at the sides of his waist.

By not giving his body enough food to sustain its functioning, it broke down muscle tissue to make up for the insufficiency of calories. And by losing an estimated 10 to 15 pounds of muscle tissue, Brad substantially *decreased* his daily energy output.

Although Brad lost 57 pounds via the scale, 10 to 15 of it was previously hard-earned muscle tissue. And the rest was a combination of fat and temporary water weight.

He was burning many calories from jogging and lifting weights—like he had done while on the mega-hype program—but he lost muscle instead of gaining it, due to insufficient nutrition.

Amphetamine-like weight-loss pills can be harmful. The side-effects that Brad experienced are common among users.

Brad's failure is an example of why crash diets never work over the long-term. He lost 57 pounds so quickly that he regained it all back shortly thereafter.

"In under a year—even though he was taking large doses of diet pills—Brad's weight swelled to 266 pounds."

The doctor's-orders diets I and II

Traumatic outside influences can have an overwhelming effect on your health, and can make losing weight difficult. Brad has endured this.

Because he was getting older—now well into his 30s— Brad was becoming concerned about his health.

Throughout the second half of the 1990s he tried many of the popular fad diets and trendy pills, but he could never generate any lasting progress. Although he wanted to lose weight, dieting continued to be an on-going source of frustration.

But he wasn't alone. Losing weight in the late 1990s was challenging. The variation of theories, fads, and gimmicks had many people frustrated.

Was it high carb, low carb, or no carb?

Was it high protein, or low protein?

And what about the hot new pill or fat burner?

Every trainer seemed to have a different opinion on what worked. And being a former personal trainer, Brad found it amazing that he was having such a difficult time himself.

He eventually found a common-sense way to lose weight. In late 1998 he put together a decent weight-loss run by severely reducing his consumption of processed food, and doing more at-home cooking without any fast food whatsoever. But, once again, the results wouldn't last long.

After getting his weight back down to 200 pounds, Brad made a career change. He began a time-consuming post in the high-stress world of real-estate finance at a large, high-pressure brokerage. It was a sink or swim, 100% commission job with brutal quotas and deadlines, and extraordinary pressure to meet the quotas and deadlines. If you didn't perform, you were ridiculed, and fired on the spot.

The comfort derived from binge eating became a necessary reprieve to help Brad make it through the nerve-racking workweek. Fast food, and all-you-can-eat buffets—his comfort-zone foods—once again became the staples of his diet.

In under a year—even though he was taking large doses of diet pills—Brad's weight swelled to 266 pounds. He took on the jolly moniker "Big Brad" in response to his newfound girth.

He was eating too much, partying too much, enduring too much stress, and popping many diet pills.

He would often lie on a couch in a cold sweat, with a racing heart beat. There were times when he felt that his heart was going to explode.

Something had to give, and Brad collapsed at work. His horrified co-workers thought he was dying of a heart attack. His heart was pounding furiously, and he felt a sharp pain deep inside his chest. He was so terrified from the anxiety that he was having a real heart attack, that he fainted.

After a night in the intensive care unit he found out that he had had a combination of a panic attack and acid reflux, which can mimic a heart attack.

The doctor said that Brad's poor diet and extreme weight-gain, among other things, helped trigger his severe acid reflux. And the sharp pain in his chest was the result of his esophagus being inflamed and irritated by regurgitated stomach acids.

The doctor told Brad that his panic attack was a response of his sympathetic nervous system as a result of a very unhealthy lifestyle coupled with living on adrenaline and experiencing far too much stress.

The panic-attack symptoms he experienced included trembling, shortness of breath, heart palpitations, chest pain and tightness, hot flashes, burning sensations in his facial and neck areas, sweating, nausea, dizziness, light-headedness, hyperventilation, and a sensation of choking. It's no wonder these symptoms are often interpreted as being from a heart attack.

Brad's blood pressure and health numbers were terrible. The doctor gave him strict orders to lose weight, exercise, eat better, reduce the partying, and cut back his stress levels, or else he would have a real heart attack.

The doctor made it simple. No fast food, no junk food, no late-night eating, and no binging. And he was told to eat a balanced diet based on normal but nutritious foods, with more realistically sized portions.

He was also told that the human body needs exercise. He was instructed to begin some walking and light jogging.

The doctor lectured Brad on the dangers of his amphetamine-like diet pill obsession. He was playing Russian roulette with his life. He was ordered to ditch the diet pills forever.

Brad quit his ultra-high-stress job and got involved with a business he always wanted to be part of. He acquired a short-track, sprint-car racing facility, by taking out a small-business loan. It was an enormous financial commitment, but the scare of the heart attack made him realize that he had only one life to live, and he wanted to take a chance in order to fulfill a dream.

His stress subsided. And he was eating better and exercising, too—just what the doctor ordered. He was down to 214 pounds by April of 2001, and feeling somewhat healthy. But this progress would be short-lived.

The outdoor-racing business is dependent on the weather. Brad ran into some bad luck and had to cancel nine consecutive events due to rain. Trying to fulfill his business obligations and loan payments with no source of income, was devastating.

To cope with his anguish, Brad wolfed food for comfort, drank beer, watched The Weather Channel, and got more and more depressed. And he was drinking dangerous amounts of alcohol— up to 12 or more beers a day.

But it was the tragedy of September 11, 2001 that finally stressed Brad past his breaking point. The monumental loss of human life devastated him. He thought the world was coming to an end. He thought World War III was inevitable.

The effects of that horrific day hampered the world's economy. And that downturn further stymied Brad's racing business, which was dependent on discretionary spending. People were now staying at home more.

Brad's business was crippled.

His failing business, and the overwhelming effects of the national tragedy, plunged Brad into a debilitating depression. And his binge eating and drinking increased yet further.

His health was in jeopardy once again. After ignoring the doctor's orders for eight months, he returned to the doctor. He weighed-in at more than 250 pounds, and his cholesterol and blood pressure readings were dangerously high.

Like a broken record, the doctor ordered Brad to eat right, exercise, drink less, and reduce stress.

It was finally time, supposedly, to heed the doctor's orders.

ANALYSIS
Why Brad struggled with his weight

The psychological issues behind Brad's weight problems mounted. By resorting to food for comfort whenever he faced a stressful situation, he was showing more symptoms of binge-eating disorder.

The level of stress that he faced following his failed business is what he called "debilitating." Stress triggers the body to release a hormone called cortisol, which reduces the body's sensitivity to leptin—the hormone that tells your brain when you're feeling full.

Studies have shown that people who secrete higher levels of cortisol in response to chronic stress tend to binge eat for comfort, and put on weight.

Stress can lead to elevated blood pressure, and chest pain, and this, coupled with the side effects from diet pills, may have contributed to Brad's collapse at work.

And stress becomes even more harmful when people resort to alcohol for relief. Instead of alcohol relieving Brad's stress, it tended to *keep* his body in a stressed state, further compounding his problems.

Many weight-loss pills and fat burners provide large doses of a dangerous mix of caffeine-type ingredients. Their use can lead to serious health risks.

The controversial diet pill that Brad was taking—an amphetamine-like stimulant, which speeds the heart rate and constricts blood vessels—was eventually banned by the US Food and Drug Administration (FDA) after it was linked to 155 deaths.

But the "no-fast-food-at-home diet" that Brad had moderate success with, did have merit. He was on the right track with that.

"Food became Brad's solace to cope with depression."

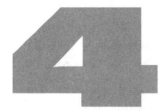

Eat, drink, and be merry!

The death of a family member can dominate your life, and lead to serious health problems. It happened to Brad.

Drinking and eating continued to dominate his life for the remainder of 2001. But, by the end of the year, he found the wherewithal to resume work. He sold his racing business and, in December of 2001, he went back to the high-stress arena of real-estate finance.

To avoid the ever-present stress of this profession, Brad tried to enjoy a more relaxed work environment. But it was the unhealthy antics of its employees that made this environment so relaxed.

He tried to follow his doctor's orders, but was surrounded by co-workers who chain-smoked cigarettes, and drank beer openly.

The co-workers lived off processed food, and ate it in front of Brad. And all company meetings were held at a local tavern that always had a tempting spread of calorie-laden appetizers, and booze.

These antics stymied Brad's weight-loss motivation. And he postponed his doctor's-orders diet yet again.

Needing a change in the spring of 2002, he found employment that satisfied his health needs and his career aspirations. Because it was a small operation, Brad told his new boss and co-workers not to parade unhealthy food around him, and to respect his efforts to lose weight and regain his health. He made this a condition of his employment.

Things were now in place for yet another weight-loss comeback. With full support from his new employer, 2002 was going to be the year that Brad would really try to heed his doctor's orders.

Because a few of his friends had lost a great deal of weight with the "no-carbohydrate diet," Brad figured he would try it, too.

But no carbs for two weeks drove him bonkers. He lost some weight, but was so lethargic and light-headed that he couldn't stick with it. He missed fries, he missed chips, he missed pizza. He missed life. This diet was the epitome of misery.

After surrendering to a three-day, binge-eating frenzy, Brad was *done* with the zero-carb plan. He lost 10 pounds, but regained 12. And he still weighed over 250 pounds.

Perhaps he was spooked by the restrictions of the zero-carb fiasco, but he was more obsessed with food than ever. Taking away his chips, fries and pizza for a few weeks made him crave them even more. And when he got his hands on any of these foods, a binge was inevitable. The "no-carb" diet messed with his psyche.

The year 2002 became a dietary hell. Brad tried almost every diet and gimmick on the market, but the weight didn't come off, and he became aggravated. It was as if he had a self-defeating attitude, and every diet failed before it had a chance to work.

Still reeling from the aftermath of his business failure, and that the US was now at war, 2002 was a wretched year.

And it ended devastatingly.

A few weeks before Christmas he was notified by his brother that their father was in the hospital in a terminal condition. But Brad had the chance to spend a few days with his beloved father before he passed away.

The sight and sound of a heart monitor flat-lining while he held his father, devoured Brad's soul, and crippled him emotionally.

He was very close with his parents, but he was especially close with his father. His father was always involved in Brad's life, and heavily involved in his racing business.

The loss of his father was the most overwhelming experience of Brad's life.

Before he passed away, Brad's father sternly lectured him, "Son, you've got to lose some weight. I'm worried about you. *Promise* me you'll lose weight and get healthy."

Brad promised that he would try. This was their final conversation. A few days before Christmas of 2002, Brad's father was buried.

Brad was so bitter and heartbroken that he cried in the seclusion of his basement for two weeks. He was paralyzed with grief.

To combat his broken heart, Brad drank heavily. And he ate a great deal of delivered pizza, usually a large meat-lover's pie every night in *addition* to his chips and other junk food.

Brad was on the brink of opening his own real-estate finance business when his father died.

Despite the motivational speech his late father had given him, Brad found it impossible to focus on anything, let alone a diet.

His profound depression continued until June, when he had to endure the back-to-back weekends of Father's Day and his late father's birthday.

Eventually, Brad could cry no more. He had to move on. He finally had the motivation to heed his late father's wishes, and get healthy.

With his enthusiasm now at an all-time high, he exercised hard, but too hard.

Because he was in poor physical condition from months of inactivity, he tore his rotator cuff while lifting weights, and severely pulled a muscle in his calf while jogging. Now he couldn't jog or lift weights, the staples of his exercise regimen.

No matter how hard he tried, he couldn't train around these injuries, and he got discouraged. And then he had an epiphany: "Screw it—eat, drink, and be merry . . . live life to its fullest . . . it's party time."

Perhaps it was a mid-life crisis, but Brad really wanted to enjoy his life. He ate out at fine restaurants, recklessly enjoyed pizza and other fast food, and partied heartily.

The non-stop party lasted all the way through Christmas of 2004.

He was fat and out of shape, but he didn't care because he was finally content. Partying and eating were a lot more fun than worrying about life's monumental hurdles—most of which were out of his control.

And partying and eating were a lot more fun than dieting.

Deep down, Brad knew he was in a state of denial, but the live-life-to-its-fullest attitude provided him with an escape.

Despite all the adversities Brad put his wife through, she was never mad at him for his stupid choices. She loved him unconditionally, even when he was depressed or angry. And she loved him just as much when he was fat as when he was slim.

Brad finally realized how lucky he was to have such a supportive wife, because he had put her through hell.

ANALYSIS
Why Brad continued to struggle

Tragedy can dominate one's life, and preclude weight-loss. Food became Brad's solace to cope with depression.

And his non-stop partying was his way of escaping emotional problems. He resorted to alcohol and comfort food as a diversion. Although he claimed he was happy, it was a facade to cover up his real issues.

Many people try to cope with tragedies in this manner. Brad should have received professional help. Many people ignore their problems, or try to solve them on their own. This can make matters worse over the long-term.

The "no-carb diet" is potentially dangerous, and nutritionally unsound. It can compound the problems of overeating. This diet has garnered harsh criticism from the National Academy of Sciences, the American Medical Association, the American Dietetic Association, the American Heart Association, the Cleveland Clinic, the American College of Sports Medicine, and the National Institutes of Health.

Among Brad's friends who lost a great deal of weight with the "no-carbohydrate diet," all of them regained their weight.

It's imperative that an exercise program is started slowly, and progress is made gradually, to avoid injury. A gung-ho attitude usually leads to injuries. The older you are, the more careful you have to be about warming up adequately, starting out light and easy, and progressing gradually.

"He abandoned the principles that had resulted in his past failures—weight-loss pills, gimmicks, fads, deprivation diets, and any expectation of fast results.

"And he sought counsel from real people who have lost a lot of weight *and kept it off*, and heeded their advice."

Finally . . . success, after a hurdle or two

The day after Christmas 2004, Brad's non-stop party lost its appeal. A new year was a few days away, and his 40th birthday was looming. The time was right for a life change.

He re-prioritized his life. His health was at the top of the list—40 was too old to be messing with his health. His late father's motivational speech was clearly in Brad's mind. His injuries had healed, and he was ready to succeed.

On January 1, 2005, Brad weighed 265 pounds. He needed a weight-loss plan that worked over the *long*-term. To get reliable answers on what really worked, Brad decided to ask successful dieters themselves—a majority of which were female—how they lost their weight *and kept it off.*

Brad became fascinated with how real dieters solved their weight problems. And after talking to many people he noticed common patterns. But these patterns weren't gender specific—the men and women essentially did the *same thing.*

He found that the only proven way to lose weight over the long-term was the seemingly archaic method of eating right, and exercising. No one attributed any of their success to a pill or a gimmick.

Patience was the key. There weren't any viable shortcuts. Brad discovered that losing more than one or two pounds of fat a week was not realistic for lasting results.

He took the input from real-life dieters, reviewed what he had done himself in the past, and cross-referenced it all with current research. He finally had a proven weight-loss model based on real-life success. And if these real people could achieve life-changing results, why couldn't Brad? He *knew* he was going to succeed now.

He was profoundly motivated.

His new exercise program consisted of a 20-minute walk or gentle jog three mornings a week, and a weight-lifting workout two mornings a week. Weekends and evenings consisted of elective activities like brisk dog walking, house chores, or bike rides—anything to avoid being a couch potato.

He kept himself busy, to help keep his mind off food. As part of this he spent many hours each day researching weight-loss.

His diet consisted of several nutritious mini-meals, or snacks, a day—normal foods in small portions.

This concept of more frequent but smaller meals was used with great success while on the mega-hype program, and Brad's research further substantiated its merits. But he replaced the severity of the mega-hype diet with home-cooked foods, and additional daily calories, to make his eating enjoyable. This home-cooked approach produced good results during his "no-fast-food-at-home diet."

Within reason, most of the successful real-life dieters enjoyed the foods they liked. And eating something every two to four hours eliminated hunger pangs and the urge to binge. This made the diet easy to follow because Brad never felt that he was dieting.

He was dreadfully unhealthy when he began his new approach. It was a struggle merely to jog a hundred yards, walk a little, jog a little, and so on. But he persevered.

Each week he could go a little farther. Within a few months he could jog a mile. And within a few more months he could jog two miles. Brad kept pushing himself, and gradually he improved.

In a little over a month, he was under 250 pounds. This was the first progress Brad had seen in years. The new program was working because it was easy for him to follow—it was fun.

He set interim goals in 10-pound intervals, instead of a daunting 100-pound overall goal. It was satisfying and motivating to achieve regular, albeit small triumphs.

As the year went by, the pounds came off . . . 240 . . . 220 . . . 210 . . . 205 . . . 202. Brad was now losing nearly two pounds a week, and the 200-pound barrier was in sight.

Regrettably, that day arrived. "Regrettably" because Brad was so thrilled that he had lost 66 pounds, he pushed his morning jog too hard and severely re-injured his calf.

With his jogging shut down, he lost his enthusiasm for lifting weights, which, in turn, foiled his weight-loss aspirations.

And now Brad would have to deal with a few weeks of temptations—Thanksgiving through New Year's. The holidays were difficult because he hosted family that demanded a spread of cake, cookies, and junk foods. He couldn't control himself around these enticing spreads.

Following the month of debauchery, he stepped on the scale and was disgusted at what he saw—219 pounds.

Despite the 20-pound regression, it was a new year with a new focus. Because he knew what worked, he knew he could return to losing weight. This boosted his enthusiasm for the 2006 comeback.

Inspired by a few middle-aged women who exercised twice a day, six or seven days a week, Brad decided to step up his training to make up for his inadvertent regression.

He jogged for 40 to 50 minutes every weekday morning. While he still jogged at a moderate pace, he interjected a few brief periods of higher-intensity exercise—running—to get his heart pumping faster. If the middle-aged women could do it, he could, too.

To prevent injuries, he began a therapy program to strengthen and stretch his calves. Injury prevention was an important part of Brad's comeback. His calf was healed, but it had to stay healed.

He shifted his weight lifting to Tuesday and Thursday evenings, when he had more energy. He reserved the other evenings, and weekends, for activities like bicycling, inline skating, house chores, or brisk dog walks. He became more active.

The biggest reason why Brad felt compelled to step up his activity level was that he felt guilty that he was sitting on his butt all day because of his sedentary career. He was enjoying exercise now that he had abandoned the gung-ho approach.

His best friend was also exercising, so Brad had a workout buddy for extra support, but only in spirit because they lived in different towns. The weekly e-mail updates were great for motivation.

Brad's diet was an enhanced version of what he succeeded with the previous year. He still ate six nutritious mini-meals a day, but this time he monitored each one closely.

Each one had about 20 to 30 grams of protein, and 200 to 400 calories, depending on the time of day. He ate a mini-meal every two or three hours. And he reduced his carbohydrate and caloric intake later in the day, and avoided nighttime snacking.

He ate normal foods like a home-cooked lean hamburger on a 100% whole-wheat bun, or a chicken breast, turkey breast, or roast beef sandwich. He ate apples, and vegetables like string beans or baby peas dressed up with tasty fat-free margarine, and pepper. And he prepared his food in a nutritious manner.

When pressed for time, Brad had an all-natural meal replacement bar, or a glass of skim milk.

His snacking was limited to nutritious foods like turkey or chicken breast slices, almonds, peanuts, pistachios, and fat-free cheese slices.

Because he ate often, and thoroughly enjoyed what he ate, Brad had a hard time calling his plan a diet.

He even enjoyed a beer or two, or a glass of wine, on occasion. He found that occasional rewards or a *little* cheating helped him to stick with the plan. Now that he had made his mental and physical health his priorities, Brad had stopped excessive drinking.

Because he was enjoying the foods he liked during the week, Brad lost his desire to eat junk food during the weekends. But he knew that he was allowed to cheat a little if the inclination arose.

He was learning how to manage his underlying desire to gorge on food. He finally cared about himself, and about his health and appearance. Eating poorly had led to feelings of guilt, and that he was letting himself down.

He no longer wanted a week's worth of progress to be wiped out by a binge.

He eventually avoided all the foods and situations that triggered his binge eating—especially potato chips, all-you-can-eat buffets, and delivered pizza.

And he voluntarily eliminated fast food and junk food from his life.

He now had sustained energy from the complete nutrition his body was receiving, and he was in a good mood all the time. He found that exercise and proper nutrition were excellent mood boosters.

As the weeks went by, the pounds disappeared.

His ultimate goal was still well down the road. He had vowed that he would return to his self-determined ideal weight—165 pounds. That would yield the century-mark of weight-loss—100 pounds.

Brad experienced no deprivation, and he realized that he could easily adhere to a version of this approach for the rest of his life. And he knew that if losing the weight was this easy, maintaining the loss would be even easier. Brad was living a normal, fulfilling life while supposedly on "a diet."

There were good weeks and not-so-good weeks, but he persisted, and the progress continued. He was down to 190 pounds by late April, and 176 by June.

He finally met his goal, and then exceeded it, by weighing in at a lean 163 pounds on July 28, 2006.

Besides the loss of weight, Brad was much healthier. All of his vital signs were in top form. He was no longer a heart attack candidate. He had reduced his blood pressure, resting pulse rate, and cholesterol levels to those of a seasoned athlete. And his unnerving heart palpitations had long since vanished.

Although he lost 102 pounds according to the scale, body-fat composition tests indicated that he had lost 114 pounds of fat because he put on an estimated 12 pounds of lean muscle tissue. And if you factor in his late-2005 fat regression (where he gained back 20 pounds), he actually lost 134 pounds of fat.

He felt like a new person. He felt healthy, and looked healthy. And his self-esteem soared. "Big Brad" no longer existed.

The best news was that his wife was no longer married to the fat guy who had been in her life for 10 years. And she was thrilled that he had regained his health and passion for life.

Life for the new Brad was fantastic now that he was healthy and fit. And his future was an exciting blank canvas without limitations.

ANALYSIS
Why Brad finally succeeded

He lost the weight on *his* terms.

He did nothing that could be considered deprivation. Although he ate primarily for nutritional reasons, he still ate what he wanted and enjoyed. And he did exercise that he enjoyed, and readily allocated the time for it in his new lifestyle.

Because he understood that it was going to take over a year to complete, he knew he had to be patient. Setting small, interim goals helped maintain his enthusiasm while he lost the full 100+ pounds. Factoring in his late 2005 regression, Brad averaged a loss of 1.62 pounds of fat a week over the 19 months it took to reach his long-term goal.

He abandoned the principles that resulted in his past failures—weight-loss pills, gimmicks, fads, deprivation diets, and any expectation of fast results. And he sought counsel from real people—men *and* women—who have lost a lot of weight *and kept it off*, and heeded their advice.

WEIGHT-LOSS SALVATION is based on this model of success.

Brad achieved his transformation well before he became aware that he's had an eating disorder for most of his life.

He's proven that vast, enduring weight-loss is possible even for people with eating disorders.

But **WEIGHT-LOSS SALVATION** includes much additional information and guidance that Brad wasn't aware of during his transformation, *to provide you with the definitive model for how to lose weight and keep it off.*

As of late 2009—just prior to the publication of this book—Brad had maintained his ideal weight for just three-and-a-half years because that's the period since he completed his transformation. But many of the real-life dieters Brad researched—who followed the same basic approach as he did—made their transformations much earlier, and thus have maintained their ideal weights for much longer.

And the approach they all used—explained in this book—will work for you, too, if you apply it as they did.

Be confident!

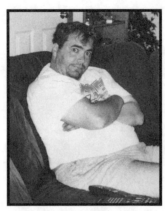

Brad, as a 265-pound couch potato, October 1999.

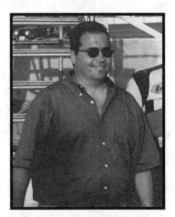

Before his second visit to the doctor, August 2001.

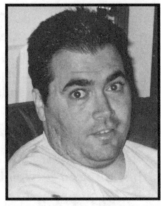

Brad's bloated face at his peak weight, October 1999.

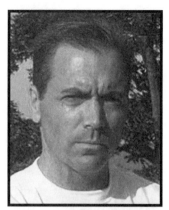

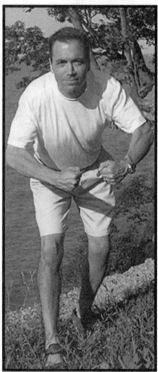

Brad, looking healthy at age 41, after his transformation, July 2006. He's mimicking a common "after" photograph of some dieters.

Part II

HOW TO LOSE WEIGHT AND KEEP IT OFF, Section A

The psychological and physiological aspects

A REALITY CHECK

How everyone gains weight

If you're heavy, there must have been a period — whether it was a few months, a few years, or even a few decades — during which you consistently consumed more calories than you used up, to produce the caloric surplus that yielded the excess stored fat. The fat didn't just appear on your body overnight.

But unlike Brad and many other once-heavy people, most people *don't* put on a vast amount of weight in a short period. According to James O. Hill in a December 2008 issue of the *American Journal of Clinical Nutrition*, typical Americans (including the initially non-overweight population) gain, on average, between about one and two pounds a year. At this pace, a five-foot eight-inch, 150-pound 18-year-old could become a 200-pound 50-year-old — and most if not all of that weight-gain will be fat. And this 200-pound person would be considered obese.

According to the Centers for Disease Control and Prevention (CDC), in 1960 the average female was about five-foot three-inches and weighed about 140 pounds. As of 2002, the average female was five-foot four-inches and about 164 pounds — just a tick away from being considered obese by BMI charts. And during the same time frame the average man grew by more than an inch to nearly five-foot ten-inches, and went from 166 to 191 pounds — nearly obese by BMI charts.

So, for many people, the cause of weight-gain isn't gluttony but, rather, a consistent but small energy imbalance that adds up year after year. Without adequate activity to burn the surplus calories off, they end up as body fat.

But no matter when or precisely how your extra weight accumulated, this book will teach you how to get rid of it, *permanently*.

Did you ever eat just one potato chip, close the bag, and were done? Probably not.

And why do many people have powerful urges to gorge on comfort foods?

This chapter will explain.

Food addiction—
why and how some
foods are *designed*
to be addictive

Processed foods are designed to be irresistible and addictive in order to stimulate your body's inborn emotional responses.

That's **why some foods are so mouth-watering.**

And that's also why many people find it so difficult to stop eating some foods.

Your innate desire for food's pleasure

According to *The End of Overeating*, by David A. Kessler, M.D. (Rodale, 2009), the human body has an inborn system that leads you to seek out pleasurable rewards.

The pleasure derived from eating is one of the rewards you're programmed to desire.

Kessler proposes that modern-day processed foods are *chemically designed* to take advantage of this pleasure-seeking programming.

The palatability of food refers to its ability to stimulate your appetite, which in turn prompts you to want more of it. While palatability includes taste, it also comprises the desire to *pursue* the taste further. It's the reason why many people crave certain foods more and more.

Although different people crave different foods, for those with a weight problem the most palatable and most craved foods are usually the chemically designed ones that contain not just added fat or sugar, but a *combination of fat and sugar coupled with salt*. And the sensory properties of these chemically designed foods—temperature, texture, color, and aroma—help to stimulate appetite. For many people, these highly palatable foods provide the most pleasure, and the greatest irresistibility.

But rather than hunger alone, it's the mental stimulation derived from these highly palatable foods that makes so many people crave them. This mental stimulation re-arouses their appetite even after they are done eating.

The insidious combination of fat, sugar and salt

The multi-billion-dollar food industry is highly competitive. Through decades of taste testing, food manufacturers have discovered that specific combinations of fat, sugar and salt—but different combinations for different foods—make consumers crave these designer foods even more. People crave them in order to get their fixes of the fat, sugar and salt combinations. And these are typically the comfort foods that many people become addicted to.

To support this view, Kessler details a host of scientific studies that show how various laboratory animals gorge themselves into obesity when fed a certain combination of fat, sugar and salt. And research on humans draws similar conclusions. Numerous studies—like one from 1995 completed by researchers at the National Institute of Health—show that when offered unlimited portions of various high-fat, high-sugar and high-salt foods, many people eat to excess. And with ongoing exposure to high-fat, high-sugar and high-salt foods, many people develop an ongoing cycle of overeating.

Engineering addiction

Food "engineers" have figured out ways to make the ideal combination of fat, sugar and salt *even more addictive*. According to Kessler, by making the designer food multifaceted—with several layers of fat, sugar and salt—it creates even more pleasure. This is what the food industry calls "layering."

Take, for example, nacho-cheese-smothered tortilla chips. They deep fry super-salty, chemically enhanced chips, and load them with a processed cheese substance that's laden with fat, sugar and salt. It's fat, sugar and salt layered on more fat, sugar and salt. And in an effort to make the food even more irresistible, the layers of fat, sugar and salt are amplified by a chemically engineered flavoring which *further* creates an addictive effect.

Just the bun for a fast-food hamburger has salt, sugar, high-fructose corn syrup, soybean oil, canola oil, and partially hydrogenated oil. Couple this with the large amounts of fat, sugar and salt that are in the hamburger patty, and you've got something that's hard to resist for many people. Add bacon, cheese, sauce and ketchup—which together add even more fat, sugar and salt—and it's easy to see why fast-food hamburgers can be so addictive for many people with weight problems.

Whether it's chicken wings, sauce-laden entrées, pepperoni pizza, or even salads with multiple toppings, most restaurant and store-bought processed foods are layered in a similar fashion. These foods are designed to "melt in your mouth" and go down with little chewing—the higher the levels of fat in the food, the easier it melts in your mouth.

The pleasure derived from the food's several layers of fat, sugar and salt can create an obsession that leads many people to want those foods again and again. And the more you eat them, the more likely you'll fuel this ongoing craving—and that's precisely what the food manufacturers want, so you'll buy the products time and time again.

As reported in *The End of Overeating*, Gerard Smith—a leader in the study of ingestive behavior at New York-Presbyterian Hospital—refers to the term "orosensory self-stimulation" to describe the process by which eating tasty foods tells the brain to repeatedly want more and more of them.

Eventually, these foods can invoke cues that are hard to break. They stimulate neurons in your brain because the foods' tastes are hard-wired to the parts of your brain that respond to pleasure. This prompts a strong emotional response to the foods. And each layer of the foods' fat, sugar and salt can stimulate different neurons in your brain simultaneously.

Ultimately, just the sight or smell of a certain food—potato chips, for example—can intensify a pleasure response. That's why so many struggling dieters can't stop at just one chip. They've been conditioned to seek out the pleasure response for potato chips to the point where it becomes a habit. These people can't control their response to this insidious pseudo-food because their brains have been rewired by their eating it.

Pavlov's dogs and their human equivalents

Advertisements for high-fat, high-sugar and high-salt foods are designed to stimulate your senses, and invoke cues to seek and eat the foods in order to get further fixes of short-lived pleasure and comfort. Even the ads alone can stimulate neurons in your brain. And for many people, this triggers desire for the foods.

This conditioned behavior is similar to that of the dogs of the famous Russian scientist, Ivan Pavlov. Pavlov signaled the occurrence of food by a variety of stimuli, including whistles, tuning forks, and ringing a bell. Once the dogs had got used to, for example, hearing a bell ring at the same time that they were given food, they would salivate at the ringing of a bell even *without* food being present.

Dopamine power, and obesity

When your senses are exposed to a certain food, bursts of dopamine can be released in your brain, which simulate the pleasure response from the food *without it having been eaten*. Dopamine is a chemical in the brain that contributes to creating the drive to eat. And it's what gives desirable foods the prominent memories in your mind. The more desirable the food, the more attention is directed to it, and the more you're likely to pursue it.

A study by scientists at the US Department of Energy's Brookhaven National Laboratory found that dopamine—which they say is involved with addiction to cocaine, alcohol, and other drugs—may also play an important role in obesity. Their research suggests that obese people have fewer receptors for dopamine.

The Brookhaven study indicates that obese people may eat more to try to stimulate the dopamine pleasure circuits in their brains, just as addicts do by taking drugs. Because eating—like the use of addictive drugs—is a highly reinforcing behavior that induces pleasure, the Brookhaven study theorizes that obese people may have abnormalities in their brain dopamine activity.

For many of you, even the sight or smell of food can motivate your reward-seeking behavior to release further dopamine. Just the smell of certain foods—like from being downwind of a restaurant—can make you crave the foods. Now you know at least part of the explanation for why watching a television ad for food can make you salivate. The ad is like the sound of the bell that made Pavlov's dogs salivate even when no food was present.

Has corporate greed contributed hugely to consumer obesity?

According to industry insiders, by capitalizing on their consumers' chemically engineered food addiction, restaurants have slowly upped their portion sizes in an effort to increase their profits. (It costs only a few cents more to create a larger portion, but the restaurants can sell it for a higher price because the customers believe they are getting increased value for money.) Generally speaking, portion sizes in American restaurants are substantially larger than in other countries.

This chapter is just an introduction to the addictive powers of food.

In the next chapter we'll go into some of the details, and let you know how real-life dieters have dealt with their food addictions— *and how you will, too.*

The guidance presented in this chapter is drawn from the success of real people—men and women—who won their psychological battles with overeating and other weight issues.

Once you've read this chapter you'll *know* that you'll succeed, too.

Regardless of how much or how little weight you want to lose, and no matter if you may think it's a ridiculous notion that you could have an eating disorder, or a psychological issue that affects your weight, *please keep an open mind, and read this entire chapter.*

You may be in for a surprise realization; but if you respond as we advise, you may leap forward in your efforts to lose weight and keep it off.

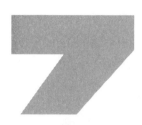

The foundation of weight-loss success for many people: *How to solve the psychological issues that are often at the root of overeating*

Losing weight is easy, right? Just eat properly, exercise, and use some willpower, and then you'll lose weight.

But if most people know that this is the formula, why do so many millions of Americans still have a weight problem?

Many people who are overweight have a root problem that "eating right, exercise, and willpower" *alone* will never fix. But most of these people aren't even aware that a root problem exists.

So what is this problem? And how do you know if you're one of the millions of people who have it? Start by asking these questions:

Do you feel that you have a lack of willpower?

Do you eat when you're not hungry?

Do you eat when you're depressed or stressed?

Do you eat until you're stuffed?

Do you eat for comfort?

Do you eat out of boredom?

Do you mindlessly snack on junk food, especially at night?

Do you feel that you're a yo-yo dieter?

Do you feel that your weight problem is hopeless?

Are you in denial about your weight?

Are you constantly thinking about food?

If you answered *yes* to any of these questions, your problem may *not* be your perceived lack of self-control, or willpower. You may be one of the many millions of people who have an addictive relationship with food.

Stay with us on this . . . *it's of huge importance.*

Brad was in denial about his addiction until he had his awakening.

The awakening

Upon Stuart's recommendation, Brad read a book by Jane R. Hirschmann and Carol H. Munter, called *Overcoming Overeating* (Fawcett Columbine, 1988).

He discovered he has a common, but often misunderstood eating disorder called *compulsive overeating*. And he has been living with it his entire life.

Previous to this awakening, Brad believed that dealing with weight was just a matter of self-control. An acquaintance of his has always said, "Just have more discipline, and willpower. An eating disorder is when someone weighs 500 or more pounds and is bed-ridden, or when a woman weighs 50 pounds and looks like a twig. You don't have an eating disorder, you just lack discipline and self-control."

Brad was tired of hearing that he lacked discipline and self-control. He had been hearing this same line for over 30 years.

He finally realized that, for himself and many people who have weight problems, the solution isn't simply a matter of self-control and discipline.

It was no wonder Brad had always had difficulties controlling his eating when certain triggers were present. And it's no wonder that millions of people have problems with their weight and are unable to follow a weight-loss plan successfully.

Brad figured out how to deal with his overeating problem by learning more about it. And once you learn more about why people overeat, you'll have the knowledge to solve your overeating problems, too.

Brad's addiction to food

Brad was brought up with the mind-set that "you must clean your plate." And he was encouraged to have second and third helpings at each meal, and obliged. When he went to college and was surrounded by unlimited temptations, he didn't put on the stereotypical "freshman 15 pounds," he put on the "freshman 40."

He had long been a chronic yo-yo dieter, and compulsive overeater, but he didn't know it. Chronic yo-yo dieting is a major symptom of a compulsive overeater.

He's *still* addicted to food. Although he has kept his weight off for more than three years, he still can't control himself in situations that trigger his compulsions.

He will still devour an entire bag of chips *if triggered*. He will still eat his wife's food, *if triggered*.

Brad always gorged and binged when he crossed his diet finish line.

If his dinner plate was empty, he routinely emptied the plates of others, especially his wife's.

He gorged on entire bags of chips and entire pizzas at a sitting.

He ate until he was sick when frequenting the all-you-can-eat food buffets.

His wife had to hide food around the house
because of his "see-food eat-food" tendencies.

Binge eating was his solace to cope with stress
and depression.

Why some people can't stop eating

The explanation is usually deep-rooted, and varies person to
person. Only you can know what your problem or struggle is.

Unless you identify why you overeat, or why you have a weight
problem, you may not know what to fix. And merely losing
weight won't necessarily resolve the root of your problem.

People with eating problems usually have weight, dieting, food,
and eating dominate their lives. And their eating problems usually
stem from multi-faceted reasons.

Many people have it much harder than others when it comes to
losing weight. For some, something goes wrong neurochemically,
and they don't feel the physical sensation of fullness like others.

And for many people, food is like a drug addiction. The reward
centers of some people's brains are like a drug addict's, but they
are stimulated by food, not drugs. The more they eat, the better
they feel. And this can cause a vicious cycle of comfort binging.

Some people are more influenced than others by the memory of
food. When the former feel hungry, a memory response spawns
cravings even more. Each binge increases the memories they have
for the comfort they derive from the food, and eventually the
overeating becomes a habit that's hard to break.

And considering that food is designed to be addictive, it's no
wonder that so many people can't stop eating.

Although it's rare, some people have chemical imbalances in their
bodies that make losing weight via traditional methods almost
impossible. They can't lose weight without medical intervention.

Obesity can stem from a traumatic event

Some women have used obesity as a cover-up from incestuous
rape during childhood. For example, a woman Brad researched

was petite and attractive at the time of the molestation, but she figured that if she put on a ton of weight, and became unattractive in her mind, it would repel further attacks.

She could never trust men again, and she overate for safety. And she hid under her obesity—and her inner secret—for decades. It wasn't until after she received professional help that she was able to put her life back together, and regain her physical and mental health.

Molestations and rapes aren't directed towards women only. A man we saw interviewed on a television show had been molested by a friend when he was a boy, and thereafter trusted no one. He buried himself in the one thing he trusted to give him satisfaction—food. After he became 500 pounds he finally addressed the cause of his weight problem. Then, by following a weight-loss plan like the one promoted in this book, he set about losing 300 pounds.

People who had severe trauma in their lives will sometimes use food as their reliable companion, like a loyal pet. If they are getting yelled at, mentally or physically abused, or are lonely or depressed, for example, food is always there. The food becomes a source of happiness and comfort that protects them from the hurtful things in life. Food becomes their safety net. And they know that food can't yell at them, or abuse them.

Other reasons why some people become obese

Many obese people don't care what they look like, provided they are allowed to eat. And many people are obese because they *can* be. It's a choice because no one is giving them a reason to be slim.

Some people are obese because it's all they know. Their entire family is obese, everyone in it overeats as a conditioned behavior, and all members of the family are enablers for one another.

Many obese people purposely hide in their fatness. It's their excuse to fail and be depressed. It serves as a shield from dealing with their real issues. These buried issues are the root of their problem.

Some people are so scared and intimidated by dating, or living life, that they stay fat on purpose. Their fatness always serves as an on-going excuse to cover something up, whether it was being passed up for a job promotion, or being single. They can't get hurt or be rejected if they don't try, so they hide in their obese bodies. They don't think of obesity as being a letdown, they think of it as a vehicle for avoiding a letdown.

Many obese people are so frustrated with diets that they write them off. Every weight-loss attempt has been a source of misery and profound unhappiness. Even the thought of starting a diet brings anguish because it takes them mentally out of their comfort zone. The happiness they derive from eating outweighs the misery associated with dieting, and the health problems related to obesity.

And with some people, failure begets shame. The would-be dieters tell their friends and co-workers they are going on a new diet—they are gung-ho and excited, and everyone has high expectations. Then when the restrictive diets end in failure, the dieters are perceived as failures, and feel shame.

Some of them are so ashamed of themselves that they would rather avoid a new diet than have to deal with the anguish of another private and public failure.

Remember, Brad had so many failed diets that he was nicknamed "the human guinea pig for failed diets." His friends commented that he was always starting a diet, but never finished one.

Repeated failure can further damage already fragile self-esteem. Dieters say to themselves, "Man, I can't do anything right. I'm a failure." And they look in the mirror, feel disgusted, and dwell on the fact that they aren't happy with their bodies, and they get even more self-defeated.

To make up for their need for satisfaction, as a result of repeated failures and self-rejection, the dieters turn to their dependable source of comfort—food. The food—via its ability to release serotonin—becomes their medicine because it feels good to eat. And the pleasure derived can help relieve stress, provide comfort, and calm them down—hence the term "comfort food."

Perhaps now you can see why food is so addictive for some people.

Comfort foods around the world

Depending on your country of origin, comfort foods can be culturally diverse. The term "comfort foods" usually refers to a variety of simple, familiar foods that are usually eaten at quick-service restaurants, or home-cooked. And comfort food may also describe certain snack foods that have emotional significance, and provide contentment and security.

While Brad has been exposed to American staple comfort foods such as chips, doughnuts, fast-food burgers, pizza, and ice cream, many people in other countries and cultures favor different items. For example, the Japanese may enjoy dishes like miso soup and ramen as comfort foods; Spaniards may favor fried eggs with fries or rice; some people from the UK may favor "bangers and mash," steamed puddings, and Indian curries; and Italians may favor spaghetti, pasta, pizza, and a chocolate spread.

But despite the culture or country of origin, most comfort foods have one thing in common: *some combination of fat, sugar and salt.* You may not think so, but if you look at the nutrition labels you may be surprised as to what you find.

The serotonin connection

A study by the University of Minnesota discovered that women are twice as likely as men to binge on food when they are depressed. And women tend to binge on sugary or starchy temptations. This can temporarily boost levels of serotonin—the chemical in the brain that regulates mood.

This is one of the major reasons why overeating and binge eating can become addictive, similar to smoking or even alcoholism.

Deep down, the overeaters know they are harming themselves—like smokers and heavy drinkers know it, too—but they are unwilling to make a change and come out of their comfort zone. The rush they get from the soothing foods, via the serotonin, is such a comfort that it makes no sense to go on a diet and take the perceived happiness away.

Why do *you* overeat or have a weight problem?

Brad often asked himself why he let himself get so fat. Besides stress and the many reasons given in Part I, the answer stemmed from a lack of patience, which led to mounting frustration and decades of failed diets. He was always searching for his weight-loss holy grail—gimmick, quick fix, or pill—that would quickly solve his battle with the bulge.

The failed diets led to more depression and more bouts with emotional eating, and overeating. But once he finally gave up on the hope for quick results, and adopted a realistic weight-loss model based on real-life success, things quickly fell into place and long-term victory followed.

But that's Brad. What about you? What are your excuses? Ask yourself these questions:

> *How did you let yourself put on the weight?*
>
> *What caused your past diets to fail?*
>
> *What's your Achilles heel that leads to overconsumption?*
>
> *Why do you eat the way you do?*
>
> *Do you use food as medicine to "soothe" your problems? If so, why?*
>
> *What's bothering you?*
>
> *What are you hiding from?*
>
> *What's your weakness?*
>
> *If you don't exercise, why not?*
>
> *What do you feel you need to change?*
>
> *If you're depressed or unhappy, why? And what's truly causing it?*

Unless you're honest with yourself, and self-diagnose what your deep-rooted problems really are, maintaining weight-loss over the long-term may be impossible. *And don't feel uncomfortable about visiting a mental health professional if you feel you need assistance in answering the aforementioned questions.*

Food doesn't solve problems

The more some people eat, the heavier they get, the lower their self-worth becomes, and the more they crave the comfort derived from food. It's a vicious cycle. And it's why so many people eat themselves into obesity.

But once you realize that food won't heal your broken heart, get your job back, bring back the loss of a loved one, or eliminate stress, for example, you'll also realize that you have to find new ways to cope. Food offers temporary comfort, but it doesn't solve the underlying problems.

The healing can't begin until the sources of your problems are addressed, and dealt with. And *you* have to find a way to alleviate the root of *your* overeating.

Is it a bad relationship?

Is it an evil boss?

Is it your out-of-control teenager?

Are you lonely?

Do you have financial problems?

Do you have a horrible neighbor?

Do you hate your job?

Are you bored with your life?

To alleviate your problems you may have to make a change in your life. It may be minor, or major. But sometimes, no matter how painful the change may be—a divorce, or a change of career, for example—it can be the catalyst that begins your healing. And if the change is a major one, sessions with a mental health professional will help move you towards your new life.

When Brad initially quit his high-stress, real-estate finance job at a large, high-pressure firm, he was able to lose 52 pounds because his daily pressures and stress subsided. But he put it all back on when he faced his next very stressful hurdle.

There'll always be more sources of stress around the corner. You must be prepared for them, and know that food won't solve the new problems.

Are all obese people depressed and unhappy?

Not all people view fatness as bad. In some cultures, being heavy is a sign of power and abundance.

But many cultures, like America's, are obsessed with body shape. America's perception of fatness and thinness is over-promoted by the media as it relates to supermodels and celebrities. And society is brainwashed in the "thin is in" mentality.

As a consequence, many people have painful relationships with their bodies, and negative self-images. But these stereotypes don't influence everybody.

Not all overweight people are sad and depressed, as stereotypes may suggest. Many heavy people are comfortable living in bodies that may be 25 or 50 pounds overweight. They are content with their lives and don't want change. And the thought of starting a diet is the last thing on their minds because it would take them out of their comfort zones, and disrupt their stable lives.

Some heavy people are so confident in themselves that they don't care what society thinks. They are strong-willed, and secure with their internal and external selves. And they know that being skinny isn't a magic bullet for happiness.

But some very heavy people live in denial about their appearance, and the consequences for their health. Perhaps they put on weight so gradually that they don't realize how heavy they've become. Brad didn't realize how fat he was until he saw photographs of himself at his heaviest. He was stunned as he commented to his wife, "Is that me? Oh my God." It was a sobering realization.

Plus-size people should take care of themselves

Although there are many happy overweight people, most can take better care of their health. And health is what we're ultimately talking about with this book—physical health, and mental health.

But physical appearance and weight are not always indicative of health. There are many skinny people who can't walk up a flight of stairs without huffing and puffing. But some overweight people are physically fit and compete in running races.

While some moderately heavy or plus-size people are healthy, obese people aren't.

Many obese people have the view that "big is beautiful," "my husband loves me curvy," or "why can't people accept me as I am?" But there's nothing acceptable about putting yourself at serious risk for a leading cause of preventable death. Heavy people should still exercise, and eat right.

Besides weight-related ailments, the better your health is, the better your quality of life can be, and the longer you may live. You can have less fatigue and fewer physical limitations in your daily activities, and you'll have more mobility.

Many people have said, "Now that I've lost weight, I can do much more with my life, and be more active." They are in a better mood, more fulfilled and in-control, and more content with their lives.

Although Brad appeared happy and content with being obese when he was on his "non-stop party," it was a facade for covering up his underlying emotions. He wanted to be slim and healthy, but he was so frustrated with repeated failure that he was too intimidated to start another weight-loss plan.

Deep down, Brad knew that being over 100 pounds overweight was morbidly unhealthy. He didn't want to be another casualty like his father, mother-in-law, father-in-law, and numerous friends.

He looked at his wife, family, and pets, and decided that he wanted to be around for them. He wanted to live. He wanted to live forever.

He's thankful that he finally stopped living in denial, and took the plunge into a healthier lifestyle.

He proved that losing a great deal of weight didn't have to uproot his life and take him far from his comfort zone.

Overeating as a psychological problem

The body is directed by the same survival mechanisms that our ancestors had tens of thousands of years ago. Back then, as a means of self-preservation, when food was available people naturally binged until they were full. They didn't know when their next meal was going to come.

But, today, many people binge on highly processed foods, with little or no nutritional value, but lots of calories.

Besides boredom, some of the common reasons for overeating are a traumatic death, loss of job, sexual abuse, or any other episode that can cause profound depression.

Brad couldn't think straight for six months after his father died. It was impossible for him to think about his health during that time. Furthermore, his collapsed business yielded profound depression that led to overeating and excessive drinking.

But the more he learned about eating disorders, the more he appreciated that there was more to these problems than meets the eye. And the huge majority of people—especially men, who may be in "macho denial"—are misinformed when it comes to eating disorders. Even Brad *used to* embrace the macho attitude of "have more self-control and discipline."

More than five million Americans have been diagnosed with binge-eating disorder, also known as compulsive overeating, and many more millions may be living with it—either in denial, or yet to be diagnosed. Its effects can vary from person to person, and be severe, moderate, or minor.

It's no wonder that many people seem to view eating disorders as a female problem—nearly every book and article on this subject seems to be about women. But binge-eating disorder isn't gender specific. Millions of men have it.

Real man, real emotions

The following real-life story, told to Brad, sums up many of the emotions Brad has experienced himself.

"How nice it would be to have a simple addiction like alcoholism—you give up drinking, and then you're recovering. But people *have* to eat. I eat when I'm hungry . . . full . . . anxious . . . happy . . . sad. Food is my friend that never fails.

"When I was a child I was conditioned that food made everything better. When we were out of money, my mom would cook even more. She was a compulsive feeder, so I became a compulsive eater.

"Every diet I've tried has failed. I'm a lifer with Weight Watchers®. I've been through Nutrisystem®. But it's not about the weight; it's about my inability to deal with feelings and emotions. It's about using a pizza or a pound of M&M's® as a narcotic to stem the pain.

"That's what compulsive overeating is.

"I cry because I'm overweight, and no one sees the real me inside. I try to show the real me, but I think that people don't like me because I'm overweight. I see my son gaining weight, and I grieve. I want out, but I realize that there's no way out. There's only control, and control is harder than being in or out."

While there are many eating disorders, this chapter will focus on the one that's at the heart of the weight and weight-loss problems of millions of people: *compulsive overeating*. For these people, only when this disorder is addressed will there be hope for a lasting solution to their weight and weight-loss problems.

What is compulsive overeating?

While overeating is generally described as eating more than your body physically requires, there's much more to it than that.

Compulsive overeating, or binge eating, is an addiction. That's why it's an eating disorder. Compulsive overeaters reach for food as a vehicle for handling difficulties, stress, or angst—much like a drug addict reaches for a drug, or an alcoholic reaches for a drink.

A binge can amount to thousands of calories at a sitting.

Compulsive overeaters are usually detached from the perspective of eating for nutritional reasons. They have the perspective that eating is for comfort, *not* to appease hunger.

Some people become compulsive overeaters in response to repeated failure with restrictive diets—this happened to Brad. Their cravings are intensified due to excessive restrictions.

Other people begin to overeat when they are unable to resolve conflicts and problems. They reach to food for comfort and security—this happened to Brad, too.

But, for others, it may just be an acquired bad habit.

Here are symptoms of compulsive overeating:

Rapid weight-gain.

Excessive food consumption.

Never leaving food on a plate.

Over-buying food in large quantities.

Eating when angry, depressed, or upset.

Feeling that eating is out of control.

During binge episodes, eating much quicker than usual.

Eating until it's uncomfortable.

Eating large quantities of food when there's little or no hunger.

Eating alone because of embarrassment over the quantity eaten.

Feeling disgusted, depressed, or guilty after overeating.

Feeling fat and not being able to do anything about it.

Feeling hopeless because of continuous failure at dieting.

Being obsessed with food, and counting calories.

Binge eaters try to use the comfort derived from eating to help them out of a difficult moment. But binging produces only temporarily comfort, and the bout is usually followed by shame, guilt, disgust, and depression.

Because some people are so conditioned to grab food for comfort, they never stop to address what's troubling them. And they blame the overeating for their weight problems. But the real issue is that the overeating is a *cover-up* for the root problem or problems.

Some compulsive overeaters aren't obsessed with the food itself. They are obsessed with the comfort they derive from the food.

Some compulsive overeaters may eat normally in front of others, but then binge in secret. And some eat all day long.

If you're a compulsive overeater, dieting may be the worst thing you can do. If your new weight-loss plan urges, "don't do this" or "you can't eat that," you deny yourself what you crave *and end up craving it even more.* The deprivation will increase the food's reward value, and a compulsive binge is inevitable.

This happened to Brad whenever he tried a restrictive diet. And this is a major reason why compulsive overeaters are usually also compulsive yo-yo dieters.

Restrictive diets are especially tortuous to the compulsive overeater, and should be avoided.

The gung-ho "all-or-nothinger"

Linda is the epitome of a yo-yo dieter. She's either fat or skinny, with seemingly no in-between.

Linda's an at-home, gourmet-chef hobbyist. She's addicted to food, and a compulsive overeater. When

she whips up her delicacies—often at nine or ten
o'clock at night, when her significant other comes
home from work—a binge is inevitable.

At some point, when she's consumed by the guilt
that she got fat yet again, Linda goes on a crash diet.
She eats nothing but baby carrots, chicken breast,
rice patties, and water—*until she self-destructs and
reverts to her gourmet overeating.*

Linda has repeated this cycle for over 20 years.

Do all obese people have eating disorders? Do you?

Do all obese people have food addictions or other eating disorders,
and deep psychological problems with eating? No. People can be
overweight or obese for many reasons.

**But many people of all bodyweights—not just the
obese—*do* have eating disorders, and psychological
problems with eating.**

Brad read a research article that showed that even some normal-
weight people have food addictions and eating disorders, *but* they
became exercise addicts to counter their excessive caloric intake.

How do you know if you have an eating disorder, or a psychological
problem with food?

**Start by reading all of Part II. Then try to self-diagnose
what your underlying problem or problems may be.**

You may find, for example, that you don't have an eating disorder
or a psychological problem with food, but you *do* have other
reasons why you put on weight, or had such a struggle to lose it.

Brad had no idea that he had an addictive relationship with food
(and an eating disorder) until he researched the material for Part II
of this book. He discovered that he had the same eating problems
when he was 190 pounds as a teenager, when he was 210 pounds
as a college student, and when he was 265 pounds as a middle-
aged man. And the same eating problems linger today, even
though he's a 165-pound, 44-year-old. They will need to be well
managed for the rest of his life if he's to maintain his weight-loss.

But no matter how heavy Brad became at certain times, other factors also contributed to his weight-gain. Like with many other heavy people, factors such as environment, inactivity, depression, and stress contributed to his weight-gain, and to how long he took between his frequent yo-yo diets.

There may be a number of issues explained in Part II that are relevant to you. Once you understand them, and apply what you learn, you'll take a leap forward in your efforts to lose weight and keep it off.

Of course, if you feel that you do have an underlying problem, you may have to visit the appropriate specialist to seek treatment.

"But people have always had psychological issues. Why have they manifested *today* in obesity for many people?"

The prevalence of obesity has exploded only over recent years. But people have always had psychological issues to deal with. Why do they contribute in a big way *today* to an obesity epidemic, but didn't 100, or just 30 years ago?

The obesity problem isn't just among adults. In the US it's of alarming proportions among teenagers, too. Two major factors have contributed to widespread obesity: *inactivity*, and *crud food*.

Inactivity

Decades ago, most children played in the yard, and rode bikes, among other activities. Now, most seem to sit almost all day long, and play video games, watch television, text, talk, and sit at a computer. Most do nothing of significance for activity or exercise. And most adults in the US, for example, are less active today than most adults were in earlier generations.

Thus, many of today's teenagers and adults in the US and some other countries have reduced caloric *output*.

Crud food

The availability of crud—primarily fast food, and junk food—has increased enormously over recent decades.

And the potential for many people to become addicted to the crud has also increased.

Many children and adults derive most if not almost all of their food from crud. Overly busy parents seldom cook healthy meals anymore. And people often skip breakfast.

Many children are provided with horrible school lunches—by their parents, or even by their schools in some cases. Then they invariably have fast-food dinners, and snack each evening on crud while they do their sedate "activities." And because many children are brought up by obese parents, they often have no chance of adopting healthy lifestyles while they live at home. But when they leave home they are likely to be fixed in an unhealthy lifestyle.

Brad sees this on a regular basis in the US. It's how an acquaintance of his feeds her teenager. Both of the child's parents live off crud, and they are both morbidly obese. The only thing that keeps the boy from being obese is that he's very active with competitive sport, at least for the time being. But if or when he becomes a typical inactive adult, his weight will take off.

Thus, many of today's teenagers and adults in the US and some other countries have increased caloric *input*.

The consistent daily caloric *surplus*—greater *input* than *output*—produces the accumulation of body fat.

Chapter 6 explained the role of food manufacturers in making processed food addictive for many people.

Although the psychological issues that drive many people to seek solace or escape through food *must* be addressed, *that needs to be combined with healthy eating, and a more active lifestyle.* But to be successful over the long-term, the changes must be *enjoyable* and *sustainable*—and *that's* what the guidance of this book is about.

Conquering overeating

Why do overeaters often turn to food for comfort? Think about your inborn response to hunger. Now take this thought back to when you were an infant. When you were hungry, you cried, and (hopefully) were fed. Your needs were met, and you were satisfied and content. And you stopped crying. Crying meant being hungry and uncomfortable, and food meant relief from those sensations.

People who don't have eating problems correlate eating with satisfying hunger. For them, eating is a necessary function for providing nutrition, and sustaining life. But overeaters often use food as a vehicle for handling difficulties, stress, or angst, *not as a source of nutrition and sustenance.* Food is used as medication, not fuel. And repeated failed diets only heighten this.

Many overeaters subconsciously revert to conditioned feelings that food is a symbol of comfort from a caring parent. And this feeling of nurturing and security soothes them as adults.

Overcoming Overeating by Jane R. Hirschmann and Carol H. Munter guides readers on *relearning how to eat.* The authors believe in restoring the correlation between food and hunger.

Food should, *primarily*, be a source of nourishment and sustenance, not a source of comfort. *You must get pleasure from your food, of course, but get the pleasure from food that's also nourishing and healthy.*

The plan of Hirschmann and Munter requires that you eat often but *only* in response to true hunger. The more often you eat in response to *a feeling of true hunger*, the less likely you are to reach out to food for comfort.

So, by eating a wholesome snack or small meal every two to four hours *only* when they felt a true sensation of hunger, Brad and most of the hundreds of real-life successful dieters he interviewed *retrained* the way they thought about food *even though they weren't aware of what they were doing at the time.*

This retraining eventually eliminated most of these dieters' compulsions for binging. And it instilled the connection of eating with hunger. They properly fueled their bodies, and satisfied their feelings for contentment and nourishment much like when their parents fed them as infants.

Do the same yourself, and remind yourself that you're strategically taking in nutrition in an attempt to nourish

your body. You're responding to physiological hunger. You're not eating just for psychological reasons—comfort or entertainment. Keep reminding yourself of this, and you'll eventually retrain your brain into thinking about food in the correct light only.

Consider your body to be a temple, and that you're taking care of it.

Internal and external psychological triggers

Overeating triggers are everywhere, but vary person to person.

Hunger pangs are physiological cues that you're hungry, but psychological cues can be triggered internally *and* externally.

Internal psychological triggers can stem from anxiety, relaxation, depression, nervousness, anger, boredom, loneliness, stress, or painful emotions.

External psychological triggers result from your environment, such as the smell and sight of food, driving by an eating establishment, walking by a vending machine, watching people eat, seeing or hearing a food advertisement, or anything else that may make you think about food.

All-you-can-eat buffets, and fast-food restaurants, were particular problems for Brad, and still are.

Food commercials are carefully orchestrated to arouse your senses, and prey on your emotions, to try to brainwash you to overeat. No wonder it's so hard for people to control their eating. Society is constantly bombarded with mouth-watering temptations.

Any of these psychological triggers—internal or external—can prompt you to overeat. This type of conditioned behavior—similar to that produced by Pavlov in his work with dogs—is extremely difficult to overcome.

But some people, like Brad, may be more conditioned to associate food with relief and comfort in response to overeating triggers.

An overeating trigger typically starts with a stressful event that provokes feelings of helplessness or anger, which leads to a binge on large amounts of starchy or sweet foods such as cake or ice cream, or foods high in fat, sugar and salt such as potato chips or pizza. This generally happens unexpectedly and unconsciously.

You may have had a stressful day at work, but devouring a carton of ice cream won't prevent the occurrence of the stress another day. But what will your emotions be like when that "few minutes of happiness" gets stored, time after time, on your body?

Generally, nighttime eating is usually comfort eating or emotional eating. And you're usually not eating for nutritional reasons at this time unless you're an athlete or a bodybuilder, for example, trying to meet pre-determined quotas for nourishment.

Most overeating triggers last for just a few minutes. If you can create a diversion in the interim, you can generally fend them off.

When you have a bad episode that may trigger you to binge, to get the desired rush from the serotonin, *create an immediate diversion to fend off the appetite-invoking cues.*

Displace your triggers to overeat

When you start a weight-loss plan, at least initially, food may consume your thoughts. You need to find a new interest to divert attention away from food. Not only will this help you with your weight-loss, it can enrich your life in other ways.

It could be devoting more time to your family and friends.

It could be a sporting hobby—golf, for example.

It could be something educational—take up a home-study course with a distance learning college.

It could be personal study of something that has always interested you but was never pursued—the history of a certain football team, or the life of a great historical figure, for example.

It could be a writing project.

It could be taking on a puppy or a kitten.

It could be joining evening classes at a college for painting, or music, for example.

It could be dance lessons, and participation in weight-loss groups.

Or it could be a home-improvement project, landscaping, or establishing a vegetable garden.

Giving and receiving emotional nourishment is very important. This is why it's vital to devote more time to

family and friends. **Many overweight people may have difficulties receiving emotional nourishment because of poor self-image due to abuse or coldness from their families. The comfort from touch isn't required by babies and young children only, but by adults, too.**

Brad used research as his main passionate diversion. For several years he spent a few hours each day researching material that, eventually, was used in the creation of **WEIGHT-LOSS SALVATION**. He also took on home-improvement projects and landscaping, and increased the care he provided for his dogs.

You can also displace your triggers with exercise

Brad found that exercise—in his case, jogging, bicycling, and lifting weights—so enhanced his mood that it helped him deal with the pressures of life. And the exercise took his mind off food.

According to a recent study by Duke University, as published in the journal *Psychosomatic Medicine*, regular exercise works just as well as many pharmaceutical antidepressants for relieving symptoms of major depressive disorder.

And a review published by Boston University found that exercise has an effect on depression on par with psychotherapy and drugs.

An invigorating workout is a great way to relieve anxiety and depression, *but it must be exercise that's safe and enjoyable.*

The "runner's high"

People who exercise strenuously enough so that their breathing is difficult for a long, sustained period — and not just runners—may experience the *runner's high*. This euphoria is due to an increase in endorphin levels in response to the exercise. And this produces an increased sense of well-being, including an improvement in the emotional attitude of the exercisers, akin to the effects of some medications.

Your brain may even relax and become highly creative during this endorphin-filled period.

The runner's high may be addictive. When Brad had a leg injury that shut down his daily jogging for several weeks, he became depressed and agitated.

Stress can wreak havoc on your waistline

The response to stress is part of our bodies' innately programmed survival mechanism—our fight-or-flight response. Stress can be triggered by many things, including worry, traumatic events, a high-energy lifestyle, long daily commutes, high day-to-day pressure, raising children, working too hard, or juggling too many things in your life.

Stress can wreak havoc on your waistline.

Stress triggers your body to release cortisol, a hormone that reduces your body's sensitivity to leptin, which is the hormone that tells your brain when you're feeling full. And this, in turn, triggers your body to consume more food, which can lead to weight-gain.

Chronic stress also makes your cells more resistant to insulin, so more insulin goes into your blood, which causes more calories to be stored as fat—perhaps especially in your abdomen. It can also cause your metabolism to downshift to help conserve energy and increase your blood sugar level, further promoting weight-gain.

And when you're stressed, the hormone neuropeptide Y (NPY) can activate receptors on your fat cells, and cause them to accumulate additional fat.

But a reduction in stress can quickly alleviate these conditions.

Alleviating stress

A healthy diet and regular exercise eventually became Brad's "medicine" to help alleviate stress. And this helped with his weight-loss and his mood.

In the book, *Calm Energy: How People Regulate Mood with Food and Exercise* (Oxford University Press, 2001), author Robert E. Thayer, Ph.D., describes how exercise can be used as a personal mood-regulator, and cites one of his studies that found that as little as 10 minutes of brisk walking can boost mood and reduce stress.

To cope with stress, be more relaxed. Take a leisurely stroll in the sunshine, listen to some relaxing music, practice deep breathing, meditate, read a relaxing book, get a massage, pet an animal, take a warm and invigorating shower or bath, or go for a swim.

And laugh more. Watch a funny movie or TV show, go to a comedy club, recall funny events with friends—anything for a daily laugh.

Laugh your ass off . . . literally

Fifteen minutes of laughing can burn 40 calories. Research published in the *International Journal of Obesity* reported that laughing increased heart rate and caloric expenditure by up to 20%.

Laughing 15 minutes a day can mean you literally "laugh your ass off" because this may equate to a few pounds of fat lost per year. And the longer you laugh, the greater the effects. Also, laughing is a great mood booster to help with stress, and depression.

Are fat-free snacks making you fat?

Stick to the "fat-free," "reduced-fat," or "sugar-free" versions of your favorite temptations. They taste similar to their more decadent siblings, but are generally less calorific. Substitute these versions of your favorite cravings, in *small* quantities, instead of eliminating them all together.

But read the labels carefully because, often, "fat-free" or "reduced-fat" foods are higher in taste-enhancing chemicals, or higher in high-fructose corn syrup and sugar (and thus higher in calories).

Conversely, "reduced-carb," "carb-free," or "sugar-free" foods may have added fat, as well as added taste-enhancing chemicals. Again, these can be higher in calories than the regular versions.

People tend to eat more of the snack if it's labeled "fat-free" or "sugar free," for example, because the product's labeling suggests it's healthier, and lower in calories.

Low-fat or fat-free labels may also make food *seem* less tasty, according to scientists at the Oregon Research Institute. And this may cause you to eat more of the low-fat version, or even lead you to crave the "real" version, which usually results in a binge.

According to the study, people who thought they were getting a low-fat milkshake had less brain activation. Knowing that the milkshake was low-fat took much of the fun out of the experience.

"This study shows that it may not be such a good idea to have all those low-fat alternatives, since people may be experiencing less of a sense of reward when they eat—and that would make these low-calorie foods completely useless," says Eric Stice, a senior scientist at the Institute.

Do you need to eliminate comfort foods?

Eventually you must stop mindless snacking on comfort foods. But eliminating them isn't necessarily the solution. "If we deny ourselves what we crave, we end up craving it even more."

You must enjoy your life. If you crave a cookie, enjoy an *occasional* cookie. If you crave chocolate, enjoy an *occasional* but *small* piece of chocolate. If you crave some pizza, enjoy *occasional* pizza.

For most people, certain comfort foods *in controlled moderation* are acceptable. It's the big picture that matters, and a little strategic cheating shouldn't derail your long-term goal.

But, for some people, enjoying comfort foods in "controlled moderation" isn't easy. Many people eat to soothe painful emotions, or to get emotional nourishment, and because of this they have big problems controlling their cravings. Brad still has this problem, especially with chips and pizza.

Comfort foods like cookies, cake, pizza, and chips are usually of the starchy variety, contain strategic amounts of fat, sugar and salt, and are highly processed. When you eat them, your serotonin levels increase, and your brain feels more relaxed and soothed. Couple this with the way they release dopamine into your brain, creating desire to eat, and it's no wonder that comfort foods can be addictive.

How to curb your cravings for comfort foods

There are tips that real-life dieters use to help fend off cravings for snacks and comfort foods. *Use them yourself*.

Many successful dieters make it a rule to have a large glass of water (preferably *ice-cold*) in lieu of a craving. This works most of the time. Alternatively, drink flavored water. Brad and his wife often mix up a gallon of sugar-free Kool-Aid®, or Crystal Light®, which are a mere five calories per serving.

Another popular diversionary tactic is the "five-minute rule." If you crave something, wait five minutes—no matter what—before you open the cookie jar, for example. You may also take a quick "cool down walk" during this five-minute break. This delay can give you a chance to rethink your actions and redirect you to a healthier decision. You'll most likely forget that you wanted the snack in the first place.

Eat *only* at the dinner table. If you eat or snack in front of the television, every time you sit in your comfort chair can be a trigger to eat. Designate an eating location at a table for all meals and snacks, *and stick to it.*

Before you grab a cupcake or bag of chips, consider how many unhealthy calories you're about take in, and how much exercise you'll have to do to burn those calories off. For example, depending on your pace, you would have to walk approximately 9 to 12 miles to burn off the calories from just six ounces of potato chips. *Then consider whether the snack is for you.* This mental arithmetic rule is one of the most effective tricks. It's a quick reality check when you know, for example, that just five minutes of snacking can nullify an entire day's (or several days') worth of weight-loss progress.

If you must grab a bag of chips, select a single-serving size. This way you'll be capped at a one-ounce, 150-calorie serving instead of gorging from a seemingly unlimited large bag. A study by the University of Illinois found that larger package sizes lead to a 22% increase in how many calories you consume, *regardless of your levels of hunger.*

Derail your cravings by having a piece of sugar-free gum, brushing your teeth, or eating something sweet or unique like a pickle spear, or a hot pepper.

If you crave frozen treats or ice cream, occasionally satisfy your cravings with 15-calorie, sugar-free Popsicle®, Fudgsicle®, or Creamsicle® bars.

In lieu of a craving, take a warm bubble bath, or make a surprise phone call to a friend.

Perhaps set up a reward system for cheating on your diet. For example, say you want to go out and have some pizza or drinks with your friends. Prior to enjoying your night out, go for a long walk, or have a workout, so you can at least feel you earned the *mini* debauchery.

Stop for a few minutes and make sure that you're actually hungry before you eat. *Physical* hunger is a basic, human need, while *emotional* hunger will generally make you feel guilty afterwards. A piece of turkey breast won't make you feel guilty like a large cookie, or a bag of chips.

To help implement this "guilt prevails effect," take a minute or two (during the "five-minute rule" break) to assess what you're considering eating. Once you realize that you're about to gorge on a chemically engineered creation loaded with fat, sugar and salt—with perhaps 1,000 or so calories that you'll somehow have to burn off—the guilt will usually prevail, and you'll most likely make a better choice.

For the most part, cravings for snacks and comfort foods are a by-product of boredom. This is why it's important to stay busy with diversionary hobbies and activities (as well as exercise) to take your mind off eating.

Keep temptations in a hard-to-reach or distant place so there's more of a challenge to obtain the treats.

The ultimate diversionary tactic is not to have any treats in the house to begin with. This may sound overkill, but it may be the only solution. And desperate times can call for desperate measures. This was Brad's solution with potato chips, because this is the one food he has no control over. He now considers that *crud* as his *enemy*.

As people improve their health and lose weight, they naturally cheat less because they don't want to let themselves down and ruin hard-earned progress. You won't want to let yourself down once you're making good progress. This was perhaps the biggest single thing that helped Brad overcome his eating disorder.

You'll eventually compile a set of tactics that will keep you from making wrong decisions. Consider the tactics as rules. Following them will become second nature as you

retrain your brain.

And like most new habits, it generally takes no more than 21 days to change your patterns *if* you practice them on a daily basis.

Crud "food"

How do you know what's crud, and what's not? *Be informed and discerning—read nutrition labels.*

If a food product has a list of ingredients that includes sugars, fats, sodium, and chemical additives, it's *crud*—unhealthy, and potentially addictive. Wean yourself off it. And review the list of the ingredients of each item you put in your home-cooked meals. Just because something is home-cooked doesn't necessarily mean that it's healthy. Make sure everything is wholesome.

What's wholesome? The food that nature provides— food *without* added ingredients or chemicals.

But even natural, wholesome, healthy food will cause weight-gain *if consumed in excess*.

Keep a food journal

A 2008 study by Kaiser Permanente found that people who maintained a daily food journal lost twice as much weight as those people who didn't keep a record of their meals.

Many dieters believe that keeping a food journal of what they eat and how much, their hunger level prior to eating, and any emotions present at the time of eating, helps them to manage their eating and snacking better, because it all fosters self-awareness.

A food journal helps you to identify underlying emotions and behaviors that can trigger overeating. Reading your food journal can become your own personal therapy session.

Most people know right from wrong when it comes to food, but they never realize how much they eat, or how bad their choices are, unless they see it all written up in their food journals. This invariably acts as a graphic reality check on why they have a weight problem.

If you feel the urge to snack, immediately write a passage in your food journal about why. Then by the time you write the passage, your urge to snack may be gone.

Many people also make a note when a nibble—like a spoonful of peanut butter, or a carrot—prevented a binge.

Even a simplified version of a food journal can work. The University of Pittsburgh found that dieters who wrote down the size of each meal (for instance, S, M, L or XL) were just as successful with their weight-loss as those who kept a comprehensive journal with nutrition specifics and calorie-counts.

Search the internet for food journals that are easy to use.

Be careful of overeating regressions

When you've acted on the guidance in this chapter you must still keep your guard up every minute of every day. When you least expect it, a trigger may materialize and cause a setback.

Months after he lost his weight, when Brad was a groomsman at a friend's wedding, he couldn't resist the all-you-can-eat buffet—his number one trigger. People looked at him in disbelief when he was on his *sixth* helping. He couldn't stop eating. Anytime Brad is exposed to an unlimited spread of food in public, he loses control. This was the first time in more than a year that he had been exposed to such temptation. His feeding frenzy finally ended only when the irritated staff removed the remaining food from the table.

Even when you think you're "cured," an inadvertent trigger can still materialize unexpectedly, and cause a binge. *Be ever vigilant.*

In late 2007, Brad and his wife were cleaning out their basement's entertainment area. He found a pristine large bag of potato chips left over from a party several months prior. He cracked the bag open for a whiff. Before he knew it he had polished off the entire bag. He still couldn't control himself with his trigger foods.

Don't feel bad if you have a problem with binging, but deal with it by keeping your guard up at all times, and avoid putting yourself in situations that may trigger a regression.

Can regressions be triggered by deep-rooted memories?

Brad was told by a doctor that certain triggers subliminally take him back to the happy times of his childhood. As a child he was happy when he ate second and third helpings with his family (provided he liked the food). And he was happy when he ate at night while watching TV with his family.

Food was the epicenter of Brad's upbringing, whether it was family cookouts, vacations, or ordinary meals. And eating was always a source of happiness. Furthermore, Brad used to help his father cook the family meals, which was a great source of male bonding.

Brad's most powerful comfort foods are those layered with fat, sugar and salt. The comfort he seeks when he eats processed foods subliminally reminds him of his joyful childhood, when he was surrounded by a loving, nurturing family, and before the pressures of adulthood made life complicated. This may be a major reason why Brad severely overate immediately following his father's death.

Food masked the pain, and provided comfort by reminding Brad of happy memories.

Help yourself by changing your ways

Brad eliminated as many triggers as he could from his daily life, and took on new activities and hobbies to serve as diversions. And he changed his environment. He stayed away from all-you-can-eat buffets, and kept potato chips out of his house.

If your temptations aren't there, you can't eat them.

Brad's wife now supports his new life, although at first she was reluctant to because she loved to go out to eat, and had unhealthy snacks in the house. Brad and his wife adapted together, and through time they changed their lifestyle for the better.

And Brad has become an expert cook. Instead of going out to a restaurant or tavern, he cooks terrific, healthy meals at home.

He now instinctively uses his eating triggers as prompts to turn to diversions like working out, walks, or mind-strengthening activities. Instead of "potato chips equal comfort," it's now "endorphins, chores, or mind-building activities equal comfort."

What works for Brad may not work for you. He went to the extreme, but you may not have to. Develop strategies that work *for you*. Extreme strategies, like Brad's, can backfire and lead to regression because unrealized temptations can become even more tempting, which can lead to a binge.

It may sound unnerving that you have to make changes and eliminate at least some of your favorite temptations.

But with time you'll learn to enjoy healthier foods, and forget why you ate the fattening crud in the first place.

Eating is a basic human function. It should be primarily viewed as a way of acquiring nutrition for sustenance, *not* as a source of entertainment or comfort. Although this mind-set change may be difficult to make, take it one day at a time and it will get a little easier each day. And after three weeks or so you'll be on your way.

If Brad can change his ways after four decades of living on processed food, you can change your ways, too. It's not as hard as you may think.

Just give it a chance to succeed.

Emotional eating in front of the television

Many families gorge on unhealthy snacks while they watch television. Children brought up in this environment tend to think that this behavior is normal, and continue it throughout their adult lives because it's a source of comfort. This was Brad's upbringing.

If people spent less time in front of the television, and did more productive, enjoyable, and worthwhile activities—hobbies and passionate interests, for example—they wouldn't have so much urge or opportunity to overeat.

Now, Brad snacks on baby carrots and turkey breast in lieu of chips, if he snacks at all. And he's spends far less time watching television than he used to. He's found more active uses of his time.

Nighttime snacking is *not* for losers

One of the dieters Brad interviewed tried an experiment based on the premise that one could lose 25 to 50 pounds in a year simply by giving up nighttime junk-food binging.

James had a healthy dinner, but whereas he would sit in front of the television and devour cookies, multiple

bags of microwave popcorn, soda, and potato chips all night, he eliminated all after-dinner eating. *And he lost 44 pounds in just under 12 months by doing nothing else but cutting out post-dinner eating. His wife followed suit and lost a ton of weight, too.*

Substitute your bad habits with good habits

Habits form when familiar stimuli trigger established neuron pathways in the brain to produce repeated behavior. Habits allow us to repeat certain responses without having to think about them, thereby conserving cognitive effort.

Bad habits are acquired patterns of behavior that usually occur automatically, and cause us to act in the same harmful way repeatedly. It's why Brad will mindlessly wolf down a bag of chips without even thinking twice about it. It's a script that has been encoded into the circuits of his brain.

Most overweight people have some bad habits that contribute to their condition.

Do you snack on starchy foods, or candy, all day?

Do you eat sugary breakfast cereal?

Do you eat fast-food combo meals on a regular basis?

Do you gorge on ice cream?

Do you eat most of your food late in the day, or in just one meal?

Do you eat until you're stuffed?

Do you starve then binge?

Is much of your socializing centered on or around food?

And do you walk straight to the fridge when you enter your house?

The latter habit is influenced by dopamine. You've trained your brain to release dopamine every time you see the fridge and reach for the handle. One dieter broke this habit by entering his house from another door so he wouldn't have to walk by the fridge.

Bad habits can be eliminated by breaking the patterns of destructive behavior by creating new patterns of *constructive* behavior, thus creating good habits.

The dieter who lost 44 pounds by eliminating his nighttime junk-food eating, previously had a bad habit of binging on junk food in front of the television each night. This was conditioned behavior he'd had since childhood—a source of comfort and mindless entertainment. He was brought up in that environment.

He eventually realized that excessive nighttime eating was unhealthy. When he changed his behavior and eliminated this habit, his health improved. He began to eat for nutritional reasons, rather than for comfort or entertainment, and soon became picky about what he ate. And because of this, his health improved even more. He now has a clean bill of health from his doctor.

Eliminating most fast food consumption can mean losing 5 to 15 pounds in a month, without doing anything else.

Changing small daily habits can amount to a big change over the medium- and long-term.

If you're stressed out from work, don't go out eating or drinking—instead, go for a walk, or go to the gym. This is one of the major changes that Brad made with his life, to cope with a stressful day. *Again, substitute a good habit for a bad habit.*

What's your weakness? What bad habit can you eliminate without upending your life? Brad voluntarily gave up his chips (and his delivered pizza, other fast food, and all-you-can eat buffets). What can you give up? And what good habit can you do instead? Think about it.

If you have the habit of snacking on junk at your desk all day, keep baby carrots or other healthy snacks in plain view, and partake of those. Given the addictive nature of processed snacks, it's best to eat *all-natural-food* snacks.

Giving up fast food and junk food is a major challenge for many people. Processed food is *designed* to be addictive—in its presentation and ingredients. But once you realize that you're wolfing down potentially thousands of calories in a short time—and calories from *crud*—it shouldn't be hard to come to a reality check.

Eating junk food and fast food can make you feel good *temporarily* (via the serotonin rush), but other things can make you feel good, too. And once you acknowledge that you're damaging your health and potentially shortening your life by binging on unhealthy food, making the effort to change becomes easier.

Change isn't as hard as you may think *provided* you approach it gradually. Retrain your brain by repeating the satisfaction-generating positive behavior. Provided the new habits are rewarding enough to replace the destructive habits, within three weeks or so you're usually home free.

But, of course, establish new, *healthy* habits to replace the old, destructive ones.

Become conscious of what you're doing to your body when you overeat. And don't look at change as negative; *look at it as positive.*

You're beginning a new life. And a healthy lifestyle will eventually become your new habit.

How to put on 100 pounds in a year

Brad has a friend who graduated from high school at 150 pounds. He got a job at a fast-food restaurant, where he was eventually promoted to manager.

A perk John had was free meals whenever he wanted, and he could take leftover food home at the end of his shift. He put on 100 pounds in just under a year as he became addicted to the high-fat, high-sugar, and high-salt fare. Eventually he could barely stand without perspiring profusely, and breathing heavily. John never had a problem with his weight *until* he was exposed to addictive fast food.

Watch out for saboteurs

Sometimes it's hard to visit family, or engage in certain family activities, because they are centered on food. You've probably seen the stereotype of a caring mother "who's just trying to make sure everyone's fully nourished." It's a common motherly instinct.

Remember that Brad was encouraged to have second and third helpings when he was a child, and many mothers never get past this mentality. And when grandma steps it up a notch, and pushes her homemade brownies on you, you're doomed.

While it may be hard to say no to mom and grandma, for example, let them know what you're trying to do, and why. More often than not they'll go out of their way to accommodate you.

Brad had this problem with his late mother-in-law because she was the ultimate "food pusher." He couldn't go more than a few minutes without having some mouth-watering temptation shoved in his face. She was a compulsive overeater herself.

But Brad's wife let her mother know how she was wreaking havoc on his psyche with her food pushing. Although she cried at first, she eventually went overboard in support. Brad was showered with turkey breast, chicken breast, and healthy sides.

A chubby girl who has a pretty face may have self-esteem problems, and is thrilled when someone is interested in her. But when a marriage ensues under these circumstances, it doesn't take much to break the delicate balance of the relationship.

If the wife begins to lose weight in an attempt to regain her self-esteem, the husband can be threatened. He may feel he'll lose his control in the marriage if she loses weight, becomes "hot," and gains self-esteem. He may try to sabotage her weight-loss.

Brad had a family friend who committed suicide because he was so distraught that his wife lost weight and regained her self-esteem. He became paranoid that she was cheating on him. "Why would such a beautiful woman stick with me?" he said. This mounting distrust damaged his fragile self-esteem to the point that he took his own life.

And don't forget about your friends who may be saboteurs.

If you tell the guys or gals that you won't be going to any more happy hours with them, do you think they'll support you? Probably not, because you would be rocking the boat. You would be creating a change that they may not be ready for.

Displays of machismo may be directed your way. Brad was called *a wuss*, among other choice words, by his beer "buddies" when he was on the mega-hype program, because he elected to forgo the weekly happy hours that were a staple of their lives.

No matter what the case, many people don't want change.

Explain to your friends and family why you're changing, and petition their support. If they care about you, they'll comply.

Weathering criticism

While criticism can merely be "the look" that obese people often get, some of it is cruel. Brad has been called many names, for example, "fat ass," "disgusting fat slob," "pig," "pathetic loser," "a potato on toothpicks," and "human guinea pig for failed diets."

It hurts to be called names.

Society has stereotypes for heavy people—for instance, they are unhealthy, lazy, unlovable, unmotivated, unstable, disgusting, and deficient in self-discipline.

There's nothing you can do to change these stereotypes. But you can change how you deal with the criticism.

Instead of letting criticism get you down—and serving as the cause for devouring a bag of chips, for example—use it as a catalyst for motivation to change your life.

While some criticism is borne out of naiveté, some is borne out of *the teasers' own insecurities.*

And some criticism, from people who know you, may be intended to inspire change. The "potato on toothpicks" and "human guinea pig for failed diets" comments were made by some of Brad's friends as ways of subliminally suggesting that he had let himself go. It was their gentle way of saying, "Brad, what the hell have you done to yourself?" He now knows that they were only trying to help, albeit in a quirky way.

One real-life dieter avoids going to her doctor for routine physicals. She knows she's heavy and needs to lose weight, but is sick of having it rubbed in her face by her doctor's annual lecture. So, she avoids the confrontation.

Brad has also been on the other side of criticism. He remembers naively teasing fat students when he was in elementary school. But, ironically, the one obese boy that Brad and his friends teased ended up as the lean, muscular star of his high school football team. And the fat girl he teased became a beauty queen.

In college, there was a girl that one of Brad's friends rudely rejected because she was very heavy. But she lost a huge amount of weight, and Brad's buddy hit on her, not knowing that this beauty was the formerly very fat student. He deserved the slap on the face. She remembered the rejection, and she couldn't wait for the moment to administer revenge.

These people turned a negative into a positive. Brad turned a negative into a positive. And if you're dealing with criticism of any kind, *you* can turn a negative into a positive. *Adopt the attitude of, "I'll show them!"*

Winning the psychological battle with your weight

Take responsibility for your own actions. Fat doesn't have to be your fate. Everyone has the ability to lose weight. Some people find it harder than others, and some people may need professional help, but if you really want weight-loss success it *will* happen *provided* you know what you're doing.

Weight-loss success begins with an honest analysis of your present condition. Accept your responsibility for your condition, and then adopt a workable plan to achieve your goal—*the model presented in this book.*

For a while, Brad was defeated as a result of three decades of failure. But once he adopted a weight-loss model based on the success detailed in **WEIGHT-LOSS SALVATION**, he knew good results were possible, and within reach. If others could succeed, why couldn't he? He made a commitment to himself to regain his health, and he began the journey. He let it happen.

Everyone has self-control; you just have to figure out how to tap yours. It's *not* about willpower, it's about commitment.

You *must* make a commitment to yourself, and you *must* commit to living in a healthier way.

And you *must* learn to appreciate how important good health is. Many people take better care of their cars than they do of themselves.

You're the only person who has to live with yourself. And if you don't care for yourself, who will?

Forgive yourself for putting on the weight, forgive people who may have acted as triggers for your overeating, and give yourself a break.

Don't let your appearance get you down.

Let it inspire change.

Go to a mirror, look into the reflection of your eyes, and say, "I apologize for letting you down."

What's done, is done. Allow yourself no more self-defeating thoughts. Let bygones be bygones, and look forward to a fresh, new life—*your future.*

No matter how you are on the outside, you're still *you* on the inside. You have to live with yourself, regardless. And you need to accept the inner you, regardless.

If you have things in your life that are causing you angst—like a bad relationship, lousy neighbor, job you hate, or a horrible boss—*deal with them.* You may have to visit a mental health professional, for assistance, and you may have to change your life substantially, *but you must bring an end to the source or sources of your angst.*

Once you take better care of your mental health, improved physical health will naturally follow.

Now, while still looking into the reflection of your eyes, promise yourself that your healthier future begins *today.* You're finally done with dieting—*forever.* You now know that the lifestyle-reform, weight-loss and health plan advocated by this book *is the way to success.* It worked for Brad, and it has worked for many men and women. And it will work for you, too. Be confident!

Brad had this confidence when he began his final weight-loss journey, in January 2005. He began with a model based on real-life success. And he *knew* that he was going to succeed, *finally.*

The journey to "enlightenment"

No matter how many pounds you want to lose, you must first lose *one.* Before you go to bed each night, be sure you did something, no matter how small, to move you towards your long-term goal.

Week after week, month after month, year after year, you'll live your new life *one satisfying day at a time.* And praise yourself for every bit of progress, no matter how small.

It took Brad 19 months to lose his weight. But every pound lost was a victory, and a reason to smile. He had more than 100 reasons to smile throughout his weight-loss journey. He was patient and persistent, and eventually super successful. Follow his example.

Get started, and plug away relentlessly. Never mind if you have a great deal of weight to lose. Many people have had far more weight to lose, but managed. *Get started!*

Remember the Chinese proverb: *"The man who removes a mountain begins by carrying away small stones."*

Never mind if you've had weight-loss failures. As Henry Ford said, "Failure is the opportunity to begin again more intelligently."

Many people say, "I can't wait to be slim, so I can begin my new life." Don't wait! Start enjoying it today. *Enjoy the ride.*

Losing weight and keeping it off doesn't have to be tortuous. That's an archaic belief. The lifestyle-reform, weight-loss and health plan works *without* sacrifice and misery, and the lost weight *stays off.*

Losing weight is a fun, rewarding journey only if you take your time and allow it to be fun and rewarding.

And stop being hard on yourself—you're allowed to make mistakes.

It's impractical if not impossible to eat perfectly all of the time. If you cheated last night or missed an exercise session, get back with the program today, and do better next time you're tempted to make a mistake. The big picture will determine your results, not the details along the way.

Some days will be better than others, and some weeks will be better than others. Start by being on track more than you're off track, and gradually increase this percentage. Eventually you'll eat well *all* of the time because that's what will make you feel at your best.

Your shiny new self

Once you start to care for yourself, and get healthier, you'll feel a greater sense of pride about yourself. Then, later on, your inner strength will not let you regress.

It's like having a new car. You clean it, wax it, and take great pride in its appearance. Now, however, it will be your "shiny new self" that you'll care for, and take great pride in.

It's not necessarily being slim that will make you happy, but the overall package of your new self.

That you may have solved your underlying emotional problems is a huge victory. And this, coupled with your improved mental and physical health, will create your sense of self-worth.

Your slimness will be the icing on the cake. You'll look better but, more importantly, you'll *feel* better—mentally and physically.

Brad finally persevered only when he got the word "diet" out of his vocabulary. He knew he could cheat in moderation, he knew he could enjoy the foods he liked, and he knew he could have some drinks. *He wasn't on a diet; but had a fresh outlook on life, nutrition, and health.*

While you can occasionally cheat, you can't binge. A binge can negate a week's worth of progress. But an occasional cookie won't.

But you must be careful when it comes to your trigger foods.

If you feel like grabbing a bag of chips, walk to a mirror instead, look at your "shiny new self," and ask, "Why am I eating this junk? Do I really *need* to eat this crud?"

By remembering the months of dedication it took to become your "shiny new self," you'll probably end up throwing the chips in the garbage can. It would have been best, however, not to have had the chips in the house in the first place.

And remember to use the tips described in the section "How to curb your cravings for comfort foods," starting on page 86.

Adopt the mind-set that you're now eating to fuel your body. You wouldn't put poor-quality fuel in your shiny new car, so why would you put poor-quality fuel in your "shiny new self"?

Caring about yourself can help you to apply restraint you may have never had. Don't let your "shiny new self" down.

You're in charge, *not* the food.

You *will* succeed!

What we can learn from Oprah Winfrey's weight struggles

"How did I let this happen again?" screamed the cover of the January 2009 issue of *The Oprah Magazine*. "Oprah on her battle with weight: A must-read for anyone who's ever fallen off the wagon."

Oprah has had a decades-long battle with her weight. Many of her struggles echo Brad's struggles, and those of many other people. When coming clean on how and why she again let her weight top the 200-pound mark, she revealed in the aforementioned article that there's no foolproof recipe for maintaining permanent weight-loss—especially for people with underlying issues.

A February 2007 doctor's visit revealed that Oprah had a problem with her thyroid, which required medication. This led to such mounting frustration and feelings of self-defeat that she once again resorted to her medication of choice—*food*. She wrote, "I use food for the same reasons an addict uses drugs: to comfort, to soothe, to ease stress." She found comfort in gorging on potato chips.

Despite following the medication and her doctor's orders, she continued to gain weight. And she was tired and listless; and everything in her life was dull. Something was wrong. Was she depressed? What was happening?

Under her doctor's advice, and in an effort to regain her health, she slowly weaned herself off the numerous medications she was taking—with the intent to overcome the thyroid problem and other health issues without drugs. She became more conscious of how she ate, and she began to work out again.

But it wasn't easy. Her life was all about work, and it didn't leave her time to have fun, to calm down, or to take proper care of herself. She seemed to have commitments to everyone *but herself*. And she was burning out from the never-ending workload.

Although she understood right from wrong concerning exercise and eating, she still struggled with her weight. But through some time off and self-reflection, she realized that she didn't really have a weight problem. She discovered she had a "self-care problem that manifests through weight." She wasn't craving food, she noted, she was craving love. Letting herself regain the weight wasn't a "weight issue," it was a "love issue." She craved balance in her life—something other than work—*and* self-care.

For 2009 and beyond, she vowed to *put herself first*. She now *makes* time for daily exercise and healthy meals. Her new goal isn't to lose weight to be thin, but to lose weight *to be healthy*. And she learned to embrace her body and be grateful for what it gives her.

What can you learn from Oprah? Love yourself, and find the *desire* you require to make yourself healthy. *Put yourself and your health first.* And find joy in your everyday life, *but don't let food be that joy.*

And, as she said on one of her January 2009 shows, she wants you to reflect and ask yourself these questions: "Why are *you* overweight?" "What can you change about yourself?" "Why have you failed at previous diets?" and "*Why* do you want to lose weight?" Perhaps some deep self-analysis can reveal the underlying issues that are the cause of your weight problem. And these issues—which must be addressed if you're to succeed with your weight-loss over the long-term—can serve as discussion points if you enlist some professional help.

Will you be cured once you've lost the weight?

No matter how much weight you lose, you'll never be cured.

People who claim that there's a "cure" for obesity are naive, or misinformed. Your weight must be properly managed for the rest of your life. If you make a major deviation from the plan that you used to lose the weight, you'll regain the weight.

About 95% of diets fail over the long-term because it's natural for people to revert to habits that are second nature—the comfort zone that they are accustomed to.

If you maintain for the rest of your life a version of your lifestyle-reform, weight-loss and health plan, your weight-loss will be permanent. But don't get complacent, or you'll soon be back where you started.

Once you've succeeded with weight-loss you may have to change your mind-set from a fat person—who may have had many limitations—to a slim, healthy person without those limitations.

Many people struggle with their new selves because they are used to being fat and being treated as fat people. Remind yourself daily that you love yourself. Your future is a blank canvas that you'll enjoy with confidence and passion.

But even slim, healthy people can't control everything.

Certain life-issues like divorce, serious illness, accidents, death, or job loss can hit you. These events will affect you whether you're fat or slim. Be prepared for any event that may test your resolve.

Brad recently experienced financial adversity that was a result of the 2008 global economic meltdown. It was an ordeal, but Brad was prepared this time.

Since Brad had already learned that physical exercise was a great stress reliever, he used it to fend off the stress that arose from the financial adversity. If he hadn't gone through his final weight-loss journey he would never have developed the psychological skills to cope with adversity. He would have buried himself in booze and binge eating, instead of exercise and nutritious eating.

Binge eating and alcohol won't solve problems. They will only make things worse over the long-term, by compounding the problems.

Are you still fat in your mind?

Many people who lose large amounts of weight sometimes struggle for a while to adjust to being thin. They are used to looking in the mirror and seeing themselves as fat people. They are used to being fat people with difficulty fitting in theater or airplane seats, for instance. And they are so used to being treated as fat people by society that it's hard to accept that they are no longer fat.

Brad knows this problem. Despite the compliments he received immediately after his weight-loss success, when he looked in the mirror he *still* saw himself as a fat person. His brain was trained to view himself that way. *But he found a solution.*

It wasn't until he saw a photograph of the "new Brad"—slim and trim—that he realized he looked good. He placed a copy of the photo on his fridge so he could constantly remind himself how far he had come.

Then he could see the man in the mirror as a slim, vibrant, and healthy person.

A reason to smile—enjoy life with a new mind-set

Many people with eating problems suffer from self-esteem issues. Their core beliefs about their looks, capabilities, and self-worth hold them back from losing weight. Their core beliefs also hold them back from enjoying life.

But it doesn't have to be this way.

A study from the Ohio State University has shown that once you start accepting yourself and your body, you'll be more likely to eat for health reasons than emotional ones. And this can help with your self-esteem.

When the dieters Brad researched began to lose weight, and get healthy, their confidence and self-worth immediately increased.

The better they felt about themselves emotionally, the better they felt about themselves physically. And the better they felt physically, the better they felt emotionally.

The more compliments they received, the more they felt a sense of achievement, and the more they cared about their health.

And because self-esteem stems from the sense of accomplishment from achieving goals, their self-esteem steadily improved.

They made an effort to eat better. The more pride they had in themselves, the healthier they ate and the less often they cheated.

They cared about themselves for a change. And they especially cared about their health.

And their healthier eating led to an increase in their energy level.

They accepted themselves, even if they didn't look like the celebrities and supermodels that many people admire.

And towards the end of their weight-loss journeys, their sense of self-worth soared.

They were new people who were at peace with themselves, and who smile whenever they look at their reflections in the mirror.

They were finally in control of their behavior. And they were enjoying every day, and living life to its fullest.

Some ladies, who once thought of themselves as "ugly ducklings," eventually became confident and sexy—*you don't have to look like a supermodel to feel sexy.* They turned their lives around.

And some men who used to feel like fat slobs, became specimens of fitness and self-confidence. They lost 50 to 100 pounds, got great haircuts, bought hip clothes, and became "chick magnets."

A sense of self-worth

Look at the photos of Brad on pages 52 and 53. The one of him on a couch was taken at two o'clock in the morning, just after he had devoured an entire pizza. He was depressed, and embarrassed about his appearance. And he didn't care about his health.

Now, look at his "after" photo. He was glowing in self-confidence. He had pride in his appearance, and even greater pride in his sense of self-worth. This is the new Brad.

For the first time in over a decade, he felt good about himself.

From now on, think only positive thoughts.

Every pound you lose will be another reason to smile, and another reason to take more pride in yourself.

A real-life triumph

Here's Jennifer's story, as an example of triumph over adversity.

Unwanted. Worthless. In the way. While I couldn't articulate those feelings as a child, they dominated my life. Many if not most people who struggle with their weight have similar feelings.

I was 16 years old when I made my first effort to lose weight. If I could go back and talk to myself as I was then, the first thing I would say to her is that the number on the scale isn't all important.

The number on the scale is one measure of the external you. It has implications for your health, but it means nothing about who you are as a person. It doesn't define your worth, intelligence, competence, or value to those who love you.

Don't ignore the health aspects of excess weight, but don't get them mixed up with your self-worth. If you don't value yourself, it will be harder to lose weight, and nearly impossible to keep it off.

As a child, when I visited my grandfather's farm he would comment on my size and that of others, especially those who were struggling with their weight. He proposed that we write our names and weights on a large poster whenever we visited. He believed that the shame would cause us to lose weight and keep it off. Wrong. Losing weight out of shame won't work over the long-term because fear and shame come from a belief that you're not worthy. Success comes from a place of believing in your worth.

I didn't recognize that I was turning to food to deal with my emotions until I became an adult, and by then the patterns were set. If I could go back and do it over, I would find hobbies, activities, people—anything to occupy my time and energy—instead of food.

One of the best things to get your mind off food is exercise. Exercise is wonderful. It accelerates weight-loss and increases fitness, but, perhaps more importantly, it helps with the negative emotions that plague those who struggle with weight issues.

My advice to my 16-year-old self would be to find an exercise that *she likes*, and stay with it. If she doesn't like one type of exercise, she should find another. The health benefits will follow later.

You don't have to join a gym, but you certainly may. You don't have to spend hours a day doing some form of exercise or activity, but you can if you have the time.

When you feel like eating the contents of your fridge, go for a walk. When you feel stressed out, go for a walk.

I swim two to four times a week—during my lunch hour I walk to the health club two blocks from my workplace. I've loved to swim since I was a girl. My colleagues encourage me. And when I return to work I have even more energy for the afternoon's tasks.

I count calories, I exercise, and I lose weight. If I falter, I gain weight. It's that simple. The hard part is telling myself that I'm worth the trouble of sticking with it. The hardest part of any weight-loss journey is keeping the weight off. To do so, you must find ways to value yourself.

Surround yourself with people you trust, and who encourage you. That may mean looking outside your family. Find a base of support—people who like you as you are—to help you through hard times. If you need professional help to sort through your issues, or give guidance on nutrition or exercise, seek it.

The key is to believe in myself, and my ability to lose weight. And when negative emotions surface, I handle them through means *not* food-related. That's my challenge. And it's probably yours, as well.

I'll always face the challenge. *So will you!*

I *am* worth the struggle. *So are you!*

I *will* maintain a healthy weight. *And so will you!*

Everyone can lose weight. But some people have it harder than others due to underlying physiological conditions.

This chapter provides awareness of the physiological issues that contribute to weight problems.

You may think it unlikely that physiological issues could have contributed to your weight problems, and difficulties with achieving lasting weight-loss.

We're confident that at least one of the physiological problems explained in this chapter *will* apply to you. *Please keep an open mind, and read this entire chapter.*

You may be in for a surprise revelation; but if you respond as we advise, you may leap forward in your efforts to lose weight and keep it off.

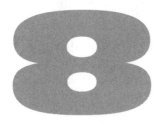

The other reasons why many people can't lose weight readily . . . *and how they can be corrected*

While overeating often stems from psychological causes, overeating and difficulties with losing weight can also stem from physiological causes—many of which are medical conditions.

But no matter what underlying problems there may be, everyone can lose weight and keep it off *if* they follow the model promoted in this book.

Chronic indigestion, diabetes, hypoglycemia, Graves' disease, manic disorder, bipolar disorder, low blood sugar level, food allergies, intestinal worms or tapeworms, and various hypothalamic diseases are common causes for overeating.

Even brain problems such as encephalitis, chromophobe adenoma, and craniopharyngioma can lead to an increase in eating.

Some people have eating disorders that can cause overeating, including bulimia, and binge eating.

Borderline personality disorder—characterized by mood swings, anger, depression, instability in one's self-image, and difficulty with relationships—can lead to overeating. And Klein-Levin syndrome—a disorder that causes recurring periods of excessive drowsiness and sleep—and hysteria, can have similar effects.

Certain physical disorders can also interfere with the body's mechanism that regulates energy use. Neurological damage can interfere with proper caloric intake, especially if the hypothalamus, which regulates appetite, is damaged.

Get a medical checkup

It's imperative that you visit your doctor before you begin a weight-loss program. You may have a medical condition that's contributing to a weight problem, and your well-being in general. Treating the condition could make a *huge* difference to your health, and your ability to deal with a weight problem.

Obesity should be treated like any chronic disease. It's a lifelong issue that may require you to seek help from a doctor or a psychologist, or both.

Your health insurance may cover treatment for these medical issues, and many medically prescribed weight-loss programs may be tax deductible via a medical deduction. And they may qualify for your employer's flexible spending account.

The flaws of the body mass index

There are mentions in this book of body mass index, or BMI. Many people, perhaps especially doctors, use BMI for medical diagnosis, but that's not its purpose. It was supposed to be a means of classifying sedentary people who have an average body composition, designed for use in social physics.

BMI is a statistical measurement that compares a person's weight and height. It's an individual's bodyweight divided by the square of his or her height. At its simplest, the formula uses kg/m² as the unit of measurement. When imperial units are used, conversion factors are required in order to yield comparable figures as in the computations using the metric system.

Pregnant women, the elderly, or people with greater-than-average muscle mass are not accurately represented by this formula. And it gives no consideration to body composition, because it's determined by height and weight.

For example, bodybuilders and some athletes, whose body-fat percentages may be under 10%, will weigh more than the average person because they have a much higher percentage of lean muscle mass. But because they may be five-foot eight-inches and weigh over 200 pounds, for example, they are considered obese by these formulas although they may be in super physical condition— fitness wise and physique wise. At five-foot eight-inches and 165 pounds, the BMI even suggests that Brad is overweight.

And although the BMI doesn't allow for body composition or gender, it's still used by the National Institute of Health, and Centers for Disease Control and Prevention, for example.

A five-foot eight-inch, 225-pound male bodybuilder uses the same index as a five-foot eight-inch, 225-pound obese woman who has never exercised. (Some nutritionists and organizations have, however, introduced a revised BMI scale that has gender and age factored in. But it's for their use only, not official medical use.)

BMI is an inaccurate, misleading tool when not used for its proper purpose. But provided its limitations are recognized, BMI can help specify some important terms.

According to this scale, if you have a BMI of 18.5 to 24.9, you have a *normal weight*. If you're between 25 and 29.9, you're considered *overweight*. If you're between 30 and 34.9, you're considered *obese*. If you're between 35 and 39.9, you're considered *clinically obese*. If you're between 40 and 49.9, you're considered *morbidly obese*. And if you're 50 or higher, you're considered *super obese*.

Fatigue

Consistent fatigue can devastate your ability to lose weight and keep it off. It's a very common problem among overweight people.

Unless you're a vigorous person you'll struggle even with the general activities of life, and formal exercise may be beyond your current abilities.

When you have a high energy level it will make general activity easy to do, and even formal exercise will be something you can do readily. And you'll be more likely to do other things that are vital for weight-loss success, such as making the effort to seek out healthier foods, and to prepare healthy meals.

A low level of physical fitness can be a major factor behind a low level of energy, but some people have such low energy that it's extremely difficult for them to put in the work to get fit.

Fatigue can simply be the result of not going to bed early enough to have sufficient sleep. It can also be the result of poor quality sleep even though the quantity may be fine. *And fatigue can be a symptom of many health problems, including some that are mentioned in this chapter.*

If you suffer from consistent fatigue, *acknowledge its seriousness*, discover the cause, and put it right. Seek appropriate help.

If you've suffered from low energy for a long time, once your energy level has been normalized you'll be amazed at how it will transform your life, *and* boost your ability to lose weight and keep it off.

Sleep and weight issues

A study by Columbia University suggests that, when you're deprived of sleep, your leptin levels fall as your ghrelin levels shoot up, thereby triggering hunger, which would encourage overeating. These hormonal changes *also* signal your body to slow your metabolism and hold on to fat stores.

And insufficient sleep affects weight control in other ways.

How many of these statements apply to you?

I wish I had more energy.

I need coffee or tea to keep me alert during the day.

Without caffeine I often have difficulty staying awake when sitting still, watching television, or reading.

I've nodded off while driving.

After I've woken in the morning I don't feel fully rested.

I often wake up earlier in the morning than I would like to.

I sometimes have a headache when I get up, albeit it a mild one.

I've been told that I snore.

I've been told that parts of my body sometimes jerk while I sleep.

I've been told that I sometimes kick while I sleep, or grind my teeth.

I've been told that as I sleep I sometimes hold my breath.

I've suddenly woken up while gasping for breath.

I sweat during the night.

My heart sometimes pounds or beats irregularly during the night.

I wake during the night and often have trouble returning to sleep.

I often feel grumpy, irritable, or impatient.

I have trouble concentrating at school, work, or home.

I often feel like taking a nap.

I have high blood pressure.

All of the above are symptoms of sleep disorders.

There are many sleep disorders—for example, insomnia, sleep apnea and hypopnea, restless legs syndrome, excessive need to urinate at night, teeth grinding, and night terrors. While many slim people suffer from sleep disorders, overweight people are far more likely to suffer from some of them. *If more than two of the aforementioned symptoms apply to you, you may suffer from a sleep disorder.*

There's *much* at stake—and not just for weight control.

If not treated, some sleep disorders greatly increase the chance of catastrophic results—heart problems, strokes, and premature death.

If you suffer from more than two of the symptoms, visit a doctor who specializes in sleep disorders (perhaps at a sleep clinic), and deal with the particular disorder or disorders that may afflict you.

Proper treatment will boost your energy level and thus help your efforts to lose weight, and it will improve your health in general, which will further help your efforts to lose weight.

Even if you feel that your symptoms of sleep disorders are mild, *still seek medical help*. If you wait until the symptoms are severe, the consequences could be grave.

As well as addressing any sleep disorders you may have, *you also need good sleep habits.* And even if you don't have a sleep disorder, if you regularly go to bed too late, and if you're regularly woken by an alarm clock, *you're going to run a sleep deficit, and then your energy level and overall health will suffer, which will undermine your efforts to lose weight.* But if you have a sleep disorder *and* bad sleep habits, that combination could lead to catastrophic results.

Here are the priority sleep habits: have a regular bedtime, allow enough time to sleep sufficiently so that you awake *naturally*, use a comfortable mattress and pillow, sleep in a dark room (fit shutters or black-out curtains), eliminate as much as possible all sources of noise that could disturb you, minimize liquid intake shortly before bedtime, be sure you're neither cold nor too warm while you sleep, and do something that relaxes you immediately prior to bedtime.

Sleep apnea

This very serious disorder is the *stoppage* of breathing during sleep. (Sleep *hypopnea* involves episodes of overly shallow breathing—but some air flow remains.) *Being overweight increases the occurrence of obstructive sleep apnea because the buildup of fatty tissue contributes to the obstruction of the breathing passages.*

The breathing stoppages can occur dozens of times during a night's sleep, and the person with the disorder may be unaware that it's happening. Symptoms, which are usually reported by an awakened partner, include loud snoring, and gasping. But apnea can occur even without the occurrence of loud snoring. Apnea can lead to cardiac rhythm disturbances, and even sudden death.

Why sleeping well is *so* important

If you don't sleep well, you'll have reduced zest for any type of activity, and perhaps be *incapable* of doing formal exercise consistently. Sleeping well is also critical for your long-term health, and your day-to-day alertness, creativity, and capacity to learn.

If our words aren't persuasive, read *The Promise of Sleep* (1999, Delacorte Press), by William C. Dement, M.D., Ph.D., one of the world's leading authorities on sleep. To quote from the book's dust jacket:

"our modern culture has become an alarming study in sleep deprivation and ignorance . . . Sleep is sacrificed to meet the demands of our endless days . . . Doctors regard sleep deprivation as a fact of life and do little to promote sleep health or awareness. Meanwhile, the physical, emotional, and psychological costs of unhealthy sleep continue to mount."

It's a modern, social disease that some people feel proud for managing on as little sleep as possible each night. You should get the sleep you need *without* any feeling of guilt for sleeping more than perhaps many of your friends do.

For many people, going to bed earlier is all that's needed, and clocking up seven to eight hours of sleep *every* night. But for many others, no matter how much they sleep they *still* don't get well rested *because the quality of their slumber is so poor due to sleep disorders.*

Dr. Dement believes that anyone who snores and has daytime drowsiness should be evaluated for sleep disorders.

Once you begin treatment for a sleep disorder, your ability to lose weight should improve.

Then, as you lose weight, your sleeping may be helped further, which in turn should help you to lose weight more readily.

And your improved sleep will greatly affect your health and well-being in many other ways.

Is a virus making you fat?

An infection with a "virus linked to human obesity" may increase fat-cell production and make fat cells even fatter. "Infectobesity" is the term coined by Louisiana State University researcher Nikhil Dhurandhar, Ph.D., and colleagues, to describe this phenomenon. Their research links a common human virus—adenovirus-36, or Ad-36—to human obesity. Their research has suggested that nearly 30% of obese people may be infected with Ad-36.

Hypothyroidism

Your thyroid plays a critical role in your health. The hormones it secretes promote healthy skin, regulate your heart rate, and play an integral part in regulating your metabolism. Your brain regulates these hormones by releasing thyroid-stimulating hormone (TSH). People with low TSH levels—a result of reduced thyroid function, or *hypothyroidism*—tend to put on weight because their body will naturally store more calories as fat.

According to the American Association of Clinical Endocrinologists, as many as 30 million Americans may have thyroid disease, but half of them remain undiagnosed.

Your risk for hypothyroidism, which can run in families, increases as you age, and women are eight times more likely to have it than men. And many people with hypothyroidism are misdiagnosed—they are prescribed antidepressants or skin creams when they really need thyroid medication.

How do you know if you have hypothyroidism? Besides weight-gain, symptoms may include depression, problems with memory, joint pain, constipation, fatigue, coarse or dry skin, thinning hair, and voice changes. If you suspect any of these, your doctor may suggest a blood test for TSH. If you're diagnosed with hypothyroidism, you'll usually end up with a prescription for synthetic thyroxine, a treatment to replace the missing hormone.

What about perimenopausal and postmenopausal weight-related issues?

Menopause is the permanent cessation of reproductive fertility in women, usually occurring between the ages of 45 and 55. Perimenopause is the transitional period leading to menopause.

The profound hormonal changes—notably in estrogen, progesterone, testosterone, and follicle-stimulating hormone—that occur during perimenopause can have dramatic effects. They can greatly influence a woman's health in general, including her ability to lose weight and keep it off. And they can affect fat storage patterns, including increased fat around the abdomen.

Studies show that many women who had profound weight-gain during their perimenopausal and postmenopausal years experienced reduced physical activity. Greatly reduced vigor is a common effect of the hormonal changes during perimenopause.

Many women are physically incapable of being very active *unless* they first receive the appropriate medical help.

Many of the successful dieters that Brad researched are *vigorous* postmenopausal women. They exercised for an hour or more, seven days a week. Some even went at it twice a day.

Research from the University of Pittsburgh found that menopausal women who reduced their caloric intake by 150 to 200 a day, and increased their daily activities, didn't gain weight.

Perimenopausal and postmenopausal women should discuss the hormonal changes with medical experts, and the possibility of hormone replacement therapy. And perimenopausal or postmenopausal women doctors may provide the most sympathetic advice on this topic.

The appropriate and correctly monitored treatment may dramatically improve the women's health in general, including their ability to lose weight and keep it off.

The male menopause

Other than in exceptional cases, and unlike in women, men don't experience a complete, permanent shutting down of the reproductive system. But what happens, generally, is that from about age 35 there's a slow, gradual decline in the production of the hormones testosterone and dehydroepiandrosterone.

The consequences of this reduction aren't dramatic, other than in exceptional cases. Loss of some muscle tissue, general fatigue, and increased difficulty with building muscle are possible effects that influence the ability to lose weight and keep it off.

Depression, irritability, and loss of sex drive are other possible consequences of male menopause, or andropause.

An increase in physical activity and exercise (if, previously, you were inactive), or maintenance of a vigorous lifestyle if you're already a regular exerciser, and a healthy diet with a slight reduction in caloric intake, will help to compensate for the effects of a normal decline in testosterone and dehydroepiandrosterone production.

If you feel that your ability to lose weight and keep it off is significantly affected by andropause, discuss it with your doctor.

The role of some other hormones in obesity

Obese people may have hormone levels that encourage the storage of body fat. Furthermore, overeating and lack of exercise can alter the hormonal processes that regulate appetite and body fat distribution, resulting in an increased inclination to gain weight.

Insulin

This hormone regulates the metabolism of glucose and other nutrients. It also helps you store excess sugar as fat. But when you have consistently high levels of insulin in your blood, you may become insulin resistant. Your pancreas then over-produces insulin, which can lead to grave consequences, possibly including cancer, dementia, heart disease, and a slowing of the metabolism.

There may be an inherited component to insulin resistance. And some researchers say that it may also be linked to excessive intake of sugary or starchy food, and high-fructose corn syrup.

Leptin

When full, fat cells release the hormone leptin, which curbs appetite. But if leptin production is hindered, the fat cells are unable to signal that they are full, and weight-gain occurs.

Leptin reduces appetite by acting on the brain to reduce the urge to eat. It also seems to control how the body manages its stored body fat. Since leptin is produced by fat, leptin levels tend be higher in obese people than in those of normal weight.

An issue being explored by research is why are obese people obese considering that they have higher-than-usual levels of the appetite-*reducing* hormone as compared to normal-weight people. One theory is that obese people aren't as sensitive to the effects of leptin. And current studies are trying to explain why leptin messages aren't getting through to the brain in obese individuals.

Studies have shown that low-calorie diets produce a decrease in blood leptin levels. Reduced leptin levels may increase appetite and slow metabolism. This may help to explain why crash dieters usually regain their lost weight. It's possible that leptin therapy may help dieters maintain their weight-loss over the long-term.

Cortisol

Cortisol is responsible for setting off the physiological responses associated with stress. Studies show that when cortisol is released into your bloodstream you become less sensitive to leptin, the hormone that tells you that you're full. People with higher levels of cortisol, whether from stress or natural disposition, are more likely to be overweight and accumulate fat around their bellies.

In Cushing's syndrome, increased levels of cortisol are secreted.

Can hormones make food addictive?

Ghrelin stimulates appetite. It may also improve perception and memory when it comes to food. And it acts on the brain to make food more appealing.

This hormonal response makes sense for mankind as a whole—it could help starving people eat food they may otherwise not consider appetizing. But during overconsumption, ghrelin may contribute to obesity.

"Obesity must be understood as a brain disease," researcher Dr. Alain Dagher, a neurologist at McGill

University in Montreal, told LiveScience.com in an interview. "Obese people eat too much, and this is likely due largely to excess hunger."

Therapies that disrupt these effects of ghrelin may help to fight obesity, the researchers conjectured. "Many drug companies are currently developing ghrelin-blocking drugs as obesity treatments," Dagher said. "However, we show that ghrelin acts on brain areas involved in emotion and motivation. A drug that suppresses this brain system runs the risk of causing depressed mood. There is a risk of side effects."

The parts of the brain linked to ghrelin are also involved in drug addiction. "It may be reasonable to think of high-calorie food as having addictive potential," Dagher added. "If food can be thought of as 'addictive,' this supports doing things like banning fast food shops from schools, and [banning] advertising junk food to children. Public policy aimed at tobacco was spurred by the science showing that nicotine was addictive."

The dangers of metabolic syndrome

Do you have a large belly that's hard and not jiggly?

If you're a woman, does your waist circumference measure 35 inches or more, and if you're a man, does it measure 40 or more?

Do you have high blood pressure?

If so, schedule an appointment with your doctor, because you may have metabolic syndrome.

A hard belly like this is made of visceral fat, which is an "internal belly" behind your abdominal muscles. It surrounds your internal organs, and produces dangerous chemicals.

Metabolic syndrome can greatly increase your chances of developing diabetes, heart problems, cancer, and liver disease. It affects nearly half of all middle-aged men.

How to deal with a medical condition

The intention of this chapter isn't to create concern. It's to help you understand what may be occurring in your body.

While you study this chapter, if you come across any condition that you think may affect you, discuss it with your doctor.

If you have a medical condition, and get it correctly treated, your life-changing, weight-loss journey can proceed without any medical problem undermining it.

And remember, no matter what underlying condition or conditions you may have, *everyone has the ability to lose weight.* Some people may require medical intervention, *but everyone can succeed.*

You should now feel further empowered to take charge of your weight, *once and for all.*

Nutritional deficiencies and obesity

When Brad was a couch potato who lived off fast food and other crud, he thought that his inactive lifestyle and intake of excessive calories were the reasons for his weight-gain. He has since discovered that this view was only partially true. Even though he was eating a great deal of food, he was suffering from *malnutrition*. And *that* was making a major contribution to his weight problem.

He was gaining weight largely because of overconsumption of the wrong foods (junk food and other nutrient-deficient crud), and the underconsumption of the right foods (nutrient-rich, healthy items).

His body wasn't getting the nutrients it required to function properly, and to help regulate its weight normally.

The correlation between nutritional deficiencies and obesity is an issue that few people know about.

How do nutrient deficiencies cause weight-gain?

Several recent studies indicate that obesity may be caused, or at least exacerbated, by an insufficiency of some vitamins and minerals. Most people eat a lot of food that has little nutritional value. And if that's coupled with a reduced-calorie diet, malnutrition is inevitable.

The insufficiency of key nutrients doesn't just contribute to weight problems in the first place. It also impairs the ability to lose weight *and* keep it off.

The insufficiency of nutrients leads to many problems, including the appetite not being sated properly, which means you may continue to be hungry even after eating.

When your body is desperate for the nutrients needed for survival, it may still crave food even after a meal. It may send signals that cause cravings for certain foods, and this can lead to food binges, especially of processed food.

This is one of the biggest reasons why some people tend to gain weight.

To prevent this problem, eat much more *nutritious* food. When your body gets what it needs—vitamins such as D, B_6, E, folic acid, and biotin, as well as minerals such as copper, manganese, and zinc—its cravings for food may be eliminated, or at least much reduced.

To ensure you're getting all the nutrients your body needs for optimal functioning, take a daily multivitamin-mineral tablet, and additional vitamins C and E. And take cod liver oil and flaxseed oil as well, to supply vital essential fatty acids.

But food supplements are never a substitute for nutritious eating—that's why *supplements* are called *supplements*. Always rely on a variety of nutritious foods as your primary source of essential nutrients.

Many people are sedentary because their energy level is so low that they are incapable of being active and vigorous. Eating a nutrient-rich diet will boost their energy levels, and add vitality to their lives.

And that will make it much easier for them to be more active in general, and to be willing to exercise.

Not eating enough nutrient-rich food is one of the biggest mistakes you can make if you want to lose weight.

Malnutrition and the obesity epidemic

There's increasing evidence that nutrient deficiency is a major contributor to the world's growing obesity epidemic.

In 2000, a Department of Hygiene Ecology and Occupational Health survey in Bulgaria revealed that many people who were obese or overweight were deficient in vitamin A and thiamin (B_1), and consumed a poor ratio of minerals *even though they consumed a great deal of food*.

And in 2007, a study by the International Food Policy Research Institute (a conglomerate arising from dozens of countries) examined the presence of micronutrient deficiencies in women. The results show a clear overlap between micronutrient deficiency and the prevalence of obesity.

Furthermore, according to a 2005 National Health and Nutrition Examination Survey report (a program conducted by the National Center for Health Statistics, which is based in America under the umbrella of the American government), even though the intake of protein, fats and oils has remained stable over the last few decades, and the intake of carbohydrates has increased, *the deficiency in critical nutrients is increasing*, with many Americans failing to ingest enough vitamins E, C, A and D, and selenium, magnesium and potassium.

These studies show a clear connection between a micronutrient deficit and excess weight. And because low-cost (and low-nutrient) processed food is generally affordable to low-income people, that contributes to their increasing obesity.

Many children today are much less active than those from earlier generations. But many studies also show that malnutrition is one of the reasons why American children have increasing obesity rates. American and British youths derive many of their calories from nutrient-deficient foods. And not enough school lunch programs offer nutrient-rich foods as part of their menus. Most nutrient-deficient food is cheaper to make, and many children have been conditioned into wanting only this type of food.

Studies also suggest that many dietary recommendations are unsound. They usually focus on *macronutrients*— carbohydrate, protein and fat—and assume, falsely, that if you follow such recommendations you'll meet your daily *micro*nutrient requirements.

"The thinking used to be that if people get enough energy in their diets, the micronutrients will take care of themselves," says Dr. Burlingame, senior officer of the United Nations' Food and Agriculture Organization's Nutrition Impact Assessment and Evaluation Group. "But increasingly, people are eating larger quantities of cheap food that fill the stomach but still leave the body without those micronutrients."

It's alleged by some nutritionists that many of menus published by the US government and medical organizations that provide an "example to the public of how to eat" are nutritionally deficient in essential micronutrients.

Vitamin D deficiency has been linked to obesity

According to research by the University Hospital of North Norway, vitamin D deficiency is associated with elevated parathyroid hormone levels, which in turn are associated with obesity. The subjects who had the highest vitamin D intake weighed the least.

Scientists have also found that vitamin D levels in the blood are lower in obese subjects than in thin subjects. A 1988 study by the Veterans Administration Medical Center in Charleston, South Carolina, found that obese subjects had dramatically lower levels of vitamin D than the non-obese subjects.

Exposure to the sunshine enables your body to make vitamin D, so get more exposure to the sun—*but without getting burned, or otherwise overdoing it.* That many people have been frightened off sunshine—almost made to think that the sun is evil, and *all* exposure to it should be avoided—has eliminated that source of vitamin D for them. In *moderation*, exposure to the sun is healthy.

An outstanding food source of vitamin D is cod liver oil.

According to research from the Pennington Biomedical Research Center, not only does vitamin D deficiency play a role in causing obesity, it also plays a role in cancer, heart disease, hypertension, diabetes, osteoporosis, osteoarthritis, periodontal disease, and even depression.

The role of genetics and heredity in obesity

Because each person is born with a unique genetic composition, losing weight and keeping it off can be more challenging for some people than others.

Your genes can influence how quickly you feel full when eating, how physically active you're prone to be, and your metabolic rate, for example. As a result, some people may be genetically more *vulnerable* to gaining weight, and certain environmental triggers can make these people more susceptible to becoming obese.

So what percentage of the population is obese because of genetics?

Some scientists claim that most obesity cases are influenced by genetics, some claim that the influence is negligible, and many believe that the right explanation rests between the polar views.

Some scientists believe that certain inherited genes don't necessarily make individuals obese. They merely give them a *predisposition* for becoming obese, but it's the *learned* or *acquired* behaviors of overeating and inactivity that *cause* the weight-gain.

While science shows that heredity is linked to obesity, it's impossible to pinpoint the degree of correlation.

There's little debate, however, over the genetic determination of body *shape*. Some people are more likely to put weight on their hips and thighs, and this is harder to lose than belly fat.

"Obesity runs in my family, and it's impossible for me to lose weight" is a classic excuse for not trying to lose weight. And it can be a convenient way of blaming others for an individual's fatness.

Obesity tends to run in some families, suggesting a genetic link. But families also share diet and lifestyle habits that contribute to obesity.

There seems to be a greater chance that people are heavy because of conditioned behaviors they learned from their family, than because of genetics.

But people still succeed with weight-loss despite a genetic predisposition to gain weight, although it may take more work and patience, and medical intervention.

Can quitting smoking cause weight-gain?

Quitting smoking can cause weight-gain. Nicotine is an appetite suppressant, and it can increase metabolism. And the act of smoking, via walking to have a smoke break, lighting up, and so on, burns calories—dozens a day on top of the 50 to 100 or so each day from the nicotine boost, depending on the quantity smoked.

Once smoking has ended, those daily activities and the nicotine-produced metabolic boost also end. And it's common for smokers to replace their smoking with increased eating—especially starchy foods—due to a reduction in serotonin.

It's usually the combination of reduced activity, and increased caloric intake, that cause a former smoker to gain weight. But exercise and a healthier diet can quickly rectify this. If you smoke, use the quitting as a springboard to begin a healthier lifestyle.

Are you on any medications?

Many people who struggle with weight-loss discover that their efforts are undermined by the medication they are on. But this is a situation can be quickly remedied, or avoided from the start. See your doctor before you begin your weight-loss plan.

Birth control pills, blood pressure medication, antidepressants, antihistamines, migraine medication, bipolar medication, medication for hypoglycemia, and corticosteroids can all hinder weight-loss, and even cause weight-gain.

Are you carb sensitive?

When you eat carbohydrates, your pancreas releases insulin. Some carb-sensitive people have a pancreas that pumps out excessive insulin when they eat refined carbs. And these insulin spikes can increase hunger and intensify cravings for sweets.

What about pregnancy weight?

Pregnancy weight creates a huge challenge for many women, but this can be properly managed under a doctor's supervision.

It's still possible to exercise while pregnant. There are many female athletes and fitness buffs who exercise well into their pregnancies. And post-birth exercise is helpful, too.

Brad interviewed several women who got back to their pre-pregnancy weights by following the weight-loss strategy set forth in this book.

And many celebrities and professional athletes quickly recapture their figures following giving birth.

Weight-loss taken to the extreme

Here's information on conditions that may cause some people to become severely *underweight*. It may help you to spot patterns in people you know who have become obsessed with their weight, and who have taken weight-loss to the extreme.

Bulimia

Bulimia, or bulimia nervosa, or binge-purge syndrome, is characterized by a (usually secretive) cycle of binge eating followed by self-induced vomiting. It may also be accompanied by abuse of laxatives, over-exercising, heavy use of diet pills and diuretics, fasting, frequent dieting, and extreme concern with bodyweight and shape.

Anorexia nervosa

Anorexia nervosa, or self-starvation, is characterized by a pathological fear of becoming fat, distorted body image, excessive dieting, and emaciation. Recognition of its symptoms can be the first step towards saving yourself or someone else from possible death:

Refusal to maintain a normal bodyweight.

Fear of gaining weight.

Talking about "feeling fat."

Difficulty with eating full meals.

Rigidity with what can be eaten.

An obsessive preoccupation with body size.

Over-exercising.

Intense dissatisfaction with physical appearance.

Personality change from outgoing to withdrawn.

Limiting food intake to a narrow selection of low-calorie foods.

Hoarding, concealing, or throwing away food.

Menstrual difficulties, or missed menstrual periods.

Anorexics may also suffer from tooth decay, or loss of skin color. And they may experience dizziness, fainting, liver damage, pancreatitis, and high cholesterol. Some may experience lanugo, where hair grows on the body in an attempt to insulate the skin because of a lack of body fat. Anorexia can also cause baldness. And men may experience decreased testicular function.

Anorexia nervosa is extremely dangerous, and it doesn't affect adolescent girls and young women only. According to an article published in *Newsweek*, of the 11 million Americans who are known to suffer from anorexia nervosa, 10% are men.

Approximately 5% to 20% of anorexics die of major organ failures. And if they don't die, they may experience heart problems.

How skinny is *too* skinny?

A "thin is in" mentality has created some twig-thin people. Woman who are skin and bone—with visible ribs, and knees larger than their thighs—are common at red-carpet gala events. But these women serve as role models for some people.

While nearly two out of three Americans are overweight, nearly 3% of American women, and almost 1% of American men, are underweight, according to the National Health Interview Survey.

Being underweight isn't always a by-product of anorexia nervosa, or bulimia. It can be an elective choice—"to look like a celebrity," or it can be the result of cachexia, a serious medical condition.

Regardless of its origin, being underweight can be unhealthy, and lead to health problems and an increased mortality rate.

You can generally tell if someone you know is underweight, and you must treat it as serious. Being too heavy *or* too light is dangerous, and seeking medical assistance may be imperative. And you may never know if an underlying medical condition is the root of the problem *unless you seek help.*

Are celebrities setting a bad example?

Many celebrities go to ridiculous lengths to be slim. Actresses have been known to spend thousands of dollars on ludicrous colon cleanses, coupled with starvation diets that consist mainly of cigarettes and ultra-high-caffeine coffee, or a bizarre blend of lemon juice mixed with maple syrup, water, and cayenne pepper, as well as salt water and a laxative tea.

Another Hollywood fad is the "baby food diet" in which actresses live off the mushy food designed for infants.

A big thing among some teen actresses is the use of "dieter's tea," which, when taken properly, has a gentle laxative effect. But these teens are drinking upwards of a dozen cups a day, which can cause excessive vomiting, chronic constipation, stomach cramps, diarrhea, and long-term health problems—and all this to lose, temporarily, a modest amount of water weight.

And some celebrities are so desperate to be slim that they check into a hospital for symptoms of "exhaustion" as a ploy so they can be attached to an intravenous drip, and avoid eating.

This "IV diet" is another reason why you shouldn't follow the example of celebrities.

Part III

HOW TO LOSE WEIGHT AND KEEP IT OFF, Section B

The step-by-step, practical guidance

Most people don't really understand what all successful weight-loss plans have in common.

When you've read this chapter you'll know the fundamentals to apply in order to succeed with weight-loss.

But if you've turned to this chapter without reading Part II, please turn back and read the previous three chapters. Following their guidance is *essential if you're to be successful with weight-loss.*

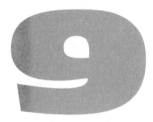

The fundamentals of weight-loss

Before you begin your weight-loss journey you must have confidence in the plan you're about to start.

For his final weight-loss journey, Brad heeded counsel from people who had been successful themselves with weight-loss. He was no longer interested in fads, gimmicks, or pills. And he had great confidence in the plan.

Because the plan he followed was based on the model of success that has already worked for countless real-life dieters—men and women—*you* should have confidence that it will work for you, too.

But before you get started, you need to understand the fundamentals of weight-loss.

Weight-loss and *fat*-loss

When people begin a diet they usually say, "I need to lose weight." It's unusual to hear someone say, "I need to lose fat."

"Weight-loss" is used in this book because that's the common term, but not all loss of weight is necessarily fat.

When you strive to "lose weight," what you really want is to lose *fat*, not just any weight. Just any weight could include muscle. Although it may look good on the scale, muscle loss is disastrous for proper weight-loss.

Crash diets can cause you to lose a lot of weight, but much of it wouldn't be body fat, but muscle and water.

The scale alone is a poor barometer for progress because it doesn't consider body *composition*.

What is body fat?

Body fat—also known as adipose tissue, fatty tissue, or fat—is your body's means of storing energy over extended periods of time that your body can use as fuel. It's your body's safeguard against starvation.

There are two main types of fat: visceral fat, which is internal fat located behind the wall of your abdominal musculature; and subcutaneous fat, which is the more visible fat located just beneath your skin.

All successful weight-loss plans have one thing in common

Contrary to some beliefs, body fat can't be melted away through plastic wraps, saunas, or steam baths; and it can't be rubbed away through massage, or vibrating and rubbing machines.

Whether you're a man or a woman, the only way to lose body fat naturally is to expend more calories than you take in. You must establish an energy imbalance, *to force your body to draw on its reserves of energy—body fat*.

To do this, ingest fewer calories, and burn more calories. Do this for long enough and you'll lose weight through a reduction in your body fat. This fundamental concept has been around since

1918 when it was introduced through the book *Diet and Health: With Key to the Calories*, by Lulu Hunt Peters.

Regardless of a diet's premise—for example, low fat, low carb, or high protein—all successful weight-loss plans have one general thing in common: *a marked reduction in overall calories.*

According to a study published by the *American Journal of Clinical Nutrition*, for weight-loss, more important than what you eat is *how much* you eat. And a reduction in overall calories is more important than the specific proportions of macronutrients—protein, carbohydrate, and fat.

What's a calorie?

The energy in food that's available through digestion is usually expressed in calories, or joules. The calorie used in nutrition is actually the kilocalorie (kcal), but the terms "calorie" and "kilocalorie" are interchangeable.

One gram of protein has an energy value of four calories, and one gram of carbohydrate also has an energy value of four calories, but one gram of fat has an energy value of nine calories.

Because fat has far more calories than the other macronutrients, eliminating unhealthy fats quickly reduces overall caloric intake. But be mindful of all excess calories regardless of their sources. Too many carbs or too much protein can still lead to excess calories.

The caloric value of body fat

One pound of body fat has the approximate energy value of 3,500 calories, but the pound isn't all fat. Almost 15% of it is other stuff, the majority of which is water. If body fat was pure fat, a pound of it—454 grams—would have the energy value of 4,086 calories (454 x 9). But because 14% isn't fat, one pound of body fat has about 390 grams of fat, not 454. That has the energy value of 3,500 calories.

To lose one pound of fat you must get rid of the equivalent of 3,500 calories by reducing caloric intake, burning more calories through increased activity, or a combination of the two.

The three fundamental ways your body uses calories is through its basal metabolism, food digestion (diet-induced thermogenesis), and your daily activities and exercise. You'll learn later on how to improve these elements, to maximize your calorie burning.

Weight-loss and your metabolism

Metabolism is the sum of all physical and chemical processes that occur in the body. The rate at which the body uses energy *at rest* (to cover the essential functioning of the organs, muscles, nervous system, and so forth) is called the *basal metabolic rate* (BMR). Beyond youth, BMR tends to decrease with age, due largely to the loss of lean body mass. Increasing muscle mass increases BMR. A closely related measurement, used under less strict conditions, is resting metabolic rate (RMR).

Some people have a higher BMR than others, but you can work to influence yours positively. A sedentary lifestyle is a major culprit for a sluggish metabolic rate.

Typically, about two-thirds of energy requirements are to satisfy the BMR. The other third covers physical activity and exercise (about 20%), and food digestion (about 10%). But the precise proportions vary relative to an individual's activity and exercise levels.

The higher the BMR, the more calories you'll burn while at rest. Weight training and cardiovascular training may rev up the metabolic rate. And the process of digesting food revs up your metabolism and uses up additional calories, which is one of the reasons why you should eat small meals often.

Determining your BMR and RMR are complex processes that vary person to person. Your genetics, gender, age, weight, height, food intake, body-fat percentage, overall health, external temperature, and overall activity levels determine your BMR and RMR.

Although there are several metabolic rate calculators on the internet, they give only a rough idea of what yours may be.

Instead of perhaps thinking about how fortunate some people are because you believe that they have fast metabolisms, make a concerted effort to improve yours.

Active people generally burn more calories than sedentary people, as many as 300 to 500 additional calories a day.

Don't thin people have faster metabolisms than fat people?

Many people assume that thin people have faster metabolisms than fat people, and that's what makes them thin. But this isn't really the case.

Thin people may burn more calories because they have a much more active lifestyle, not from faster metabolisms. Because heavier people have more bodyweight to sustain and move around, they usually have more active metabolisms than thin people.

And because very overweight people have to cart around a lot of excess weight, doing any activity is harder for them than it is for a lean person, and requires more energy. It would be like if a normal-weight person had to wear a 100-pound vest while trying to do daily activities. Brad was exhausted all the time trying to move his 265-pound bulk around. And going up a flight of stairs was an ordeal. No wonder he was such a couch potato. (And imagine the ordeal of dragging around a body that weighs over 300 pounds.)

Heavy people can expend more energy per minute of a given activity than thin people, *but they are less likely to do so because of the effort involved.* And when their weights decrease, the energy output for any given activity will decrease because less weight is being carted around.

But it will be easier for them to do more activity, and the resulting increased energy output will burn more calories. **This is what happened to Brad.**

Gender, energy expenditure, and weight-loss

Comparing a man and a woman of the same age, height, weight, and activity level, the man will nearly always have a greater energy expenditure. Due to the effects of the hormone testosterone, the man will have a substantially higher percentage of muscle mass than the woman. His greater muscle mass means that he'll burn more calories than she will.

Then, consider a 220-pound man and a 180-pound woman, for example, of average body compositions for their bodyweights. Because of his higher percentage of muscle mass, and his much higher overall muscle mass, the man will burn substantially more calories per unit of activity, *and* while at rest.

Furthermore, because he has a heavier body to move around, the man will burn even more calories than the woman, at the same activity level.

And men, generally speaking, may be more active than women, so they will burn yet more calories each day than women.

Men, generally, are better calorie burning "machines." So, everything else being equal, men may find weight-loss easier than women, because they can consume more calories but yet still maintain a sufficient caloric imbalance between input and output to produce weight-loss.

But women can still be hugely successful with long-term weight-loss, as countless women have proven, *provided they follow the right approach.*

And especially if they are very active in general, and do strength training to build some additional muscle, women can substantially increase their ability to burn calories, and make weight-loss easier to achieve.

Then, once they have reduced their body-fat percentage substantially, and provided they maintain an active lifestyle, they can sustain the weight-loss with ease.

Gain muscle to help lose fat

Muscle is much more metabolically active than fat. Muscle uses more energy, even when you're at rest, than does an equal amount of body fat. But precisely how many calories is uncertain. Some people claim no more than about 10 for each additional pound of muscle, while a few claim around 100, which is probably way exaggerated.

Let's adopt a conservative estimate that a single pound of additional muscle requires about 20 calories a day to sustain it. If, for example, you add five pounds of muscle, you'll increase your daily energy output by about 100 calories, or about 700 a week, or about 9,000 every three months.

But this is offset to some degree by a reduction in caloric needs if you lose a lot of fat. Even body fat has a small caloric requirement. But by having a lighter body to move around you'll find it much easier to burn calories because you'll be more active in general, be more inclined to exercise, and be more likely to build muscle.

And the health benefits from building extra muscle extend far beyond the aforementioned benefits.

The additional benefits will be explained in detail later.

So, adding some muscle to your body is important to a weight-loss program for many important reasons. And this isn't just for men. Most of the women Brad interviewed were adamant about the multitude of benefits they experienced from the extra muscle they developed.

Which is more important, dieting or exercise?

In a plan to lose weight, most of your success will, by far, come from changes to your food intake. A lesser contribution will come from your activity level, and formal exercise.

This is because it's *much* easier to establish an energy imbalance through a suitable reduction in caloric intake than through a suitable increase in energy output through increased activity.

So, you must eat healthily *and* reduce your caloric intake. These are the most important things you can do to lose fat. Exercise alone won't make up for an overly calorific diet *unless* your exercise is on par with a triathlete, or long-distance runner or cyclist, for example.

Nevertheless, nutritious eating of a suitable caloric intake, *and* sufficient activity (including formal exercise), work *hand-in-hand* to produce the most effective weight-loss plan.

The wrong way to establish an energy imbalance

An adequate energy imbalance is required. But adopting a severe energy imbalance is a huge mistake. Severe caloric reduction can slow your metabolism. This is why crash diets must be avoided. Severe caloric reductions can also reduce your muscle tissue.

The innately programmed starvation effect

Various versions of this theory—each with a different name, and perhaps different interpretation—have been around for decades. While this theory has been the subject of numerous research articles, and referred to in some books written by doctors, it doesn't have an established scientific name. We'll refer to it as *the innately programmed starvation effect.*

Physiologically, when you go too long without eating, or if you severely reduce your caloric intake, your body slows its basal metabolic rate as a means of self-preservation. Your metabolism slows because your body saves its energy for the most essential functions like breathing, circulation, and maintaining tissue.

Our bodies are complex and adaptable, and our genes have been working the same general way for thousands of years. Back in the Stone Age, humans were hunters and gatherers, and it was common to go days without food, and when they ate, they gorged. The people with greater stores of body fat and slower metabolisms were able to endure these periods of famine.

Crash diets automatically help preserve body fat stores as a means of defense for what your body construes as an impending famine, but if you eat every two to four hours, this effect won't occur.

To prevent the starvation effect, don't reduce your daily caloric intake by more than 250 to 350 calories *every few days* until you get down to your target daily caloric quota.

For instance, say you're currently consuming 4,000 calories a day. Drop to 3,700 calories for the first few days, then to 3,400 for the next few days, then to 3,100 for the next few days, and so on. Eventually you'll be at your target daily caloric quota which may, for instance, be 2,000 calories.

Don't "dive bomb" to 2,000 calories from 4,000, or you'll be at risk for reducing your BMR, and initiating the starvation effect.

A simple way to reduce your daily caloric intake is by eliminating soda, sweets, unhealthy desserts, and excessive dietary fats. And then by avoiding fast food, junk food, whole-milk products, butters, calorie-laden sauces and condiments, fruit juice drinks *and* 100%-pure fruit juices, and fat-laden meats, and by reducing nighttime snacking, you can cut calories with little struggle.

For example, by reducing or eliminating your nighttime junk-food snacking (to the tune of 250 to 500 daily calories), you can lose as much as 25 to 50 pounds of fat in a year. A small change can have a big effect over the long-term.

Adopt the attitude that eating is a necessary task to make sure your body is getting the nutrition it needs to function properly. You must separate this reality from the almost romantic love some people have for food. Many people eat for psychological reasons instead of physiological reasons—*they eat for entertainment and not for nutritional reasons.*

But don't think that eating will become boring while on a weight-loss program. You'll enjoy the tasty, nutritious meals that you'll prepare and eat, and eventually you'll lose the taste for processed foods.

You can still enjoy your favorite foods, but you must learn to eat primarily for nutrition, *not* for entertainment.

And make sure that your reduction in calories creates an energy imbalance.

For instance, let's say a woman currently consumes 3,000 calories a day, and has about 1,000 of them while snacking in front of the television each evening. If she gradually eliminates her late-night snacking, she'll reduce her daily caloric intake to 2,000. But if she requires only 1,400 calories (for her daily activities, BMR, and diet-induced thermogenesis), she's still 600 in excess, and thus she'll *gain* weight, albeit at a slower rate than before.

Although she'll have made terrific progress by reducing her caloric intake substantially, she won't have established the energy *imbalance* necessary for fat-loss.

Remember, to lose body fat, you *must* expend more calories than you take in. Only by creating a caloric *deficit* will you force your body to draw on its energy reserves—body fat.

An *average* daily energy imbalance rids weight

A sustained, daily reduction of just 250 calories can yield a fat-loss of 26 pounds in a year, but *only* if this reduction establishes an average daily *imbalance* or *deficit* of 250 calories.

Increase the average daily energy imbalance or deficit to 500 calories, and this can become a 52-pound loss of fat in a year.

Add some daily activities, some metabolism-enhancing techniques, and some formal exercise—to increase the average daily energy imbalance to 1,000 calories—and a 100-pound loss of fat in a year is possible.

The next time you eat excessively, what will your plan be for burning the excess calories off?

If you don't burn off the extra calories, where will they end up—on your butt, hips, or belly?

Make an energy imbalance a daily rule to live your new life by, until you reach your target weight.

Calories and weight-loss, *clarification*

When we give illustrations of how many pounds of fat a certain reduction of calories produces, and how many calories a certain activity uses up, they are *approximations*. The precise quantity of weight lost, or calories burned over a given time, varies from person to person.

Many factors—such as your age, weight, height, food intake, body-fat percentage, muscle-mass percentage, overall health, external temperature, and overall activity levels—affect your rate of energy expenditure, and weight-loss.

For example, a 300-pound man will burn more calories when walking than will a 160-pound man, comparing the same distance covered. And, generally speaking, men burn more calories for a specific activity than women, due to several of the aforementioned factors.

Furthermore, how much fat you lose, and how much muscle you gain (or lose), will have an influence, too.

But the principle of creating an energy *imbalance* or *deficit*—fewer calories consumed through food and drink, than expended—of a sufficient degree, and for a sustained period, is *sound*, and *required* for weight-loss.

"But I really don't eat a lot"

Brad has encountered several middle-aged people—who have put on 50 to 100 pounds over the last several years—yet say, "But I really don't eat a lot," or "I only have one meal per day."

Upon analyzing what they do, they all starve then binge, and they rarely eat breakfast, and hardly ever exercise. They may not consume a huge number of calories, but they have all or most of their calories (sometimes 1,500 to 2,000 or more) in one binge session—whether it's a fast-food biggie meal for lunch, or a huge late-night dinner.

By starving and then eating all or most of their calories in a single meal, they are training their bodies to store fat when they gorge—the *starvation effect*.

But if they would spread those same calories over the day, they would be well on their way to losing weight. And once they replace unhealthy meals with healthy ones, they'll be even further on their way to losing weight.

How many calories should you eat per day?

Feedback from most successful dieters indicates that it's up to you to find the daily number of calories that works for you. And, generally speaking, women need fewer calories than men. While there are energy expenditure calculators on the internet, they can only be approximate because of all the variables at play.

To determine your daily caloric needs, begin by analyzing how many calories you currently consume each day. Do this by keeping a food journal for your *usual* food and drink consumption.

For a week, write down everything you eat and drink— measure quantities *precisely*, and be honest. *Use a kitchen weighing scale, and volume measures.*

Become familiar with your portion sizes, especially as they relate to those referred to on food labels. A "cup," for example, isn't necessarily the size of an ordinary glass or cup. Once you use a set of proper measuring cups, or a single all-in-one measuring cup, you may discover that you've been underestimating how much you actually eat of some items. If you measure a one-cup serving of cereal, for example, you may be surprised by how little it is because your actual serving size is much larger and thus has many more calories than the label says for a one-cup serving.

And when you get a proper measuring cup (or set of them), buy a set of measuring spoons so that you don't get tablespoon, dessertspoon and teaspoon measures mixed up. These measuring items are inexpensive, and commonly available at grocery stores.

Compute the total number of calories consumed over seven days. An excellent website to help you is www.calorieking.com. Then divide the total by seven to produce your current daily average caloric intake. *Then start making changes.*

But remember not to reduce your daily caloric intake more than 250 to 350 calories every few days, until you get down to your soon-to-be-determined daily caloric quota. It's important that you don't make big, instant reductions in your intake.

Start by gradually cutting out processed food—including soda, sweets, unhealthy desserts, and fast food—and replace it with healthy foods.

Then gradually eliminate fruit juice drinks *and* 100%-pure juices (eat whole fruits instead), and fried food and other unhealthy fats.

Make further reductions of 250 to 350 calories by reducing your intake of butters, calorie-laden sauces and condiments, fat-laden meats, whole-milk dairy products, and nighttime snacking (even if it's of healthy food). You may need to eliminate all of these items, eventually.

Once you've made those changes and you consume *only* healthy food, if you *still* haven't reduced your caloric intake sufficiently to lose weight, you'll have to reduce your intake of healthy food gradually until you start to lose weight.

Although it's much easier to overeat on processed food, it's possible to overeat even on an intake of exclusively healthy food.

CalorieKing.com: *king* of calorie-counting websites

This free website makes it easy to compute caloric values for any given quantity of almost any food— even restaurant food and fast food. And it makes counting calories fun.

The company that hosts this site, CalorieKing Wellness Solutions, Inc., also has a pocket-sized reference book, *The CalorieKing Calorie, Fat and Carbohydrate Counter*, which is the best resource of its type that Brad and Stuart have encountered.

It's an up-to-date book of food counts.

It has food data that's not available elsewhere.

It has 11,000 food listings.

It includes 200 fast-food chains and restaurants.

It contains international foods, carnival foods, and fair foods.

It uses color coding to make it quick and easy to find what you're looking for.

It's rated #1 by many health professionals and many consumers.

It has been used as a resource for numerous government studies on obesity.

It's used by diabetics, and health educators.

CalorieKing.com also has a number of neat free tools.

Approaches to avoid

Many diets go by portion sizes, and don't involve calorie counting. This can be confusing because you may never know precisely how much food you're taking in, and you can easily go overboard.

At the time of Brad's weight-loss transformation, one of the most popular diets in America was a restrictive one created by the doctors behind a popular made-for-TV weight-loss show.

It advocated that the number of calories to consume each day may be as simple as multiplying your weight by 7—for example, 200 pounds x 7 = 1,400 calories.

While this approach produces weight-loss, it's easy to feel miserable and deprived from so few daily calories. This is one of the major reasons why many diets fail.

Another problem is that you could be in danger of restricting calories too much and thus initiating the *starvation effect*. Furthermore, severe diets can also trigger catabolism, which depletes muscle tissue, and

is disastrous for multiple reasons—including appearance, physical fitness, and health in general.

Follow Brad's example of what to do

Some diets promote a greater number of nutritious calories than more restrictive alternatives do, to prevent the metabolism slowing down. This can work well for people who have a higher caloric expenditure—for example, due to sufficient exercise, or a high level of activity from their work.

To honor a version of the low-level caloric intake *as well as* a version of the higher-level caloric intake, many dieters use a compromise. This is a great way to achieve permanent weight-loss without feelings of deprivation.

The compromise utilizes a modified version of the "seven-times-bodyweight caloric intake" approach one day, *and* it honors the higher-caloric approach by having you eat a few hundred extra calories on the next day. Alternate between the two approaches.

To illustrate this, let's look at what Brad was doing when around 200 pounds, and losing between 1.5 and 2 pounds of fat a week.

Partly following the "seven-times-bodyweight caloric intake" approach, Brad consumed approximately 1,400 to 1,500 calories on Sundays, Tuesdays, and Thursdays. And utilizing the other approach, he consumed 1,800 to 1,900 calories on Mondays, Wednesdays, and Fridays (which were his more active days). He went a little over 2,000 calories on Saturday, which was his treat day (but *still* a highly active day, from chores).

His approach worked because he maintained the *average* caloric deficit he required for fat-loss. And his approach also included substantial activity and exercise, enhanced basal metabolism, and diet-induced thermogenesis, which combined to increase his energy output substantially relative to what it would have been on an approach that relies on reduced food intake *only*.

Brad could have lost weight faster if he kept his daily average caloric intake at the 1,400- to 1,500 mark, but he wouldn't have tolerated the ongoing feelings of deprivation. And this would have led to long-term failure due to a reversion to his comfort zone of overeating.

To follow this approach, you'll have to adjust your calories depending on your gender, and overall size and activity levels. For example, a moderately active 150-pound woman may vary her calories from 1,100 to 1,300 on lower-calorie days, 1,300 to 1,400 on moderate-calorie days, and 1,400 to 1,600 on her higher-calorie days. But other factors influence these daily counts, and no two people are the same. Experiment to find what works best for you.

If the caloric intakes in this segment are too low for you, choose to lose weight at a slower pace, *or* increase your activity levels to compensate for the extra few hundred daily calories you need in order to feel satisfied.

Don't like counting calories?

Many people dislike counting calories because they think it's too much to think about as part of a busy day. And it tends to make them obsess about food. If this is the case for you, you must still be aware of what you're taking in, and roughly how much, by reading nutrition labels.

Be in the ballpark, calorie-wise, and you can still make the reduction of 250 to 350 calories every few days, and be on the right track to weight-loss without having to count the calories of every morsel you consume.

But if that approach doesn't yield weight-loss, you'll need to count calories to some degree, or else you're not going to be successful.

Brad didn't count calories obsessively during his transformation, but he understood what he was eating, and how much, and he kept his caloric intake within a precise range each day.

Some successful dieters weigh their food with a kitchen scale to help them determine caloric content, but this may be too demanding to adhere to as part of a busy life. Some people love it, and some people hate it. But if it helps you, by all means do it.

Reduce your calories as you reduce your weight

According to a study from the Laboratory of Human Behavior and Metabolism at Rockefeller University, as you lose weight, your body's caloric needs go down. This means that it takes fewer calories to support your lighter weight, and you'll need to reduce your daily caloric intake as you lose weight—by around 70 calories for every 10 pounds of lost weight.

Leptin changes

As you lose body fat, your levels of leptin may go down. Then you may not feel full as easily, and you may tend to eat more.

This drop in leptin may also slow your metabolism—so, as you lose weight, be even more mindful of the importance of your exercise program, and of being active in general.

Permanent weight-loss takes time—be patient

Weight-loss failure often occurs because the would-be dieter sets an overambitious goal, or tries to reach an unachievable target weight. And many people give up because they are frustrated they don't look a certain way—or like a certain person—overnight.

Establish your goals in baby steps. Set one small goal, achieve it, set another small goal, achieve it, and so on.

Brad's first goal was to weigh 250 pounds. After he achieved that victory, he had another when he cracked 240 pounds, another when he cracked 230, and so on.

Achieving 199 pounds took a while, but it was a thrilling milestone.

Although his long-term goal was to lose 100 pounds, the short-term goals of 10 at a time made the overall process manageable. And he knew from the onset that it would take over a year to meet his long-term goal.

By taking your time and setting small, short-term goals, you'll greatly increase your chances for success over the long term.

Each 10 pounds lost is an exciting, rewarding milestone because it's another mental and physical barrier broken.

Before you can lose many pounds, you must first lose *one*. You'll have a reason to smile and feel good about yourself with each pound you lose. Brad had over 100 reasons to feel good about himself.

Set your sights on what your life will be like in a year, or even two years from now. Do you want to be heavy because of a failed diet attempt or two (or three or four), or do you want to be where you desire—slim and healthy?

All of Brad's failed diets had one thing in common—quick weight-loss. He lost more than 50 pounds on several occasions, but each time—because he was so deprived—he quickly put the weight back on, and ended up fatter than when he first started.

Many studies have confirmed that the quicker you lose weight, the quicker you'll usually put it back on. And feedback from real-life dieters substantiates this.

You didn't get heavy overnight, so don't expect to get slim overnight, either. Take it one step at a time—day-by-day, week-by-week, month-by-month, and, ultimately, *one pound at a time.*

Don't cross the finish line

Many diets promote a specific weight-loss period—for example, "Get in shape in nine weeks," "The sixteen-week, Brand-X Diet," or "The twelve-week, miracle shape-up plan."

It's good to have a goal for a certain period of time, but these short-term plans have a finite weight-loss period.

Too many people see the twelfth or sixteenth week, for example, as the finish line, and they have a celebration after their final weigh-in, and quickly revert to their old ways—the ways that got them heavy in the first place.

The lifestyle-reform, weight-loss and health plan that **WEIGHT-LOSS SALVATION** showcases has no finish line because it's a sustainable plan that will continue for the rest of your life.

How quickly can you expect to lose weight?

Many gimmicky plans promote fast weight-loss that's not realistic. Losing nine pounds of *fat* in a week, for example, won't happen.

It's improbable for most people to lose more than two pounds of fat a week in a healthy way, even under the most aggressive of plans. If you rush your weight-loss, you'll lose muscle and create even more problems over the long-term.

If you lose a seemingly modest 2 pounds of fat a week, that's an *outstanding* 104 pounds over 12 months.

And even a "mere" pound a week would be 52 pounds over the course of a year. Most people who want to lose weight would be thrilled to lose 52 pounds of fat over 12 months.

Of the hundreds of successful dieters that were researched for this book—who *maintained* their weight-loss *long-term*—the average fat-loss was just under *one* pound a week. It was 3.84 pounds *a month*, which is almost 50 pounds of fat lost in a year.

But some did better. Brad averaged a loss of 1.62 pounds of fat a week over the 19 months it took to reach his goal. His speedier weight-loss, without any deprivation, was due to his minimum of 45 minutes of daily exercise coupled with a lifestyle that's much more active than most people's.

Several people lost two pounds a week, on average. But only one person (a middle-aged woman) averaged three pounds a week over the long-term. That yielded an astonishing 156-pound loss of fat in a year.

Some of the success stories of two and three pounds of fat lost per week were among a handful of middle-aged ladies who exercised with great tenacity for 60 to 90 minutes a day, six or seven days a week—and sometimes twice a day—and who were strict with their food intake.

Much of your initial weight-loss will be through a reduction of superfluous *water* weight. Some obese people lose as much as 8 to 12 pounds in their first week or so, and then get frustrated that their weight-loss comes to an apparent standstill.

Many obese people are bloated from food intake that's high in sodium and processed fare, and this bloat is what they initially lose in the first few days of the plan.

Many farcical plans claim a huge initial weight-loss, but this isn't from a loss of fat.

If you can average a seemingly snail's-pace loss of one pound a week—52 pounds of fat in a year—you're doing better than most.

So, what's your hurry?

Made-for-TV weight-loss boot camps

For those people who lost a huge amount of weight at made-for-TV weight-loss boot camps, losing weight was their full-time job. They exercised six to eight hours a day, and were on ultra-restrictive, medically supervised diets.

Some contestants lost 150 to 200 pounds in under a year, but this is unrealistic for everyone else. And for many people it's much easier to lose vast amounts of weight when motivated by huge prize money rather than health or personal satisfaction alone.

These television shows set a dangerous precedent for fast weight-loss. And many of the show's former contestants put much of their weight back on because the boot camp regimen was too restrictive to continue under normal conditions. Some of them put even more weight on than they lost.

For example, one winner lost 214 pounds during his stint at the boot camp, but then put most of it back on when he resumed his normal life.

When interviewed on a January 2009 *Oprah Show*, he admitted that losing a lot of weight was achievable when caught up in the intense atmosphere of the contest, and with the financial incentive. But the ultra-rapid weight-loss never dealt with the emotional issues and food addiction that were the causes of his profound weight-gain in the first place.

Although people can lose massive amounts of weight under supervised instruction or gimmicky diets, they will never maintain the lost weight unless the root of their problem (whether psychological, physiological, or both) is addressed and treated.

What's *your* ideal bodyweight?

Eventually, you'll end up at *your* ideal bodyweight. This is the realistic, achievable weight that works for you.

Your weight-loss goal may be unrealistic, because it may not be possible for you to be as slim as you desire. Not everyone has the genetics to look like some of our "perfect" celebrities.

Your body is predisposed to be a certain weight, within a range of, perhaps, 20 pounds. Your lowest adult

weight—which may be what you weighed in your late teens, or early twenties, *provided* you were slim at that time—may be a good indication of your lowest achievable target. Getting below that point may not be possible because you can't overcome your bone structure and internal predisposition.

Goals

A goal of how much weight you want to lose is an important element of your weight-loss plan *provided* it's attainable.

Brad's realistic, attainable goal was to return to his high-school graduation weight of 165 pounds. But while he reached this goal—a weight where he was happy and healthy—he knew that "being ripped," like some guys in the magazines, wasn't realistic.

Trying to obtain the look of a supermodel, or a ripped athlete, is unrealistic for most people. Many of those people have won life's genetic lottery, or are so ultra-disciplined that severe training and highly restricted eating obsesses them.

And forget about duplicating the ultra-fast results you see on made-for-TV weight-loss boot camp shows. Do you have the discipline to exercise for eight hours a day? Your ultimate goal must be set in a reasonable time frame.

So, with all of that in mind . . .

What's your goal weight?

Is it realistic?

What degree of leanness do you want?

Is it realistic?

Now, what's really your goal weight?

If you set an outrageous goal that you'll never be able to attain, you're going to be frustrated, and have a sense of failure *even though you may have produced a great success story.*

For example, if a woman who currently weighs 195 has a goal of being 110 pounds with visible abs, but "only" makes it to 125 without visible abs, she's going to be dissatisfied with a body that most women would be thrilled to have.

And if a man who weighs 240 pounds wants to be 160 with a ripped six-pack, yet "only" makes it to 170 with a slightly-visible six-pack, he'll be dissatisfied even though he has a physique that most men would be thrilled to have.

Regardless of how much you want to lose, there's a series of step-by-step goals that must be achieved in order to reach your ultimate goal.

Your first goal should be to get today right—one meal at a time, and one walk at a time.

Anyone can get one day right.

And if you can get one day right, you can get the next day right, and then the next, and then the next, and so on.

It will quickly become a habit.

Then you'll lose one pound. And if you can lose one pound, you can lose another, then another, and then another, and so on.

Make one day at a time, and one pound at a time, your weight-loss creeds.

Remember the Chinese proverb:

"The man who removes a mountain begins by carrying away small stones."

Apply that to weight-loss.

This chapter explains how real people found the motivation to lose weight and keep it off.

When you've read this chapter *you* will have the motivation to lose weight and keep it off.

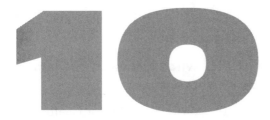

What's your motivation for losing weight?

The first step in the process of losing weight is to admit that you need to lose weight. Once you've done that, ask yourself these questions:

Are you ready to follow the plan that transformed Brad and hundreds of other real-life dieters?

Are you ready to eat better, and be more active?

Are you ready to change your life for the better?

But just because you answered *yes* to these questions doesn't necessarily mean that you're ready to succeed. To succeed, you need strong motivation.

Obesity is a leading cause of death

For Brad to make his transformation, he needed strong motivation so that he would persevere.

Besides his late father's deathbed motivational speech, Brad's biggest motivation came from having just turned 40. He had reached the age where he felt he could no longer mess with his health. Obese people in the over-40 bracket are especially at serious risk from life-threatening health problems.

At five-foot eight-inches and 265 pounds, Brad was morbidly obese, and finally aware of the gravity of the situation.

You have only one body to live your life in. Take care of it. It's your most important possession.

Remember the old adage: "He who has health has hope, and he who has hope has everything."

According to a recent study by the National Center for Health Statistics, 62% of Americans are overweight or obese. And this percentage is projected to climb to 86% by the year 2030 if current trends continue, according to a study by the journal *Obesity*.

Relative to normal-weight people, overweight and obese people are much more likely to develop type II diabetes, have a heart attack, develop heart disease, have a stroke, develop high blood pressure, sustain liver damage, have high cholesterol levels, be more susceptible to cancer, develop sleep apnea, and be vulnerable to many other weight-related ailments.

And according to the Centers for Disease Control and Prevention, the result of an unhealthy lifestyle, including obesity and physical inactivity, is the second leading cause of preventable death in the US—a close second to smoking—with more than 400,000 annual deaths. And by the time you read this, the result of an unhealthy lifestyle may be *the leading cause* of preventable death.

Do you like life? Staying alive and healthy should be monumentally motivating.

Healthy people generally live a longer and fuller life. A study from the University of Cambridge suggests that those who follow a healthy lifestyle live an average of 14 years longer than those who don't.

Millions of people want to lose weight, but most of them aren't willing to do anything about it until they have begun to suffer serious health problems.

It was the fear of dying that finally got Brad off his lazy butt.

Make your health a top priority. And make it a priority to be healthy for your family and loved ones, too. Many of you are caregivers for your family. But how can you care for those people if you die or get sick?

Brad finally realized that being obese and unhealthy was unfair to his loved ones, irresponsible, and unnecessary.

Make a commitment to yourself, and *follow through*.

Don't let yourself down.

And don't let your friends and family down, either. It's your obligation to be around for the people who rely on you, and care about you.

You have just one life. Don't shorten it by living in an unhealthy body.

Health risks from being overweight

The following should make you think twice about being overweight:

Mobility

When you have to cart around a lot of bodyweight, your mobility is impaired—in effect, the extra weight incapacitates you to some degree. It restricts your activity level in general, and makes formal exercise very difficult to do. You'll burn far fewer calories than if you were active, your poor physical conditioning will undermine your health, and you won't have the vigor required to enjoy life fully. Many obese people become couch- and seat-bound.

Heart

You could accumulate additional fatty plaque in your heart's blood vessels, which would increase your risk of high blood pressure, high cholesterol levels, and a heart attack. Heart diseases promoted by obesity include:

coronary artery disease

myocardial infarction (heart attack)

angina (cardiac chest pain)

abnormal cardiac rhythms

cardiomyopathy (disease of the heart muscle)

congestive heart failure

sudden cardiac death

Joints

Being overweight can lead to arthritis, and gout. You may develop osteoarthritis in your hips, knees, and ankles due to the excessive wear and tear on your weight-bearing joints. Eventually you may need to have hip or knee-joint replacement surgery. Furthermore, the bones and muscles in your back can be damaged, and this can result in undue pain, a decrease in mobility, and disc problems.

Liver

You can develop a fatty liver, which is the build-up of fat in the liver cells. This can lead to inflammation of the liver, which can cause scarring and hardening of the organ. When scarring becomes extensive, it's called cirrhosis—a very serious condition.

Brain

Besides depression and a host of psychological problems, extra weight can suppress your brain's response to leptin, the hormone that makes you feel full. This can cause you to overeat even more.

Lungs

Excess weight leads to heavy chest walls, poor breathing, decreased lung expansion, and poor oxygenation. And this can interfere with normal daily activities. This shortness of breath can prevent many people from exercising, and can be disabling. Obesity is also a major risk factor for asthma.

Digestive system

Being overweight can cause chronic heartburn, acid reflux disease, and constipation.

Gallbladder

Excess weight can lead to gallbladder disease and gallstones, which can cause abdominal pain, infection, and jaundice.

Sleep disorders

As explained in Chapter 8, overweight people are more likely to suffer from some sleep disorders than normal-weight people. If you suffer from a sleep disorder—apnea, for example—the minimum consequence is that your energy level will be impaired substantially, which can hugely undermine the quality of your life.

But if not treated properly, sleep disorders can greatly increase the chance of catastrophic results—heart problems, strokes, and even death.

Type II diabetes

This occurs when your cells have diminished sensitivity to insulin, and sometimes when there's impaired insulin production. Insulin is necessary for your body to be able to use glucose for energy. When you don't produce enough insulin, glucose can build up in your blood (hyperglycemia) instead of going into your cells, and your cells may be starved of energy. Over time, unless treated successfully, the high blood glucose may harm your eyes, kidneys, nerves, and heart, with grave consequences.

Cancer

As many as 20% of cancer deaths can be directly attributed to excess weight. Overweight men and women have an increased risk of death from cancer of the pancreas, colon, liver, rectum, esophagus, gallbladder, and kidneys. Overweight women have an increased risk of cancer of the ovaries, cervix, uterus, and breasts. And overweight men have an increased risk of prostate cancer.

Find *your* motivation

You need strong motivation so that you'll persevere, like Brad did. If you aren't motivated to change, you'll most likely continue your current ways. Find *your* motivation!

A common trick is to write down your motivating factors and goals on a piece of paper, and place it on your refrigerator or vanity mirror, for daily inspiration.

You may also place a photograph of yourself during your glory days, perhaps together with one from when you were at your fattest, to remind you of why you want to lose weight.

Some people place a photograph of a child or family member, to remind them of who they *need* to be alive and healthy for.

Next to where he stored his running shoes, Brad had a collage of his 265-pound couch-potato photograph, a few photos from during his lean days, and one of his wife, for motivation to make him use the shoes each day.

When Brad looked for "before" pictures for this book, there were few to choose from because he always hid from the camera due to embarrassment with his appearance. He even avoided mirrors because he was ashamed to look at himself.

What about you?

> *When you look at yourself in the mirror, do you like what you see?*
>
> *Are you happy with your body and health?*
>
> *Do you hide from cameras?*
>
> *Can you look at your naked body and be proud of what you see?*

If you aren't satisfied with your body and health, decide to do something about it.

Each day, visualize yourself as the person you want to be. This will help motivate you to become that person.

Losing weight isn't about "I'll try to do it." It's about "I'll *do* it."

But *doing* produces results only if you *stick with the plan.*

The epic promise

One of the dieters Brad interviewed tried something unusual. Ed promised everyone he knew—wife, family, friends, co-workers—that he was going to change his unhealthy habits for one month in an effort to lose weight and start to regain his health.

The promise was the foundation of Ed's plan. His plan had a support group, with dozens of caring people to remind him on daily to stick to his guns.

To fulfill his promise, he eliminated processed food, reduced his caloric intake, and exercised. After completing the plan for a month, he pledged that he would continue for another month, and so on.

After a year—one month at a time—Ed had lost 50 pounds. He has since maintained a healthy weight for several years. His plan started as a promise, and became a way of life.

Don't be pre-defeated, or intimidated

Many people say they are fine with being overweight, and don't care to lose weight.

But deep down they would much rather be slim and healthy, and in better shape. They may not be lazy, but they may be overly frustrated with successive failure, or too intimidated even to start a weight-loss program.

They are overwhelmed with the prospect of changing their lifestyle and moving out of their comfort zone. Losing 50 or 100 pounds, or just 15 or 25, is intimidating and overwhelming, and they are pre-defeated and won't make the change.

Brad was pre-defeated for many years, but one day he woke up *and decided to change*. It was 19 months until he met his goal, but Brad's life has changed for the better in many ways. He regained his health and self-esteem, and he now feels like a 25-year-old again.

You don't have to be gung-ho to achieve results. If you upend your life too much, you probably won't stick with the plan.

There are hundreds of tips in this book to choose from. But you don't have to follow every one of them to lose weight. Start by following a handful of tips that you think will work best for you, and incorporate more and more of them as you progress.

Do what you can do for now—*starting* is the priority. *And good things take time.*

This chapter explains how people are duped by a manipulative industry.

When you've read this chapter you'll know the scoop on weight-loss scams.

11

Watch out for weight-loss scams

The Federal Trade Commission (FTC) has estimated that in 2007 alone, 4.8 million Americans were victims of weight-loss scams.

The term "snake-oil salesman" originated from the travelling "doctor" with questionable credentials who sold medicine (the "snake oil") with boisterous marketing hype, often supported by bogus pseudo-scientific evidence. To enhance sales, an accomplice in the crowd (a "shill") would often "attest" the value of the snake oil in an effort to provoke buying enthusiasm.

The "doctor" would promptly leave town before his customers realized they had been duped.

Snake oil is a derogatory term applied to something that's fraudulent, fake, or ineffective. The term is also applied metaphorically to any product with exaggerated marketing claims, and questionable or unverifiable quality.

In the unregulated, multi-*billion*-dollar dietary-supplement industry, snake-oil peddling is endemic via scams and rip-offs.

Be forewarned about this part of the weight-loss industry, so that you don't fall for any of the scams. Then you can focus on proper eating and exercise—the real way to lose weight and keep it off.

An example of a scam

"Lose 22 pounds in one week. No gimmicks, no exercise. Amazing tea melts fat like magic!"

Is there really a magical pill that could burn the equivalent of 77,000 calories in one week without exercise? Is this "magic tea" the weight-loss holy grail? Of course not.

One could theoretically lose "22 pounds in one week" if it's almost entirely superfluous water weight, but that could easily lead to cardiac arrest if not done properly. Some weightlifters and wrestlers do this sort of thing to make weight for competition, but it's usually done under a doctor's supervision.

Note that the ad says, "Lose 22 pounds," but didn't say, "Lose 22 pounds of *fat*."

Have you fallen prey to snake-oil scams?

Most of the snake-oil products sold by the dietary-supplement industry have a huge markup. Some pills and potions that can be manufactured for less than a dollar are sold for $60 or more.

Whether a product is effective or not, the manufacturer has one agenda: to promote and sell a product that must make money.

But whereas many noble industries promote their products in an admirable fashion, a large segment of the dietary-supplement industry promotes their products in a ruthless, manipulative manner that preys on the gullible.

Gullible victims aren't necessarily naive; they are misinformed and manipulated (just like Brad was with the mega-hype program).

And the more victims who fall prey to the scams, the more the snake-oil salesmen are encouraged to keep scamming.

If a product sounds too good to be true, *it is* too good to be true.

As an illustration of the severity of the problem, a recent women's health magazine had ads for 37 different diet pills and fat burners, of which each one claimed to be the best or fastest.

Some magazines are propaganda vehicles for the products that the publication (or parent company) has a financial interest in. Not only do these magazines take on the appearance of a catalog for a specific brand of products, they also provide editorial bias for the associated product line. This is a highly effective form of consumer deception.

Most weight-loss-pill ads contain fine print: "Claims and statements have not been evaluated by the FDA," and "Results not typical." (The FDA is the US Food and Drug Administration.) The "Amazing 22-pounds-a-week magic tea" ad has these disclaimers.

Greatly exaggerated claims are cleverly crafted to catch the attention of gullible readers. They are supported by fictitious testimonials from the weight-loss subjects *and* the highly compensated medical "experts," biased or bogus "clinical studies," and manipulated before-and-after photos. In fact, one prominent internet ad has a fine-print disclaimer that says, "Testimonials of individuals shown may be of fictitious persons or paid models, and are not necessarily users of these products."

And a recent high-profile ad for a product that's "endorsed by a doctor's testimony"—complete with a picture of the stereotypical white smock and stethoscope, of course—has a fine-print disclaimer that the doctor in question is but a pen name, and the photograph is of a model not the doctor. *What a sham. Buyer beware!*

We've discovered that many doctors' endorsements are fake. For example, Brad saw a news story in which a doctor was paid $10,000 to endorse a weight-loss product for an infomercial. She fabricated bogus claims without ever even reviewing the product.

Sometimes, simple arithmetic can help you determine if a claim is legitimate or not. The ads for the mega-hype program Brad followed (explained in Chapter 1) claimed a fat-loss of 100 pounds in as little as 12 weeks. Simple arithmetic suggests that this would be an average of eight pounds lost per week—which is 28,000 calories worth of fat-loss. This is highly unlikely unless your exercise is on a par with an ironman triathlete, for example.

The manager of a local nutrition franchise told Brad that the most-returned products—by a large margin—are the high-profile pills and fat burners that have advertised claims of "miraculous benefits" or "fast" results. The duped customers returned the products because the miracles never materialized.

Brad's feedback from real-life dieters substantiates this. None of them attributed any of their results to a pill, fat burner, or high-profile weight-loss supplement.

And if any results do materialize from a pill or potion, it's most likely from a placebo effect. This was the reason the mega-hype program worked for Brad. He believed the pills were doing something, so he trained and dieted harder as a consequence.

There's no magical weight-loss pill or fat burner that will *alone* cause you to lose 10, 20, or 40 pounds of fat. It just doesn't exist. Your doctor will confirm this.

Any better-than-average results arise from strict diet and intensive exercise. Some pills may help a few percent, but no more.

What about "colon-cleanse" pills?

Misleading advertisements claim various "colon-cleanse" potions to be a magic bullet for weight-loss, often with a celebrity endorsement. These ads claim that you can lose 15 to 30 pounds in a matter of weeks by the ingestion of the cleansing pills, but with no dieting or exercise. This is a scam based on half-truths. While they may create a short-term reduction of weight by temporarily ridding fecal matter and superfluous water, colon cleanse products contribute nothing to fat-loss.

While proponents believe colon-cleansing provides health benefits—by removing toxins, and boosting their energy levels and immune systems—doctors view this differently.

According to the Mayo Clinic, most doctors don't recommend colon cleansing for better health, or to prevent disease:

It's unnecessary. Your colon doesn't require enemas or special diets or pills to eliminate waste material and bacteria. It does this naturally, on its own.

It may be harmful. Your colon absorbs water and sodium to maintain your body's fluid and electrolyte balance. Some colon-cleansing programs disrupt this balance, and cause dehydration and salt depletion. And excessive cleansing programs can lead to problems such as anemia, malnutrition, and even heart failure.

How did snake-oil peddling get so out of hand?

Because the Dietary Supplement Health and Education Act of 1994 (DSHEA) *deregulated* the dietary-supplement industry.

After this act, manufacturers no longer had to prove that their supplements were safe and effective.

If the FDA wanted a product off the market, it had to show conclusive proof that the product was unsafe and ineffective. As of 1994, the FDA regulates supplements as foods, not drugs.

Without regulation, the modern-day, snake-oil business took off, with an abundance of worthless products, and deceitful ads.

The "before-and-after" scam

Look closely at the before-and-after photos used in some of the high-profile snake-oil ads. Don't they look suspicious?

The typical "before" photos show the subjects hunched over, with frowns on their faces, men often unshaven, and their relaxed stomachs pushed out.

The typical "after" photos show the subjects tensing their stomach muscles, smiling, and with ideal overhead lighting. The men now have nice haircuts, trimmed facial hair, and shaved, tanned bodies.

Not only do many of the "after" photos look suspicious, some of the "before" photos seem to have been tinkered with. General bone structure, especially shoulder girth and cranium width, sometimes seem to have been altered.

And if they really did lose a ton of weight, why are some of the subjects wearing the same outfit in the "before" *and* "after" photos. Can the same bikini or shorts still fit in such a perfect manner on someone who lost 50 pounds?

The documentary, *Bigger, Faster, Stronger*, (Magnolia Pictures, 2008) reveals that most of the before-and-after photographs prevalent in today's magazines are manipulated, digitally altered, or even completely faked by substituting torsos and other parts of the body from other subjects.

When confronted about the suspected manipulation, one high-level photographer confided, "There are all kinds of techniques to manipulate the body. In fact, some of the before-and-after pictures can be done on the *same* day."

When confronted about whether he has created phony before-and-after photos for an ad on the same day, he confided with mischievous laughter, "I have, actually."

With the camera still rolling and his laughter mounting, he asked, "Is this the self-editing part where I should keep my mouth shut?"

In the same documentary, Rick Schaff, a fitness-industry photographer, and author of the book *Misled*, was quoted as saying, "Probably 80% or 90% of all the stuff I see in the magazines is complete hogwash, it's ridiculous to me."

He then noted, "I can take *anybody*, take a picture of them and make them look their worst [for the "before" photo]. Then through all kinds of ways, make them look their best.

"People fall for this . . . all the time. It's beyond what I can understand because it looks so silly to me, but, of course, I'm someone who's had sort of an 'inside backstage pass' of what is *really* occurring. I've been part of some of these scams."

The insider's view

Did you ever notice that many ads say, "Individuals have been remunerated"? This means that the test subjects have been financially compensated for their participation, which further undermines credibility.

To substantiate his suspicions about a certain product, Brad had a conversation with the proprietor of a large health-food chain—an "insider." The proprietor revealed that the manufacturer of a popular weight-loss supplement that promises "quick" results, runs want-ads in their local newspaper, seeking fit women—who just had a baby, and are still carrying postnatal weight—to participate in a paid weight-loss experiment.

The post-pregnancy ladies are put through a strictly controlled, weight-loss boot camp, where they lose large amounts of weight, but they are also coaxed into suggesting that the weight-loss supplement was responsible for their quick weight-loss, not the strict regimen of diet and exercise.

In other cases, the "magical" pill being advertised in some ads made little or no contribution to the claimed astonishing transformations. More times than not, it's the use of diuretics and bodybuilding drugs (according to sworn statements from several before-and-after models as part of a multi-million-dollar lawsuit) that were responsible for the results outside the scope of severe diet and exercise.

Through a first-hand, inside-backstage-pass involvement at many of these photo shoots, the book *Misled* chronicles similar acts of before-and-after deception.

What you see isn't necessarily what you get

In an effort to inform the public about these acts of deception, ABC News ran a revealing story on their "20/20" television show. The story, entitled "What You See Isn't Necessarily What You Get," exposed the aforementioned postnatal before-and-after scam—where the "before" photos were taken immediately after giving birth—as well as a scam in which the athletes in the "before" shots were purposely fattened up.

Furthermore, when hired by the manufacturer of a high-profile fat burner, a seasoned bodybuilder was paid to gorge on ice cream and doughnuts, and told, "You've gotta fatten up. Eat like a pig. Gain as much weight as you can. Stop working out." And for the "before" photo, "They told him to stick his stomach out, to have a frown on his face. They told him to pull his shorts down below his belly button, to make it look like his belly was hanging out. And they told him to stand there like he was a slob."

In the same exposé they showed that some ads had a different person in the "after" photos. The show's producers "checked out the commercial for a product that showed what seemed to be an unbelievable transformation. The commercial promised, 'You can go from flab to rock-hard abs.' But if you looked more closely, as the '20/20' producer did, one guy in the ad had a birthmark and the other didn't. They were two different people."

In January 2007, the FTC levied fines of $25 million against four high-profile companies for their bogus claims of unreasonably rapid weight-loss, under the grounds of "false advertising with *no* evidence to back up their claims."

When describing some of the misleading tricks these companies use, FTC Chairman Deborah Platt Majoras revealed, "The personalities hired by the diet-pill companies are often offered diet coaches and personal trainers to guarantee weight-loss."

In fact, the FTC showed that one of the companies named in this lawsuit concealed research proving that members of their placebo group lost more weight than those who were using their fat-burning supplement.

In a statement announcing this landmark lawsuit, Ms. Majoras stated, "You're *not* going to find weight-loss in a bottle of pills."

But despite the fines, all four of the manufactures who were successfully sued for false advertising were allowed to continue marketing their hokey products.

Most weight-loss claims and before-and-after photos that accompany most weight-loss pills and potions are not to be trusted. And neither are their products.

Now that you know what's truly going in this industry, you should never waste your money on the sham products.

Shouldn't society be smarter?

Here's something else revealed in the documentary *Bigger, Faster, Stronger*: When confronted about the fact that he admitted that he was on steroids when training for his "after" photo, one of the fitness models—who was the poster boy for a popular weight-loss supplement that promises "quick" results—was quoted as saying, "But it doesn't necessarily mean I *don't* take something else [steroids and other bodybuilding drugs]. If they [society] choose to believe that [the weight-loss supplement] is the only thing that I'm taking to look like that, then so be it, they should be smarter than that. Is it misleading? A little bit, yeah."

Watch out for internet snake-oil scams

Deceitful internet sites are one of the major reasons why many people are lured into legitimate-appearing weight-loss scams.

The internet has a spawned a new breed of cyber snake-oil salesmen—super ruthless, relentless and manipulative. Without regulation, the internet has become a free-for-all for crooks.

Many internet sites that promote or review certain weight-loss products are doing so with misleading research via unsubstantiated or bogus hype that's riddled with fake testimonials from subjects and "medical experts."

Many if not most of the "weight-loss-pill review" sites are propaganda attempting to steer you towards specified products, or platforms for sponsored links that promote other snake-oil potions.

It's foolish to ingest a weight-loss product purchased via the internet. Remember, the FDA is powerless to regulate these products to verify that they are safe and effective. If you purchase and ingest a "magical" pill or potion via an enticing internet pop-up ad, your doctor will vouch that you're putting your health at risk and, in extreme cases, even your life.

And the same goes for sponsored links or pop-ups that claim accolades like "2009 Diet of the Year." This is part of a scam that has been going on for over a decade. What legitimate source actually voted on this honor? None. It's made-up propaganda attempting to steer you towards a deceitful site.

Don't fall for any of these scams.

And be leery about buying any weight-loss product through the internet, or from a toll-free phone number. The Attorney General is uncovering weight-loss scams that are really credit card scams.

Certain "acai berry," "colon cleanse," and "detoxifier" products, as well the "fast results" products that appear too good to be true, are the enticements set up by crooks to get you to use their websites. If you fall for their hokey pitch, or "free trial offer," you're the kind of victim they are looking for to hack your credit card and steal your identity.

The "free trial offer" sounds like a good deal, but you have to pay for the shipping to get it, which means you have to give out your credit card number and pertinent information. Even if the crook who created the site doesn't steal your identity, you'll see a recurring charge on your credit card each month until you figure out how to stop it.

Some of these internet sites are loaded with malicious code that automatically infects visitors' computers. This would allow the hackers to take over your computer remotely.

These scams are difficult to stop because the source or location of the websites may be untraceable, and overseas. And if they do get shut down by the authorities, they reappear under new websites the next day. The FTC and authorities can't keep up with these crooks.

Astonishingly, the credible news story that reported this "acai berry" credit card scam had a sponsored link section that had three variations of links that would lead you to the same scam it was exposing.

Never buy any weight-loss product unless your doctor tells you to. And purchase the doctor-recommended product only from a trustworthy source.

Never buy the doctor-recommended product via the internet because even legitimate-appearing products can be counterfeit and contain hazardous ingredients.

Nausea, dizziness, and a racing heart

Most "magical" pills and fat burners provide high doses of a dangerous mix of caffeine-type ingredients that will most likely make you nauseous, lightheaded, irritable, uncomfortable, anxious, and unbearably moody.

While soaked in a cold sweat, Brad has experienced the terrifying feeling that his heart was going to explode, from using these pills.

Obviously, these products are terrible for your health. Remember, Brad's doctor forbade him to ever take these things again.

Like Brad, most dieters tried these products at some point, but after a bout of frustration, and experiences of nausea, dizziness, and a racing heart with unnerving skipped beats, the bottle of "magical weight-loss pills" ended up in the garbage can.

Common fat-burner horror stories

On a whim, Brad searched the internet for a popular weight-loss supplement that promises "quick" results. He quickly found many complaints and horror stories about this product that echoed his own experiences. Here are three examples:

"I suddenly became very dizzy, and sick to my stomach. My heart would beat incredibly fast, and then skip beats. I thought I was going to have a heart attack. And after two weeks I haven't lost any weight."

"My kidneys began hurting, and once I went to the doctor I was told that I had a bad urinary tract infection, was peeing blood, and my kidneys were not doing good because of this pill."

"The pills gave me incredible headaches, my hands shook, at times I became very dizzy upon standing or while walking. I spent my last day on the pills on my sofa in tears, unable to stand, and feeling sick to my stomach each time I moved. Don't buy it, don't even sample it. Save your money and your health. I really feel that these pills could kill someone."

What about "appetite-control" pills?

Many of today's popular weight-loss pills claim to control or suppress appetite. But don't believe the hype.

While most diet pills are worthless, some do more harm than good, and some are very dangerous. Some high-profile appetite-suppressant drugs from the 1990s and 2000s were pulled from the market after they were linked to grave side effects, and even deaths.

Forget diet pills in general.

Instead, focus on what's safe and what really works over the short-term *and* the long-term—the lifestyle-reform, weight-loss and health plan promoted in this book.

"Lose nine pounds a week— *every* week!"

This lie was on the cover of a popular women's grocery-store periodical. It means, supposedly, that the plan yields a loss of nearly 40 pounds a month, and 115 pounds in just three months. Let's get real!

To lose nine pounds of fat in a week, one would have to create an energy deficit (difference between caloric *output* and *input*) of 31,500 calories during that week.

It's not possible to achieve this by diet alone, even if no food was eaten during the week. Assuming the minimum food intake for health and basic energy requirements, the typical ladies would have to use up the equivalent of 4,500 calories a day, *which would be comparable to 45 to 65 (or more) miles of walking each day, depending on the speed and the individual.*

About 90% of weight-loss ads are targeted at women. And because of this, women's periodicals have become the breeding ground for the absurd.

But no matter how absurd or far-fetched they are, catchy headlines sell magazines. One headline claimed that "Anyone can drop 85 pounds in two months," and another claimed that anyone can "Lose 37 pounds in two weeks with *no* dieting and *no* exercise."

Over-the-top claims, lies, and deception, and unscrupulous individuals and companies, are endemic in the weight-loss industry.

Caveat emptor—*let the buyer beware.*

Be leery of quirky books, and diet fads

There's a book that claims it has a "protocol" for the cure of obesity. It suggests that the government and other powerful entities have been covering up this "miracle weight-loss cure." The book supposedly guarantees that anyone can lose 30 pounds in 30 days.

Its bizarre multi-phase plan is hopelessly severe. And it gives you no liberties to deviate from the ultra-strict steps and phases. It would be impossible for the great majority of people to adhere to this plan for any period of time.

The plan is also very expensive. It must be performed under a doctor's supervision, with daily colonics, and injections of a peculiar substance derived from a pregnant female's urine.

But will this "cure" cause you to lose lots of weight?

Of course it will. But to achieve the extraordinary results it promises, you'd better be financially secure, and have discipline far greater than that of a professional bodybuilder. And much of your lost weight will be from the daily colonics and loss of superfluous water weight— *not* from loss of body fat.

There are also many diet plans promoted through books that have multiple phases with varying degrees of detoxification practices, and complex procedures.

Almost all weight-loss plans work over the short-term, but most of them are impractical over the long-term.

Some once-popular fads like the "cabbage soup diet" and the "spinach diet" work because they are low in calories. No miracles are happening there.

And if you see a weight-loss book with a photo of a ripped celebrity on the cover, you may have a better chance of winning the lottery than looking like the celebrity who "wrote" the book.

Celebrity scams

Be leery of any weight-loss plan endorsed by a celebrity. Celebrities are compensated handsomely for their roles as spokespeople for the plans.

And just because you see before-and-after pictures of the celebrities as part of the advertising campaigns, that doesn't necessarily mean that the particular plan was responsible for the celebrities' weight-loss.

And the immediate results don't mean that the celebrities kept their weight off over the long-term. There have been instances in which some celebrities regained all of their weight once their stints as spokespeople for the diet plans were over.

One high-profile celebrity recently regained 83 pounds following her stint as spokesperson for a popular weight-loss plan ended.

The FTC's weight-loss red flags

The FTC has posted red flags to make the public more aware of potential weight-loss scams.

If the product makes one of the following claims, or something similar, don't waste your money:

"Lose weight without diet or exercise."

Achieving a healthy weight takes work. Take a pass on any product that promises miraculous results without effort.

"Lose weight no matter how much you eat of favorite foods."

Beware of any product that claims you can eat all you want of high-calorie foods and yet still lose weight. Losing weight requires sensible food choices.

"Lose weight permanently. Never diet again."

Even if you're successful in losing weight, permanent weight-loss requires permanent lifestyle changes. Don't trust any product that promises once-and-for-all results without ongoing maintenance.

"Lose 30 pounds in 30 days."

Losing weight at a pound or two a week is the most effective way to take it off and *keep it off*. At best, products that promise very fast fat-loss are bogus. At worst, they can ruin your health.

"Lose weight with our miracle weight-loss patch or cream."

Don't believe the ads for patches or creams that are claimed to melt away the pounds. There's nothing you can wear or apply to your skin that will cause you to lose weight.

The FTC is there for your protection

The FTC, a government agency, has said, "Claims of anything over three pounds per week can land a company in court. Fast and easy fixes undermine the reality of what it takes to lose weight. People are buying empty promises."

Here are the links for two of the FTC's publications. They are fun to read, informative, and free. Please take some time to review them.

The FTC's *Red Flag* brochure:
www.ftc.gov/bcp/conline/edcams/redflag/index.html

The FTC's *Deception in Weight-Loss Advertising* workshop:
www.ftc.gov/os/2003/12/031209weightlossrpt.pdf

And check out the FTC's ad for a fake weight-loss product:
www.wemarket4u.net/fatfoe

This chapter explains where your calories should come from if you're going to lose weight and keep it off.

It will also explain how protein, and certain carbohydrates and fats, can help promote fat-loss.

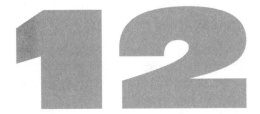

Where your calories should come from

There are five fundamental constituents of food: the three macronutrients (protein, carbohydrates, and fats), water, and fiber. The macronutrients provide *your caloric intake.*

Healthy nutrition is also about *micronutrients* —vitamins, minerals, essential fatty acids, and phytochemicals.

Getting the right caloric intake for you is *essential*, but, as explained in Chapter 8, getting sufficient micronutrients is *also essential*—for your health in general, *and* to make it easier to lose weight and keep it off.

Eating healthily is a vital component of a weight-loss plan.

Protein

Protein is utilized for body tissue repair and growth. There are two types of protein: complete, and incomplete.

Complete proteins are usually derived from animal sources, and contain all the essential amino acids. Incomplete proteins are usually derived from plant-based foods, and lack one or more of the essential amino acids.

According to a 2004 study by the Department of Nutrition, Harvard School of Public Health, as published in the *Journal of the American College of Nutrition*, there's evidence that protein increases the thermic effect. Over the long-term, this effect may be significant in total weight-loss, and the percentage of total fat lost.

According to the *Testosterone Advantage Plan*, by Lou Schuler et al (Rodale, 2002), it takes more energy to digest protein compared to other macronutrients. This can be as much as two-and-a-half times greater than what it takes to digest carbohydrates.

So, by eating more protein on a daily basis—substituting protein for some carbs—your body may burn more calories than it would if less protein but more carbs were eaten (while keeping total calories the same). This is called *diet-induced thermogenesis*.

A study from the University of Illinois found that those who followed a "protein emphasis diet" had less body fat and improved blood fat profiles. And the higher-protein approach also slowed the rate at which carbs become blood sugar.

Protein may also increase the feeling of fullness. And according to a study by the University of Washington School of Medicine, high-protein foods suppress the release of the hormone ghrelin, which helps to decrease appetite. This may improve your ability to maintain a reduced caloric intake over the long-term.

If upwards of half the calories you consume come from foods that are rich in protein, you'll give yourself a chance to achieve these added benefits.

Furthermore, you'll be more than supplied with the protein required for maintenance of muscle mass, recuperation from exercise, and possible muscle growth.

Protein sources

Eggs, meat, fish, low-fat cheese, cottage cheese, and skim milk are rich in complete protein. (Meat, however, isn't a necessity. Stuart hasn't eaten any for over 30 years.) Shrimp, scallops, lobster and crab are also sources of complete protein. Be cautious with deli meats because many are highly processed.

Some protein sources are expensive, so do what fits your budget.

Protein shakes

Provided you eat a nutritious diet that includes foods rich in complete protein, you're unlikely to be deficient in protein even if you exercise regularly.

Bodybuilding hokum has encouraged people to overdose on protein in general, and to think that commercial protein supplements are essential. But even people who lift weights seriously are better off getting their protein from regular food.

Protein shakes are overrated because they aren't essential, many upset the digestive tract and thus aren't digested well, many are expensive and highly processed, and it's easy to overdose on calories through shakes.

"Spend" your calories on proper foods, rather than on shakes. And proper foods are more satisfying and enjoyable than shakes, and richer in micronutrients.

A pint of skim milk is a cheap, nutritious and easily available protein drink, provided you're not lactose intolerant.

Brad used protein shakes during his final weight-loss journey, but he now realizes that other choices would have been better.

Account for every calorie

Just because you may be able to consume more calories than someone who's having only 1,700 a day, for example, doesn't mean you can afford to waste some of them on junk food and other crud.

Even when you can have more calories once you're in your maintenance phase (because you'll no longer be trying to lose weight), you should *still* eat healthily. The healthier your fare, the healthier you'll be, and the easier you'll maintain your weight.

When you're losing weight, and thus are on a reduced caloric intake, it's even more important that every calorie originates from nutrient-rich healthy food, to help you with weight-loss and your health in general.

As Brad and every other real-life dieter discovered, healthy food can taste great. Eventually it will become all that you'll want to eat.

Sooner or later the crud will taste yucky, and make you feel lethargic, bloated, and even sick, while the nutrient-rich, healthy food will make you feel energetic. You'll also feel better mentally.

Carbohydrates

Carbohydrates are the body's primary source of energy. They are divided into two categories: simple, and complex. Simple carbs are, more or less, sugars. They digest quickly and provide a fast energy boost. Complex carbs provide energy for a longer period, and should be a staple of your diet to prevent the highs and lows of the "sugar rush."

Certain types of carbs may help you lose weight faster.

The glycemic index (GI) is a ranking of carbohydrates on a scale from 0 to 100 according to the extent to which they increase blood sugar levels after consumption—70 and above means a high GI, while 55 and below means a low GI. The concept was developed to find out which foods were best for people with diabetes, but it has value for other purposes.

According to the GI theory, by focusing on low-glycemic foods—for example, most fruits and vegetables, grainy breads and cereals, pasta, and legumes—you can prevent rises in blood sugar level, control appetite and delay hunger, lower your levels of insulin, and help to allow stored fat to be burned. And there are other health benefits arising from focusing on low-glycemic foods.

High-glycemic carbohydrates—for example, corn flakes, watermelon, most white rices, white bread, extruded cereals, and glucose—can create a rush of insulin, which can block the release of stored fat. And meals rich in high-glycemic carbs can produce other harmful effects.

Supporters of the low-glycemic approach claim you can lose weight faster on it than on a low-fat approach. Thousands of dieters, including Brad, endorse the proper use of this index.

Visit www.glycemicindex.com for GI ratings of foods.

Carbohydrate sources

Sources include whole-wheat bread, whole-grain breads (and bagels) in general, whole-grain pasta, oatmeal and other whole-grain cereals, brown rice, wild rice, oatcakes, potatoes, sweet potatoes, yams, broccoli, corn, beets, beans, peas, lentils, avocados, pineapple, prunes, dates, figs, bananas, peaches, grapes, strawberries, blueberries, mangoes, oranges, pears, and apples.

Most fruits and vegetables are also excellent sources of vitamins, minerals, phytochemicals, and fiber. They can decrease your chance of heart disease and various cancers, and reduce blood pressure. Many experts feel that the more colorful the produce, the better.

Obtain your vegetables fresh or frozen, rather than canned. Steaming is usually the best method of cooking, to preserve nutritional content. And obtain your fruit fresh or frozen, too. Be wary of canned fruits because they are usually packed in sugary liquids, and contain chemicals. Read the label before you decide whether or not to buy something in a can.

Stay away from processed or refined carbohydrate sources — generally, the ones with a high glycemic index. And some common carbohydrate sources have hidden or refined sugars.

Fat-burning carbs?

Research from the University of Colorado found that *resistant starch* — a naturally occurring constituent of many carbohydrates, and a type of dietary fiber — can have fat-fighting properties, and can increase fat burning.

Resistant starch resists the digestion process. While normal starch is easily broken down, and absorbed by your body as blood sugar, resistant starch passes through your digestive tract undigested and eventually begins to ferment. Researchers believe that this fermentation process is involved in explaining why the resistant starch helps burn fat, and may lead to lower fat accumulation.

Furthermore, because resistant starch is a type of dietary fiber, it also helps to promote a lasting feeling of fullness, and stable blood-sugar levels.

Foods high in resistant starch include bananas, navy beans, lentils, potatoes, pasta, corn, oatmeal, and whole-grain bread products.

Fats

Not only are some fats not bad, they are essential for good health, *and may even help with weight-loss.*

While the weight-loss industry has made almost everyone believe that fat makes people gain weight, it's the *extra calories*, no matter what the source, that's the true culprit.

You can lose weight with any diet as long as you control your caloric intake correctly. But people who eat a lot of fat-laden foods tend to gain more weight because fat is much more calorific, ounce for ounce, than protein or carbohydrates.

Some fats are harmful, and should be avoided, such as refined vegetable oils, hydrogenated oils (for example, in margarine and shortenings), and trans fats.

Healthy fats are necessary for many important reasons, including the health of the skin and other organs, proper insulin function, red blood cell formation, and the lubrication of joints.

Omega-3 fatty acids, like the kind found in fish and fish oil, can trigger enzymes that may help lower body fat.

The University of Missouri-Columbia proposes that omega-3 fatty acids can stimulate fat oxidation in the liver. And according to Harvard University, omega-3 fatty acids can help the body secrete leptin, a hormone that can raise the rate of metabolism and boost feelings of satiety.

Essential fatty acids (EFAs) are also extremely important for good health. Deficiencies in EFAs are linked with cancer, diabetes, cardiovascular disease, arthritis, weakened immune functions, and other health problems. Many people have taken the "fat is bad" opinion and applied it to all sources of fat and oil, *even the good ones.*

There are two major *families* of EFAs—the omega-3 fatty acids, and the omega-6s. Many common foods contain omega-6s in small quantities, and a few contain omega-6s in large quantities, such as corn oil, safflower oil, and sunflower oil, which many people use for cooking. Furthermore, lots of packaged and processed foods contain hidden omega-6s.

Few foods in the typical diet contain omega-3s in anything other than small quantities. Therefore, the typical diet has few omega-3s, but many omega-6s, and usually poor-quality omega-6s. This produces a serious imbalance between the EFAs.

Flaxseed oil is rich in the most important member of the omega-3 family—from which other omega-3s can be produced .Through consuming sufficient flaxseed oil you can correct an EFA imbalance. Oily fish doesn't contain the entire family of omega-3s. No matter what your consumption of oily fish, you may still be deficient in the primary member of the omega-3 family unless you have a rich source of it in your diet. This is where flaxseed oil is helpful.

Flax seeds themselves can be consumed. They must be ground first, and eaten immediately (before they go off upon exposure to air).

Consume fish oil or oily fish, *and* flax seeds or oil, for the best all-round intake of omega-3s.

According to Drs. Udo Erasmus and Donald Rudin, two experts on fats, two or three tablespoons of flaxseed oil a day for a month or two or three may be needed to correct a deficiency of omega-3s, but much less is needed thereafter. A sustained high intake of flaxseed oil can produce an imbalance, and should be avoided.

Dry hands, feet, and elbows indicate insufficient consumption of omega-3s. Once your skin is smooth and no longer dry (without using skin creams), consume just sufficient flaxseed oil to maintain that condition—perhaps just one dessertspoon (two teaspoons) a day. Keep the oil refrigerated once a container has been opened, and use it within a few weeks. If it tastes off, don't use it.

Stuart eats fish most days, has a dessertspoon of flaxseed oil each day, and a dessertspoon of cod liver oil most days. And Brad and his wife take 3,000 mg of omega-3 fish oil daily, via softgel caplets.

In *moderation*, and when cooked *in a healthy way*, saturated fats aren't harmful like some people make them out to be. Saturated fats were an important part of traditional diets that kept many societies healthy for generations *until* the effects of modern farming, refining, and processing were felt, including the addition of refined sugar and oils (and products containing them), refined grain products, and the use of processed vegetable oils.

If you eat only healthy foods, and a broad variety of them, your fat intake should naturally work itself out. About 25% of your total calories should come from healthy fats.

Getting most of your fat intake from fish high in essential fatty acids (such as herring, mackerel, salmon, and sardines), along with other healthy fat from avocados, olive oil, nuts and seeds, flaxseed oil and butter in moderation, and boiled or poached eggs (low-temperature preparation relative to frying and scrambling), is vastly different from getting the same total quantity of fat from fried food, margarine and shortenings, refined vegetable oils, omelettes, and scrambled eggs. Over the long-term, the different effects on your health from the two approaches may be dramatic.

Extra virgin olive oil

Olive oil isn't rich in EFAs, but in healthy, mono-unsaturated fatty acids, and many nutrients and valuable substances unique to olives. It has many health benefits.

According to a study published in *Clinical Cardiology*, olive oil may cut your risk of coronary heart disease almost in half. It offers protection against heart disease by controlling the low-density lipoprotein level (the "bad cholesterol") while raising the high-density lipoprotein level (the "good cholesterol"). And its antioxidant polyphenols have been shown to reduce blood pressure by dilating arteries.

Spanish researchers concluded that regular olive oil consumption may also help prevent colon cancer. And the oleic acid in olive oil can help enhance fat metabolism.

Use extra virgin olive oil daily, on salads, and fish, for example, or spread a spoonful of it on a slice of bread, perhaps with some tomato paste, Mediterranean style.

Make your own salad dressing rather than buy inferior, ready-made ones that contain dubious ingredients, and poor oil. Mix olive oil and cider vinegar in proportions of about four to one, together with some herbs and mustard paste.

Buy only *extra virgin* olive oil—oil that's been extracted without using heat or chemicals.

More on monounsaturated fats

Monounsaturated fats from all sources, not just from extra virgin olive oil, have numerous health benefits, and can help with weight-loss. According to a study published in the journal *Diabetes Care*, monounsaturated fats may help prevent weight-gain— especially the accumulation of visceral belly fat.

Besides in extra virgin olive oil, monounsaturated fats are found in nuts, seeds, avocados, and olives. Brad eats peanuts, almonds, and pistachios as his snacks of choice, and he cooks with extra virgin olive oil as his oil of choice. Stuart consumes extra virgin olive oil, olives and almonds daily, and avocados from time to time.

Cod liver oil

This has long been a traditional remedy for joint pains and stiffness, and an aid for strong bones, good vision, healthy skin, and resistance to coughs and colds.

Cod liver oil is rich in omega-3s, and fat-soluble vitamins A and D, which are commonly undersupplied. Cod liver oil is potent, and may be toxic in large amounts. Two teaspoons a day is sufficient for adults, and one is enough for children.

Should you follow specific macronutrient ratios?

Among the many dieters Brad interviewed, the *average* macronutrient ratios were approximately 40% to 50% of calories from protein, 25% to 35% from carbohydrates, and about 25% from fats. A few had 60% protein, 20% carbs, and 20% fats. But some succeeded with ratios that were roughly 50% to 60% carbs, 20% to 30% protein, and 20% fats.

While many had an emphasis on protein, a disproportionate amount of protein is *not* a prerequisite for losing weight. It worked for many people, but not everyone. Some people can't stand a protein-rich diet, so they ate what they liked.

Regardless of the percentages, everyone who lost weight had one thing in common—*a marked reduction in overall calories.*

You must keep your caloric intake in check. Regardless of what you eat, you must establish an *energy imbalance* (a *caloric deficit*) to force your body to draw on its energy store—body fat. That's the priority. It's how it's carried out that varies, including the ratios of macronutrients.

The best approach is the one that you enjoy, can stick with over the long-term, and is healthy.

Most of your meals should have some high-quality protein, complex carbohydrates, and healthy fat. This will stabilize your blood-sugar levels throughout the day because it will slow the rate at which carbs are converted to blood sugar, and reduce the production of blood-sugar hormones (and sugar cravings).

How to prepare food

Baking, broiling, grilling, frying, steaming, poaching, boiling, and microwaving are the common alternatives.

Avoid frying in general, other than perhaps occasional low- to medium-heat stir-fry with extra virgin olive oil, or a little butter, or non-stick cooking spray.

Deep frying is especially harmful because, in addition to the high heat, unhealthy oils are invariably used *and overused*. And not only are unhealthy oils used in the first place, but they are often still used even after they have become rancid.

The high heat used in baking, broiling and grilling can also damage food at the molecular level—but food cooked by these methods is still better than fast food or junk food, as is microwave cooked food.

Because they use the lowest temperature, steaming, poaching and boiling are usually the best methods of cooking—they do the least damage to food, and they preserve its nutritional content.

Invest in your life

Nutritious foods may be more costly than crud. But you have just one body to live your life in. Invest in it and you'll be more productive in everything you do, *and* you'll look better and feel better about yourself.

But consider how much money you'll not waste on processed food. And by having cut back on eating out in general, you'll make a big saving there, too.

Furthermore, by investing in your health you'll probably reduce your medical bills.

Brad has an acquaintance who often complained that "it costs too much to eat healthy." But after suffering a heart attack and having to pay a $10,000 insurance deductible, he no longer makes that complaint. His refrigerator, cupboards, and pantry are now stocked with nutritious foods only.

Although Brad buys only nutritious foods now, his grocery bill is *less* than what it was when he was eating unhealthily. He used to spend a small fortune on processed food, and frozen, microwaveable short-cut meals.

Chicken breast, fish, and fruits and vegetables, can be costly, but if you use coupons and follow sales, you can often buy these items for much less than their original price. For example, when chicken breast is on sale for a "buy one, get one free," Brad buys in bulk and freezes most of it.

Are hungry shoppers fat shoppers?

Because hunger accompanies increased ghrelin activity, hungry shoppers tend to fill up their shopping carts with food they crave rather than the nutritious food they need. The hormone ghrelin heightens perception and memory when it comes to food, which makes food seem tastier and more attractive.

According to Alain Dagher, a neurologist at McGill University in Montreal, "When you go to the supermarket hungry, every food looks better. Now, we've found that it is ghrelin that acts on the brain to make food more appealing."

Prepare a shopping list ahead of time, of healthy food *exclusively*. *Don't* shop when you're hungry. And purchase only the food that fulfills your menu plan, and don't be tempted to buy anything unhealthy. *Stick to the list.*

By showcasing the eating strategies that real people used to lose weight and keep it off, this chapter will teach you *how to eat*.

13

How to eat for weight-loss

It's very important that you enjoy eating, but *what* you eat and *how* you eat it are very important, too.

Some people seem to think that the only food they can enjoy is unhealthy food. While unhealthy food can be tasty, so can healthy food.

But while unhealthy food *erodes* health, healthy food *builds* health, makes you feel and function better, and makes weight-loss easier to achieve *and* maintain.

Many obese people are the result of excessive eating in general, and excessive unhealthy eating in particular. And many parents pass unhealthy eating habits to their children, which produces generation after generation of obese people due to conditioned behavior.

Eating together at fast-food restaurants, eating fried chicken for dinner at home, devouring delivered pizzas, and junk-food snacking in front of the TV, has created some very obese families.

And many people have friends and acquaintances whose poor eating habits can be contagious.

Many social events are centered on or around food. Many people congregate at restaurants and taverns where they gorge on plates of greasy chicken wings, or large portions of deep fried specials. It's no wonder why so many people who routinely behave in this manner put on a ton of weight.

But it's not just *what* you eat and *how* you eat it that affect your health and weight. Your health and weight are also a reflection of *what you do in order to eat*. You need to walk to get your food, for example. How your gait is affected by your posture and physical condition plays a major role in your health, well-being, ability to exercise, and what types of activities are safe for you, *all of which influence weight-loss and your ability to keep the weight off*.

Eat often but reduce your portion sizes

For most people, "Eat often but reduce your portion sizes" is likely the single most important strategy for weight-loss.

Extensive research, many books, and many real-life success stories have concluded that, for weight-loss, it's best to eat something every two to four hours. And all the real-life dieters that Brad interviewed agreed with this.

Instead of eating three large meals a day, redistribute the same caloric intake (or less, if you're currently overeating) into five or six mini-meals so that you get a more steady supply of nutrition.

Each mini-meal, or snack, should be 200 to 400 calories, depending on your body size and activity levels. If you get each normal meal and cut it in half or thirds, you'll get the concept of mini-meals. For example, instead of having a normal dinner at 6:30 pm, eat half of it at 5:30 and the other half of it at 7:30.

Then you'll have more energy. And your metabolism will get a boost each time you eat—from diet-induced thermogenesis—because energy is required to digest your food.

And by eating smaller meals you'll also give your body a better chance to assimilate what you eat.

A recent study conducted in Sweden concluded that those people who ate five or six mini-meals a day lost 45% more weight than those who ate three square meals, *even though they all consumed the same daily caloric intake.*

A study published in the *American Journal of Epidemiology* found that men who ate three or fewer times a day were twice as likely to become overweight than men who ate three meals and two healthy snacks a day.

And a study published in the *European Journal of Clinical Nutrition* showed that men who adhered to three principal meals *and* two or three healthy snacks a day lost more weight than those who ate three larger meals and no snacks.

While the five or six mini-meals approach works for most people—and is a great way to help overcome binge eating and compulsive overeating, and control hunger—it doesn't work for everyone.

For some people, eating five or six daily meals tends to result in overconsumption of daily calories. In some studies, a number of people found it too challenging to consume a 200- to 400-calorie mini-meal—they wanted more normal-sized meals for breakfast, lunch and dinner. (And then the two or three additional snacks would add too many calories.) For these people, they lost more weight with the three square meals approach *provided* it yielded the necessary energy imbalance to produce weight-loss.

Although a given eating pattern won't work the same for everyone, *all* **successful weight-loss plans have one thing in common—***a marked reduction in overall daily calories.*

But, again, for most men and women, "Eat often but reduce your portion sizes" is likely the single most important strategy for weight-loss. Try it properly, and you'll probably see that it will work for you, too.

Never eat to the point where you're stuffed. Eat the nutritious foods you like, but make your portion sizes smaller.

When you get familiar with the foods you eat, and their caloric values per serving, determining your portion sizes will become second nature. But to begin with, always choose a *smaller* portion size until you've mastered the art of portion control.

Unless you're aware of what you eat and drink, it's easy to overshoot your daily caloric intake goal. Most people underestimate the calories in their meals, especially at restaurants.

When *a little* means *a lot*

If you were to consume a mere 100 extra calories a day on a sustained basis, or 100 fewer calories a day on a sustained basis, (and provided you do nothing different physically), this apparently little change can have a big effect over the long-term.

It would be equivalent to 36,500 calories over a year, which could be 10 pounds gained or lost—and 50 pounds over five years, and 100 pounds over ten years.

You may have seen someone at an event like a high-school reunion who was perhaps 100 pounds heavier than 10 years earlier. Chances are that he or she did just a little to get that heavy, but on a daily basis for year, after year, after year.

Small but daily bad eating habits, especially when coupled with a waning metabolism, and inactivity, add up to big changes. Something as little as mayonnaise on a daily sandwich could be the difference between gaining or losing 100 pounds over 10 years.

Be aware of the true size of your mini-meals

Let's review some illustrative arithmetic:

200 x 6 = 1,200; 300 x 6 = 1,800; 400 x 6 = 2,400

If you eat six mini-meals a day, which is common among the dieters Brad researched, the difference in effect between 200 and 400 calories per meal is huge.

Even with the mini-meals approach *you must stick to your required average daily caloric intake.* Adjust the size of your mini-meals accordingly.

For example, if you're striving for an average of 1,600 daily calories, six 300- to 400-calorie mini-meals will put you over your daily quota, and you'll gain weight. Be aware of every morsel of food you eat, and in a food journal track the calories you consume.

Rather than mini-meals of a fixed caloric value, let some of them average around 400 calories, and others average around 200. In that way you can still

**average about 260 calories per mini-meal for the
1,600 example. This will help break up the monotony
of eating the same portions throughout the day, and
let you feel that you're still eating some larger meals.**

Don't "bulk up" by overcompensating

The *International Journal of Obesity* published a study that indicates
that half of all dieters overcompensate. They eat too much when
they begin an exercise routine because they think they need more
nutrition or, specifically, more protein, and thus more food. This
negates any help with weight-loss that the exercise should provide.

Don't assume that you can eat anything you want just because
you're exercising regularly. Your body may, however, need more
nutrients—and not just because you're exercising. But if you create
an unfavorable energy imbalance via an overconsumption of
calories, you'll gain weight despite the extra exercise.

By improving the quality of your food intake, not the quantity of
it, you can easily increase your nutrient intake.

An hour of exercise is easily nullified by a post-exercise drink. For
example, don't chug a sports drink or a protein shake after a
workout, even if you think you've earned a treat as a reward.

The hunger scale

Studies show that many obese people eat beyond the point of
satisfying hunger, and because of this they eat significantly more
throughout the day than people of normal weight. To help curtail
this, some people use a hunger scale to help them gauge when they
are full. Formulate a scale from 0 to 10, in which 10 is "stuffed," 0 is
"starving," 5 is "comfortably satisfied" and 7.5 is "full." This is
based on *your* feelings of hunger.

Never exceed a feeling of five. Anything more than a five would
mean that you'll probably be overeating, and overeating usually
leads to fat storage.

You may want to use this hunger scale as part of your food journal
entries, to note your hunger levels. And remind yourself that
you're no more than "comfortably satisfied" after each meal—this
helps with reinforcement, and the establishment of the new habit.

You'll eventually realize that being "comfortably satisfied" will make you feel much better than being "stuffed." Then, being "stuffed" would make you feel lethargic, and perhaps miserable.

Control your hunger with soups and salads

Focus on foods that have fewer calories per bite, or a lower energy density. And start at least some of your meals with a low-calorie soup or salad, and eat main dishes that are full of vegetables and fruits. Fill yourself up on foods that are low in calories.

This approach is substantiated by a Penn State University study, which found that adults who had vegetable soup before a meal consumed 20% fewer calories during the meal than those who didn't, because the soup tended to make them feel full sooner.

Eliminate processed foods

Knowing that processed foods are chemically "engineered" to be addictive, should make you think twice about eating them.

And if you check out the nutrition labels on junk food and fast food, you'll see that that crud is high in calories, but low in nourishment.

Get rid of processed foods. If you can't go cold turkey, wean yourself off the rubbish over a few weeks. Have a little junk food as a treat on *one* designated day each week. Over time you'll acquire an intensified taste for nutritious foods, and gradually lose your desire for rubbish. This happened to Brad and many other people. Stuart hasn't eaten any crud for many years. But he doesn't discipline himself not to eat it. He simply doesn't have any desire to eat it.

Having healthy snacks at your desk or in your purse can serve as a great diversion. For example, instead of vending-machine chips or candy, grab an apple, carrot, cheese stick, or peanuts.

Processing removes vitamins, minerals, and other valuable nutrients, and usually replaces them with rubbish such as sugar, high-fructose corn syrup, and chemicals.

Eating processed foods can cause your insulin levels to spike, which triggers your body to store fat. If some food doesn't exist in nature, it's probably a processed food and you should avoid it.

If you see "high-fructose corn syrup," "hydrogenated vegetable oil," "refined or enriched," "trans fats," or mysterious chemicals on the label, the item is a processed food, and you should avoid it. *Be informed and discerning—read nutrition labels.*

Many dieters swear by the mass-marketed, single-serving frozen meals with labels that state, for example, "280 calories and seven grams of fat per serving." But be careful of these microwaveable, short-cut meals, because many of them are high in sodium, sugar or high-fructose corn syrup, and are highly processed. Look for the all-natural varieties. *Be informed and discerning—read nutrition labels.*

Brad's snacks include selected fruits or vegetables, almonds, pistachios, peanuts, turkey breast, and chicken breast. You'll get to love your own selection of healthy snack foods, like Brad did his.

Don't enhance your food's taste with high-calorie dressings. Eliminating a few daily pats of butter, or dollops of mayonnaise, for example, can add up to many pounds of lost body fat per year.

And ketchup, steak sauce, barbeque sauce, and other tasty condiments can contain a lot of high-fructose corn syrup. Find healthy brands, or use alternatives. *Be informed and discerning— read nutrition labels.*

Many ordinary appearing foods can be high in sugar and high-fructose corn syrup. For example, cereals, deli meats, canned fruit, desserts, and breads can have hidden surprises. *Be informed and discerning—read nutrition labels.*

But many of these foods belong to the category of "processed," and shouldn't be consumed in the first place.

Salad dressings can have hundreds of calories per serving. Fat-free salad dressing can have sugar or high-fructose corn syrup added to salvage its taste. Stick with vinaigrette or lo-cal dressing served on the side. *Be informed and discerning—read nutrition labels.*

And watch out for refined sugar, brown sugar, corn sweetener, sucrose (table sugar), fructose, glucose, lactose, maltose, fruit juice concentrate, syrup, or dietary sugars of any kind. Stay away from these sugary foods because they can cause your insulin levels to spike, which triggers your body to store fat. *Be informed and discerning—read nutrition labels.*

And even healthy sweeteners such as pure honey, maple syrup, date syrup or molasses should be consumed in only small quantities.

According to the US Department of Agriculture (USDA), the average American ingests 150 pounds of sugar a year, and about a third of it may be converted to stored energy—body fat. And according to research from the University of Texas Southwestern Medical Center, fructose can turn into fat with "surprising speed."

Used in *tiny quantities*, sugar substitutes are acceptable. From the dieters that Brad knows, sucralose—sold under the name Splenda®—is preferred to aspartame, better known as NutraSweet®. (Sucralose is about 600 times as sweet as table sugar, twice as sweet as saccharin, and about three times as sweet as aspartame. The sugar substitutes have zero or almost-zero calories.)

Avoid the white stuff

This means that you should avoid processed or refined foods that are white, which includes most bagels, biscuits, pizza doughs, pasta, pretzels, pancakes, crackers, rice, and types of bread.

White flour can be disguised as "enriched wheat flour" or "wheat flour," so be careful. *Be informed and discerning—read nutrition labels.*

Most of the white stuff has a high glycemic index. And some refined carbohydrates—such as those in refined pasta—can stimulate the activity of SCD, an enzyme that signals the liver to store calories as fat.

There are, however, many whole-grain and whole-wheat alternatives, as well as oat or maize alternatives. These also have more fiber and antioxidants, which can help control insulin levels, and result in a greater loss of abdominal fat.

Oatmeal (porridge), although white, is great food if it's whole-grain and prepared without the addition of any crud.

High-fructose corn syrup, the *death* of any diet

High-fructose corn syrup, or HFCS, is a man-made sweetener that became prevalent about four decades ago. It creates a sugary flavor that many people find almost addictive. And it's in almost all pre-packaged foods.

Many studies have shown a compelling link between HFCS and obesity. According to the USDA, the annual consumption of HFCS has gone from half a pound per

person in the 1970s, to an average of 63 pounds per person today. (And some other reports indicate an even higher consumption.) The percentage of the population that's obese has nearly doubled during this period.

According to *The Sugar Fix*, by Richard J. Johnson M.D., and Timothy Gower, HFCS is "metabolic poison." It can elevate your blood pressure, reduce your liver's ability to detoxify your body, impede your memory, make your skin sag, and lead to a high blood sugar level, insulin resistance, and diabetes. And it can also increase the risk of heart disease.

HFCS can impair your body's ability to control appetite and hunger. It can also impair your liver's ability to break down fat into fuel, and disrupt your body's ability to regulate blood sugar.

Some research has concluded that HFCS bypasses the normal energy balance systems, which causes your brain to trigger you to eat more food because your brain never fully registers the calories of the HFCS. Furthermore, HFCS may even turn on gene signaling that promotes fat formation and fat accumulation.

While some studies have suggested that HFCS is no worse than ordinary refined sugar, ordinary refined sugar is bad, too. HFCS and refined sugar should be avoided by everyone, not just those who want to lose weight.

Be informed and discerning—read nutrition labels.

One real-life dieter claims she lost 54 pounds in less than a year by the simple elimination of anything that contained HFCS.

Chocolate *alert*

Some people have created the illusion that dark chocolate is a healthy alternative to ordinary milk chocolate. While milk chocolate is highly processed candy that should be avoided, most dark chocolate products—even those that have a high percentage of cocoa—are *still* highly processed candies that are usually sweetened with sugar. They should be avoided, too.

The dark chocolate products that offer minor health benefits have at least 70% cocoa content, but preferably 100% cocoa and without any added sugar. These are higher in monounsaturated fats, which are beneficial to your health. But they don't taste like the sweetened chocolate that most people have become accustomed to. And they may be more calorific than ordinary milk chocolate.

But like any snack food, if you crave chocolate and must have it, have *a little* of it. (But even a small piece of dark chocolate can still be high in calories.) A small piece of chocolate is fine on your treat day, but if it would open the floodgates—like even a couple of chips would with Brad—or cause you torment to have only a little when you want lots, avoid it totally.

Don't starve yourself, or eat too little

Your body *needs* food for proper sustenance.

Severe caloric reductions can cause your body to *store* fat when you eat. And severe diets can trigger catabolism and deplete your muscle tissue.

When Brad temporarily lost 57 pounds on his wedding diet, 10 to 15 of it was probably lost muscle tissue.

Don't try to make up for a few missed meals by having a big "make-up meal." Much of such a meal—especially when your body is already leaning towards the starvation effect—would likely be stored as fat.

Starvation can stymie your willpower

Florida State University researchers showed that men with the lowest blood sugar levels performed the worst on tests that evaluated self-control. Their self-control was stymied by periods of starvation.

When your brain is deprived of its primary fuel, glucose, you may struggle to control your cravings. Keep your blood sugar level steady by eating something nutritious every few hours, and then your cravings will be kept in check, or at least will be much reduced.

The "starve-then-binge club"

A common habit, because of an overly busy schedule, is the practice of skipping breakfast, not eating much all day (or snacking on junk food and fast food), and then eating a huge dinner—sometimes as late as ten or eleven o'clock. This is a sure way to put on fat, and is a prime reason why so many busy parents and workaholics become overweight. And it's a prime example of how the starvation effect affects your body.

One of the dieters Brad interviewed claimed that all of her work associates shared this same predicament, and blamed their ultra-busy schedule for their weight-gain. They were forced, she said, to starve all day due to back-to-back appointments, and they ended up gorging on a massive dinner to try to make up for their caloric deficit.

She eventually realized that she could make the little time required between appointments to have a pint of skim milk, a meal replacement drink, an all-natural meal replacement bar, or a single-serving yogurt. She now keeps her office's miniature refrigerator stocked with single-serving snacks, and single-serving milk drinks and yogurt, and she has one of them every few hours. She now has much more energy and better focus at work, *and* she's losing weight.

Pocket meals

Don't think that you'll have to cook and prepare meals all of the time on your new schedule. You can be busy and yet still keep to the plan. All-natural meal replacement bars, skim milk, almonds, peanuts, pistachios, pre-made sandwiches, and "100-calorie" or "portion-control" snacks can substitute for meals when you're busy.

An all-natural meal-replacement bar is a mini-meal you can enjoy daily. Brad calls it "pocket food," and "purse food" (for women).

Many people think that all-natural nutrition bars taste like cardboard. While this is the case for some, many of them have a terrific taste. Find some that taste good to you. Brad's wife hated them at first, but she eventually found bars she likes.

Some protein drinks, meal replacement drinks, protein bars, and energy bars are high in sugar or high-fructose corn syrup, and are no more nutritious than candy bars. Opt for the all-natural and healthy variety only.

Be informed and discerning—read nutrition labels.

The importance of breakfast

A Harvard University study concluded that people who skip breakfast are four times more likely to be obese than those who eat breakfast.

It's *essential* to eat a nutritious breakfast. It *is* the most important meal because it's the first one.

"Breakfast" is named so because it follows a period without food. The "fasting" period is broken by the first meal of the day—thus, you "break" the "fast."

Low blood sugar levels due to a skipped breakfast not only hamper memory and concentration, but can also impair physical performance. Children who are fed a nutritious breakfast perform better in school. And adults who have nutritious breakfasts perform better during their days, too.

Many studies have showed that skipping breakfast leads to overeating later in the day by raising your ghrelin levels, which, in turn, stimulates your appetite at a time when your metabolism is already in a slowed state.

Even if you're in a crunch for time, find just two or three minutes to have a glass of skim milk, or a granola bar.

The importance of meal timing

Many weight-loss experts feel that you should reduce carbohydrate intake later in the day. While this is a theory that not everyone agrees with, most real-life dieters agreed on the benefits of it.

Many prominent weight-loss books and nutritionists also promote the benefits of this principle, and a study published in the *Journal of Nutrition* backs it, too. It helps not just because it usually leads to a reduction in overall caloric intake, but because it also reduces the amount of insulin your body produces, which decreases the amount of fat your body stores.

If you eat carbs too late, or by themselves, your body must release more insulin to put your nighttime carbohydrates to use in your body, which can decrease fat burning and increase fat storage.

Cut back on carbohydrates during the last one-third of the day. Instead, have some protein-rich foods to help your body to repair itself while you sleep.

Many nutritionists and books suggest cutting back on all eating for a certain period prior to bedtime. Have a "cut off time" whereby you stop eating two to three hours before bedtime.

As noted earlier, a real-life dieter lost 44 pounds in just under 12 months solely by eliminating post-dinner eating. He and his wife now put a "Sorry, we're closed" sign on their refrigerator in the evening, to remind themselves *not* to indulge at night.

Learn from their example and be more mindful of how bad nighttime eating can be to your weight-loss aspirations.

In a study with obese females, the *Journal of Nutrition* reported that people who ate larger breakfasts and lunches lost more body fat than those who ate larger dinners and had nighttime snacks.

But some old-school nutritionists believe that there's nothing special about the timing of the largest meal or meals each day. They feel that if people simply stop eating at a specified time, they will consume fewer overall calories, and that's what's required for weight-loss.

Most real-life dieters that Brad researched support the view that having larger meals earlier in the day helped them to lose weight.

This means that if you were to have three meals each day—and nothing else—reserve the larger ones for breakfast and lunch.

Coined by Adelle Davis, a famous nutritionist during the 1950s and 1960s, the adage "eat breakfast like a king, lunch like a prince, and supper like a pauper" is still smart. In fact, some diet plans are based solely on this premise—and they work.

Recent findings from Virginia Commonwealth University confirmed that to lose weight and keep it off, you should eat a big breakfast packed with carbohydrates, fiber, and protein. The "big breakfast diet" works because it helps to control appetite, and satisfy cravings for sweets and starches.

According to the findings, women who ate a larger breakfast reported feeling less hungry, especially before lunch, and having fewer cravings for carbs than women on a low-carb diet.

Don't, however, go to the extreme of preparing huge meals for breakfast, and diminutive meals for dinner.

"Let's go out to eat after the game"

Many people eat late at night at sports-themed restaurants or taverns. This usually serves as dinner—as many as 2,000 calories (or more), right before bedtime. Generally, restaurant food of this type is unhealthy, and laden in fat and calories.

This is a conditioned behavior that's based on social influences because many people have learned to go out to eat after a game, or for reasons similar to this. This is another sure way to put on weight—often a lot of weight.

You don't have to refrain from these social gatherings, just keep the portions to a minimum, and keep your food choices healthy.

Vary your calorie levels *day-to-day*

If you drastically reduce your daily caloric intake in one step—rather than gradually—*and* eat the same number of calories each day (for example, dive bomb from 3,000 calories a day to 1,200), your body will think a famine is occurring. Then, by initiating the starvation effect, it will slow its metabolism in an effort to preserve its fat.

As explained in Chapter 9, to prevent the starvation effect, don't reduce your daily caloric intake by more than 250 to 350 calories *every few days* until you get down to your target daily caloric quota.

And once you've *gradually* reduced your caloric intake sufficiently, to then keep your metabolism revving, vary your caloric (and carbohydrate) intake day-to-day, but while *averaging* the daily caloric intake that will produce gradual weight-loss.

For example, while he was losing weight, Brad varied between 1,400 and 1,900 calories (and 2,000 or more calories on his "treat day"), but *averaged* around 1,700 a day, which, coupled with his high activity level, maintained the caloric deficit necessary to lose up to two pounds of fat a week.

Here's a typical week's caloric intake for Brad when he was losing weight: 1,400 on Sunday; 1,800 on Monday; 1,500 on Tuesday; 1,800 on Wednesday; 1,600 on Thursday; 1,900 on Friday; and 2,100 on Saturday.

By varying your calories day-to-day, you're essentially outwitting your body's innate survival mechanism so that it doesn't "think" it has to store calories (in body fat) for a famine.

This strategy has been around for decades. It goes by a number of names, including "zig-zag dieting," "carb cycling," "calorie cycling," and "up-day down-day." A few books are based on this premise. Brad and most real-life dieters believe this strategy works.

Have a weekly treat day

If you wish, allow yourself *one* treat day each week to satisfy *some* of your cravings, and help to maintain a positive attitude because you won't feel that you're always on a diet.

But use prudence, because a whole week's worth of progress can be eradicated by a day of cheating. This routinely happened to Brad during his wedding diet.

By varying your daily caloric intake, and having an occasional "treat day," you'll satisfy yourself psychologically and physiologically. Most of the successful dieters that Brad interviewed incorporated this strategy, to enjoy their favorite snacks. *But, once again, use caution, and enjoy it in moderation.*

Prevent a see-food diet

One of Brad's biggest problems has been that if he sees enticing food, he'll eat it. And it's common among most real-life dieters. Research shows that many overweight people want to eat all of the food they see, but normal-weight people eat only what satisfies them regardless of how much food is in front of them. The overweight people don't have the ability to exercise restraint.

To remedy this problem, don't stock your home with any foods other than those that are nutritious and healthy. Obviously, if you can't see the irresistible temptations, you can't eat them.

But this solution won't work if your roommates, spouse, or family members are not on a nutritious plan themselves. If the people you live with support you, it's *much* easier to succeed.

Prepare nutritious meals ahead of time

It may seem convenient to forgo meal preparation in exchange for a trip to a drive-thru restaurant. A way to avoid this is to cook large batches of nutritious foods once or twice a week, refrigerate them, and then use them up gradually. These foods can be frozen in single-serving portions ready for a quick microwave re-heat.

But by the time you get in a car, drive to a burger joint, return home, and then eat, how fast was the fast food?

Pack your lunch and take it to work. If you already pre-prepared some healthy sandwiches, or pre-cooked some chicken breasts, fish cutlets, or lean hamburger patties, for example, that should be quicker and more nutritious than what you'd get from a trek to a fast-food joint.

People who pre-plan their meals and pack their lunches are much less likely to stray from their eating plans.

By having a pre-prepared lunch rather than a trek to a fast-food restaurant or tavern, you could easily cut your caloric intake by about 500 a day, which would add up to a great deal of lost fat over the course of a year. *And* you could save up to $2,000 annually.

Many real-life dieters, including Brad, take their lunch to work in a small cooler.

When you mass-prepare your food ahead of time, don't give in to any "see-food" temptation (like Brad used to) and eat the entire batch of food in one massive serving.

Do pre-packaged meal plans really work?

Americans are bombarded by commercials with athletes and celebrities claiming that they lost many pounds from following certain weight-loss plans that provide pre-packaged, processed meals of the right portion sizes.

The plans can work because they remove human decision-making, but you must tolerate a limited variety of meals every day. Many people can do this over the short-term, but not over the long-term.

Everyone Brad talked to who temporarily succeeded with these plans couldn't wait to return to their normal fare—the food that made them heavy in the first place.

Brad has tried these plans, but eating pre-packaged meals every day wasn't satisfying, and he couldn't stick with it for more than a few weeks at a time.

These plans can also be expensive, costing as much as $400 to $600 a month for the pre-packaged food, plus hundreds of dollars more for the "real food" that compliments the system.

Although the principles of these pre-packaged meal plans are fine, they need to be applied to a better approach. For instance, the pre-packaged meals could serve as snacks or occasional meals, but you should primarily eat the normal foods you're accustomed to if you're to stick to a weight-loss program over the long-term.

Eat slowly

Savoring your food stimulates the "brain phase" of digestion by stimulating your hypothalamus to trigger the release of cholecystokinin (CCK), which, in turn, slows the production of fat-accumulating cortisol.

Thorough chewing is the first step in the digestive process. By slowing your eating, you get a chance to enjoy and experience your food more. And because you tend to be satisfied longer as a result, it also helps reduce your chances of snacking between meals.

Cut your food into much smaller pieces—this makes your portions seem bigger, and more satisfying. Furthermore, take smaller mouthfuls, and chew the food more thoroughly. This forces you to eat slowly.

Someone that Brad interviewed said she spent several months using chopsticks to eat her food. She ate slower, and ate much less per bite compared with the spoon-and-fork method, and as a result she greatly reduced her overall caloric intake, and lost weight.

If you're right-handed, hold your fork or spoon with your left. The fumbling that this creates will slow your eating, and probably reduce your caloric intake. You may also use cutlery designed for children, which will probably also reduce your caloric intake.

And many dieters set their fork or spoon down between bites—this can slow your eating significantly.

Many people don't stop eating even when their stomachs are full. According to Brian Wansink, Ph.D., director of the Cornell University Food and Brand Lab, it takes about 20 minutes after starting a meal before your brain can indicate satiation—the signal that you're full. And by that time you may have already wolfed too much food.

And according to new research from the University of Rhode Island, eating fast can cause you to eat more. In the study, women who ate slowly (as compared to those who ate quickly) consumed about 70 fewer calories per meal, *and* felt satisfied for longer.

The researchers from the University of Rhode Island also found that if you slow down and consciously breathe between bites, you can reduce your caloric intake by as much as 10%.

Pretend you're a food critic examining the food's flavors. This can boost your enjoyment of a meal and reduce your caloric intake. *Take your time, and savor your meals.*

Eat more fiber

Dietary fiber, or roughage, is the indigestible portion of plant foods. The term is a misnomer, however, because some types of so-called dietary fiber are not fibers. Fiber can be insoluble (not able to dissolve in water), or soluble (able to dissolve in water). Resistant starch, mentioned in Chapter 12, is another type of dietary fiber. It can provide some of the benefits of insoluble fiber, and some of the benefits of soluble fiber.

Fiber slows your rate of digestion, which keeps you feeling full for longer. When saturated with water, the fiber swells in your stomach, and creates a sensation of fullness. Fiber also increases the calories burned as a result of diet-induced thermogenesis. Furthermore, fiber helps to control blood sugar levels and decrease insulin levels. And fiber has a brooming effect because it helps to sweep waste out of your body.

It's a good idea to have the majority of your fiber early in the day, especially at breakfast. Early-day fiber—along with fat, carbohydrates, protein, and plenty of water—can make you less likely to snack by giving you a prolonged sensation of fullness.

Adult women should consume 25 *or more* grams of fiber a day, and adult men 40 *or more*. Sources of fiber include 100% whole-grain products (including cereals), fruit, vegetables, nuts, and legumes. Figs, dates and prunes are especially rich in fiber.

If you have a digestive tract problem such as irritable bowel syndrome (IBS), insoluble fiber in large quantities may irritate your colon. Rich sources of insoluble fiber include whole-*wheat* bread and cereals. If you have IBS, consume more *soluble* fiber—oats, white rice, barley bread, and corn bread are rich in it—and reduce your intake of insoluble fiber, especially whole-*wheat* products.

But for fiber to do its important work, you must drink sufficient water. Merely not being thirsty doesn't mean you're adequately supplied with water. Drink enough to produce at least four *clear* urinations a day (in addition to colored ones.)

Oh, those embarrassing beans

Beans contain oligosaccharides. To digest them properly, an oligosaccharide enzyme is required. Since a normal human digestive tract doesn't contain oligosaccharide enzymes, bacteria act on the undigested oligosaccharides, and produce flatulence.

To make the beans digestible, put the dried beans in a bowl and cover with warm water. Stir in some lemon juice, and leave in a warm place for 12 to 24 hours, depending on the size of the beans. Then drain, rinse, place in a pot, and cover with water. Bring to a boil and skim off the foam. Reduce the heat and simmer covered—for several hours if necessary—until the beans are very soft. Check occasionally, stir, and top up the water when necessary. Then add other ingredients and simmer for whatever additional time is required.

Another possible way to improve the digestibility of beans is by using a product called Beano®. It's a natural food enzyme dietary supplement that helps with the digestion of complex carbohydrates.

www.beanogas.com

The benefits of nuts and peanuts

Peanuts aren't nuts, but legumes. Peanuts and almonds are highly nutritious foods that make a good snack. They are high in protein, fiber, and key nutrients, but naturally low in carbohydrates. But eat only *unsalted* nuts and peanuts.

Researchers from Harvard University found that people who snacked on peanuts kept weight off, while those who didn't, gained the weight back. This is attributed to the type of fat in peanuts that maintains a feeling of fullness that can stave off cravings.

Furthermore, recent research on peanuts and nuts has found them to be high in antioxidants that may provide health benefits.

Research conducted by a team of University of Florida scientists, published in the journal *Food Chemistry*, shows that peanuts contain high concentrations of antioxidant polyphenols, and that roasting can dramatically increase the peanuts' p-coumaric acid levels, boosting their overall antioxidant content by over 20%.

Peanuts and almonds can help lower your cholesterol levels, and reduce your risk of cardiovascular diseases. And peanuts are a great source of resveratrol—a chemical that has potential anti-aging effects, and can help reduce the risks of cardiovascular disease and cancer.

Peanuts are not, however, for everyone. Some people have allergic reactions to them, from mild to severe. For people with a peanut allergy, exposure can cause a fatal anaphylactic shock—from eating just a single peanut, or merely breathing in peanut dust.

And some peanut particulates are hard to avoid. An allergic reaction can be triggered by eating foods that have been processed with machines that have previously been in contact with peanuts.

The digestibility of nuts—problem, and solution

While most Americans have convenient access to a variety of pre-roasted nuts that are easily digestible, it may not be so elsewhere.

Nuts are nutritious, but difficult to digest in their raw form if consumed in anything other than tiny quantities, because of the enzyme *inhibitors* they contain. If you don't have easy access to digestible nuts, make them digestible yourself. If the nuts are put in warm water and mixed with some salt, and soaked overnight, the enzyme inhibitors will be neutralized. This makes the nuts much more digestible.

Stuart does this to the almonds he eats—he prepares enough in one soaking to last about 10 days. The three-stage process costs him no more than five minutes in total: to prepare the nuts for soaking, then the following morning to rinse them and spread them out to dry, and a few hours later to gather them and put them in the refrigerator. He has a handful of the almonds every day, with his breakfast oatmeal (or porridge, as it's called in its home country, Scotland).

The soaked nuts—once they have been removed from the brine, rinsed and left to dry naturally for a few hours—must be stored in a refrigerator, or otherwise they will go bad after a few days or so. If the soaked nuts aren't to be kept in a refrigerator, they should be thoroughly dried in a warm oven.

Another way to make nuts and peanuts digestible is to roast them.

Why you should you eat peanuts in shells

Eat dry-roasted, peanuts that come *in their shells*, rather than ones without their shells. The former are commonly available in the US.

When you grab a handful of peanuts in their shells, you grab fewer peanuts per handful because of the volume the shells take up—24 ounces of peanuts in shells equals about 16 ounces of just the peanuts themselves once the shells have been removed. And the act of removing the peanuts from the shells, and the fumbling it creates, diverts time and attention away from the act of eating.

Brad used to eat peanuts without their shells straight out of a jar, and all too often he would empty the jar in a sitting. Since he switched over to eating peanuts that come with their shells, and eating them out of a bag, he eats far fewer. So, he now gets the nutritional benefits, but without overeating.

Vinegar

According to a study published in the *European Journal of Clinical Nutrition*, some vinegar sprinkled on your food may increase satiety (the feeling of fullness), and thus may reduce the quantity of food you eat by suppressing appetite somewhat.

Vinegar and lemon juice are used in the traditional Mediterranean diet, which is noted for its healthful qualities. Stuart has lived in the Mediterranean area for over 25 years—in Cyprus—and has incorporated some local dietary customs into his daily fare, including cider vinegar, olives, extra virgin olive oil, and cheese made from the milk of goats and sheep.

Phytochemicals

Phytochemicals are chemical compounds that occur naturally in plant foods, including fruits, vegetables, whole grains, nuts, and legumes—but processing reduces their supply. The term usually refers to those chemicals that seem to be healthful. There are many phytochemicals, for example, carotenoids (in carrots), resveratrol (in grape skins), tannic acid and catechins (in tea), and flavanones (in citrus fruit). *Be sure that you have plenty of plant foods in your daily diet.*

Most people underestimate the number of calories in restaurant meals by around 600.

When you've read this chapter you'll know all you need to about eating out.

14

Eating out

Eating out is a major culprit in America's obesity epidemic. If you curtail your eating out, or at least implement better choices, you may be amazed by how much weight you can lose, readily.

A sit-down restaurant meal can be laced with hundreds if not thousands of hidden calories. And by the time fixings are added to a sub or salad, their advertised caloric values may be doubled or even tripled.

Fast food and "quick-service" food *alert*

Fast food consumption is one of the major reasons why many people eat excessively. *Fast food is designed to be addictive.*

The USDA found that men eat an average of 500 additional calories on the days they eat fast food as compared to the days in which they prepared their own meals.

Research by the NPD Group, a global market research company, claims that 77% of all meals purchased in the US (and eaten *at the time of purchase*) are from "quick-service" restaurants—better known as fast-food restaurants.

Fast-food eating is often a ticket to binge sessions. If you read the content in a typical fast-food value meal, you may be shocked with how many calories, and how much crud, it contains.

Be informed and discerning—read nutrition labels.

If you must indulge in this pseudo food for the time being, save it for your "treat day," and have it in moderation. But once you've been on the lifestyle-reform, weight-loss and health plan for a while, you'll probably lose your taste for crud.

If you stay clear of greasy burgers and fries from drive-thru restaurants—and do nothing else—you may be amazed by how much weight you'll shed.

Pizza used to be the staple of Brad's eating. Now, of course, he knows how many calories are in pizza. Just one slice can have 600 calories (including 30 grams of fat), which means that an entire pizza can have 5,000 calories (including 250 grams of fat).

Brad still eats pizza, but in moderation. And he creates his own tasty pies on 100% whole-wheat crust, and makes them small, thin and nutritious. Pizza *can* be healthy. For Brad, unhealthy delivered pizza is a distant memory.

If you're traveling, be aware of the establishments that provide healthy food. Subway® restaurants are known for healthy alternatives to burgers, but there are other good possibilities, too.

And it may even be possible to obtain a decent meal from some fast-food restaurants that have a reputation for providing crud, *but be selective, and watchful of your portion sizes and caloric intake.*

People have still lost weight while enjoying fast-food wraps, and healthy sandwiches and salads. But we aren't aware of people losing weight by regularly devouring bacon double cheeseburgers, and large fries.

Be skeptical when a quick-service restaurant claims that its food is a "healthy alternative." This statement isn't recognized by the FDA, and could be the basis of a misleading lure to get you in the restaurant's door. Take a minute to read the nutrition labels to see whether the "healthy alternative" is healthy. And find out whether the described portion size is what you're going to be served.

A study published by the *Journal of Consumer Research* found that people are likely to underestimate their meal's caloric content by as much as 35%. And a University of Mississippi study found that you're likely to consume 54% fewer calories if you review the restaurant's nutrition guide before you order.

Be informed and discerning—read nutrition labels.

Drive *past* the drive-thru

One of the dieters Brad interviewed is a sales rep who almost lives out of his car. Todd's daily fare used to consist of nothing but fast food, and his rotund physique showed it.

After he realized how much money he spent on his fast-food bill, he started to use his local grocery store to stock up on lean deli meats, 100% whole-wheat bread, fruits, vegetables, and all-natural meal replacement bars. He packed a small cooler with ice-cold water, nutritious meals, and sandwiches, which he consumed every three hours while on the road. As a result of that change alone, Todd lost 22 pounds in just over three months. And he still enjoyed his meals.

Whenever you travel by car, pack a little cooler with nutritious foods. It can take away the temptation to visit a drive-thru.

Too much of a good thing

Even when the only sandwiches and subs you eat are healthy, don't assume that you can eat them to your heart's content. Although these items can be healthy, you still must adhere to your prescribed portion sizes and caloric allocation per sitting.

While Brad's favorite sub is turkey breast on a 100% whole-wheat bun, he used to eat an entire foot-long sub several times a week, and wondered why he didn't lose weight. He now knows that he ingested too many calories per sitting. Even too much of a good thing is bad.

Even a modest six-inch sub can have too many calories if you aren't careful with the extras it contains.

Restaurant *alert*

Most restaurant food is loaded with calorie-laden enhancers that contribute to the mouth-watering taste. And as you learned in Chapter 6, this type of food is purposely layered with a combination of fat, sugar and salt in an effort to make you addicted to it, and "condition" you to revisit restaurants repeatedly.

Some dishes have multiple sticks of real butter melded into them. Mashed potatoes, rice, and vegetables taste great because they ooze with extra calories.

The butters, marinades, or calorie-laden sauces used to help flavor your meals at even fine restaurants can add more than 1,000 additional calories to a single meal.

You would probably be astonished if you knew what you were ingesting, even at fine restaurants.

To keep to a weight-loss and health plan at a restaurant, insist that your food is prepared to your liking—for example, without the butter or calorie-laden enhancers. And order smaller portions if they are available, or otherwise eat half of the meal at the restaurant, and take the other half home. Most restaurants serve double or even triple the quantity of food you should eat at a sitting.

According to the New York City Department of Health, 9 out of 10 people underestimate the number of calories in restaurant meals by around 600.

While most dieters generally pass on white bread or appetizers, some of them intentionally reduce their appetite by eating a whole-wheat bun or two before the main course, and then are satisfied with a reduced main course. This decreases their overall caloric intake.

Because most restaurant appetizers add too many calories to the overall meal, you should save your calories for the main course— the reason you're at the restaurant in the first place.

Perhaps have a nutritious salad in lieu of an appetizer. It's a good way to reduce your appetite before the main meal. But make sure your salad doesn't have excessive croutons or calorie-laden toppings.

Many low-fat or fat-free salad dressings usually make up for their lack of flavor with added sugar or high-fructose corn syrup. They should be avoided. Instead, enjoy a salad dressing that's low in calories, like the house vinaigrette, served on the side. The vinegar in the vinaigrette may even be an effective appetite suppressant.

Some dieters take their own single-serving salad dressing packets with them to restaurants.

Most desserts are loaded with calories and would take hours of exercise to work off. Do you really need a fattening dessert after all the calories you ate with the main course?

According to Brian Wansink, Ph.D., director of the Cornell University Food and Brand Lab, people tend to overeat when dining in a fun, comfortable social setting among friends. Many people may eat twice as much in such a setting as they would normally, mostly due to spending a longer time in the restaurant than usual, and while paying more attention to the fun atmosphere than the food.

And according to research from the University of California, the dim lighting of a restaurant can relax your inhibitions, and cause you to eat more.

Avoid "shared food" — for example, at sports-themed restaurants and taverns. Research from the State University of New York at Buffalo found that men who ate with a group of male friends — via plates of calorie-laden appetizers, nachos, wings, or pizza — consumed 60% more calories than when they ate with a woman. And food of that type is very unhealthy.

If you're trying to lose weight, why eat at a sports-themed restaurant or tavern in the first place? The atmosphere there can be fun and exciting, but you may be hard pressed to find anything healthy to eat, and the portion sizes are usually excessive.

Many compulsive overeaters, like Brad, should avoid these situations. The temptation to overeat, and undo possibly weeks of good weight-loss work, is too great. And many compulsive overeaters must forgo the binger's paradise, and Brad's Achilles heel — all-you-can-eat buffets.

Another benefit of cutting down on outings to restaurants is that they are expensive. By not regularly dining at restaurants with his wife, Brad saves nearly $4,000 a year. Eating out regularly adds up even more if

you're feeding children, too. If you eliminate most of your eating at restaurants, you'll easily be able to afford nutritious foods so that you can eat better at home. *And* you'll probably still have a lot of the savings left over.

And watch your snacking at entertainment venues. A large tub of buttered, movie-theater popcorn can have 1,750 calories (including 115 grams of fat). Some movie-theater candy can contain over 1,000 calories (including 160 grams of sugar and high-fructose corn syrup).

While they can be alluring and tasty, carnival fries, nachos with oozing cheese, cotton candy, corn dogs, foot-long stadium dogs, gigantic pretzels, pizza, fried steakburgers, and many other stadium staples are terrible for your weight-loss aspirations.

Don't assume all salads are healthy

Many people assume that a salad is a healthy alternative to a side dish, or a healthy alternative to a meal. But many fast-food or restaurant salads are not healthy. For example, McDonald's® Premium Southwest Salad with Newman's Own Creamy Southwest Dressing has more calories than their fat-laden Quarter Pounder. And many restaurant salads are well over 1,000 calories, if not 2,000 or more. While the lettuce has hardly any calories, be aware of the high-calorie dressings and toppings that make these salads so tasty.

Watch your multi-course meals

If you're not careful, you can ingest several thousand calories in a single, multi-course meal.

Who needs to eat a burrito the size of a large shoe? And do you really need a triple- or quadruple-decker cheeseburger with double-bacon?

A huge bowl of spaghetti with heavy sauce can exceed 2,500 calories, and a 22-ounce ribeye steak can contain 2,200 calories (including 110 grams of fat). Add a side dish, a drink, and an appetizer, and you may end up with 3,000 to 4,000 (or more) calories.

"Emergency" fast-food choices

Stuart and Brad don't endorse conventional fast food, but here are some acceptable "emergency" choices available at fast-food providers for when you're stuck on the road with no other options. These are much healthier than the crud that most people associate with fast food.

Subway®

Six-inch oven roasted chicken breast (310 calories)

Six-inch roast beef (290 calories)

Six-inch Subway Club® (320 calories)

Six-inch turkey breast (280 calories)

Six-inch Veggie Delite® (230 calories)

Six-inch cheese breakfast omelet sandwich (410 calories)

Cold cut combo salad with fat-free Italian dressing (285 calories)

Turkey breast wrap (380 calories)

Veggie Delite® Wrap (330 calories)

Wendy's®

Ultimate chicken grill sandwich (320 calories)

Grilled chicken go wrap (260 calories)

Jr. cheeseburger (270 calories)

McDonald's®

Egg McMuffin (300 calories)

Hamburger (250 calories)

Cheeseburger (300 calories)

Filet-O-Fish® (380 calories)

Chipotle BBQ Snack Wrap® Grilled (260 calories)

Premium grilled chicken classic sandwich (420 calories)

Southwest salad with grilled chicken (320 calories)

Newman's Own low-fat balsamic vinaigrette (40 calories)

Burger King®

Tendergrill™ chicken sandwich without mayo (400 calories)

Tendergrill™ garden salad without dressing (240 calories)

Hamburger (330 calories)

Cheeseburger (330 calories)

Ham omelet sandwich (290 calories)

Taco Bell®

Grilled steak soft taco (260 calories)

Spicy chicken soft taco (170 calories)

Bean burrito (330 calories)

Zesty Chicken Border Bowl® without dressing (350 calories)

Arby's®

Regular roast beef sandwich (320 calories)

Grilled chicken fillet sandwich (396 calories)

Ham and Swiss melt sandwich (268 calories)

KFC®

Oven Roasted Twister® without sauce (330 calories)

Tender Roast® sandwich without sauce (300 calories)

Roasted Caesar salad with light dressing (260 calories)

Don't assume that just because something *sounds* healthy, it actually *is* healthy

In certain countries, many McDonald's locations now put nutrition information on some of their product packaging. Many locations also have have nutrition information for popular items on their paper placemats (although it may be on the *underside*), and on their websites.

So, if people are being made aware of what they are eating, why do so many people continue to eat unhealthy, high-calorie, processed food?

Because people are oblivious of this posted information.

A Yale University observational study published in the May 2009 issue of the *American Journal of Public Health* showed that only 6 out of 4,311 people (0.14%) looked at on-premises nutrition information at fast-food restaurants—including McDonald's—before purchasing their food.

Are you aware of what you're eating at McDonald's, for example? Which has more calories, a Premium Grilled Chicken Club Sandwich, or a Quarter Pounder®?

If you chose the grilled sandwich, you guessed wrongly. The Premium Grilled Chicken Club Sandwich has 530 calories, while the Quarter Pounder® has "only" 410 calories. And their Premium Crispy Chicken Club Sandwich (which has fried chicken) has a whopping 630 calories.

There are some deceptively "healthy sounding" options on the menu at McDonald's—like their five-piece Chicken Selects® Premium Breast Strips—but which have 660 calories and 40 grams of fat, for example. *So, not so healthy, really.*

From now on, don't make assumptions about food. *Be informed and discerning—read nutrition labels.*

Did you know that 92%-fat-free burgers may still have 50% fat?

Most people don't really know what they are eating.

This chapter will educate you on hidden surprises, and how they affect your ability to lose weight.

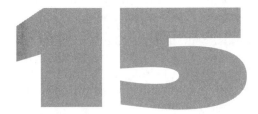

Know what you're eating

Most people don't understand what's on a product's label. And there are many deceptive things about food packaging you may not be aware of.

Understand the words on the label

Be informed and discerning—read nutrition labels.

The ingredients listed on the food's nutrition label are in the order of significance. Pay particular attention to the first few, especially the first three, because these are the most predominant.

Be especially leery of high-fructose corn syrup, corn syrup, sugar, hydrogenated and partially hydrogenated oil, trans fats, chemicals, or anything that says "enriched." That crud is bad for your health *and* your weight-loss aspirations.

According to the FDA:

> *"Free" contains insignificant calories, fat, sodium, or sugar.*
>
> *"Reduced" has at least a 25% reduction in calories, fat, sodium, or sugar relative to the regular version.*

"Light" has at least a 50% reduction in calories or fat relative to the regular version.

"High" means the item contains at least 20% of the daily values for the specified nutrient, per serving.

Furthermore, *low-calorie* has fewer than 120 calories per serving, while *low-fat* has fewer than 3 grams of fat per serving—based on a 3.5-ounce serving size. And *nonfat* and *fat-free* have under half a gram of fat per 3.5-ounce serving.

If a food is labeled *healthy*, it must contain under 3 grams of fat per serving—with less than a gram of saturated fat, fewer than 480 grams of sodium, fewer than 60 mg of cholesterol, and must contain at least 10% of the recommended daily values for vitamin A, vitamin C, iron, calcium, protein, or fiber.

When buying organic foods, the US Department of Agriculture (USDA) says that *100% organic* is verified to be free of pesticides, antibiotics, hormones, or artificial ingredients. *Organic* means that it's at least 95% organic. And *made with organic ingredients* means that the food contains at least 70% organic ingredients.

Just because a food manufacturer includes *good source, wholesome, natural, free range, antibiotic-free* or *hormone-free* on a product's label doesn't guarantee that the food is nutritious. Many of these claims aren't recognized by the USDA, and are advertising hype.

Most people don't understand how to read a Nutrition Facts label. To help rectify this, the FDA has created a web page entitled "How to Understand and Use the Nutrition Facts Label."

Please take a few minutes to review this web page at www.cfsan.fda.gov/~dms/foodlab.html

Deceptive serving sizes

Some normal-sized drink bottles contain two-and-a-half servings, but how many people drink an exact serving size of a beverage and put the rest back in the fridge?

What may seem to you to be a normal portion of food or drink may actually be two or three servings in terms of the serving sizes used on food labels. *You must know precisely how much food or drink you consume in order to know its true caloric value.*

A container typically has *multiple* serving sizes. Many snacks, for example, are misleading in their caloric content. While some are truly single-serving sizes, many small bags of potato chips, for example, may have two-and-a-half servings per bag even though they appear to be the same size as a bag that *has* a single serving.

Be informed and discerning—*read nutrition labels*. And understand the serving sizes referred to on the labels.

Odd-shaped foods, such as a wedge-shaped piece of pizza, can often lead to a miscalculation concerning how big the serving size is, and how many calories you're consuming. Be aware of this, and always eat *less* rather than more if you're unsure of the serving size you're eating.

Why 92%-fat-free burgers may have 50% fat

The leanness of meats is determined by weight, *not* caloric value. Consider the nutrition label from a 92%-lean-ground beef patty. A four-ounce patty has 160 calories and nine grams of total fat. A gram of fat has the energy value of 9 calories, so nine grams of fat has 81 calories, which comes to 50% of the total caloric value of the burger.

Watch your sodium intake

While sodium is necessary to help transport vital nutrients around the body, send nerve messages, and contract muscles, many people ingest far more of it than they need.

Because many people consume a lot of processed food, they consume a lot of salt, and hence sodium. Although some foods may not taste salty, they can still be loaded with sodium. And many people sprinkle salt on their already salty meals.

While dietary guidelines say that children under 13 should have no more than 2,200 mg of sodium a day, many fast-food child meals can have two to three times this amount in a single serving.

Common meals at popular restaurants can have more than 7,000 mg of sodium per entrée. Add in the appetizer, sides, and additional salt sprinkled over the food, and the grand total of sodium per sit-down meal can be huge. Then factor in the other sodium-rich meals that are consumed during the day, and it's no wonder why many people are so bloated due to excess water retention.

Excessive sodium intake may contribute to dangerous conditions such as high blood pressure, stroke, osteoporosis, and exercise-induced asthma.

According to msnbc.com, the American Heart Association (AHA) and some other medical entities want stronger labels on foods with high-salt content, and are calling for a 50% reduction in the amount of salt in packaged and processed foods. Cutting sodium intake by half would prevent 150,000 deaths from cardiovascular disease each year, according to estimates from the National Heart, Lung, and Blood Institute.

To reduce the negative effect of sodium on blood pressure, load up on healthy, potassium-rich foods. Oats, wheat, potatoes, nuts, legumes, corn, squash, tomatoes, bananas, oranges, and dates are rich in potassium, for example, but with very little (if any) sodium.

Look for foods that are low in sodium. According to the AHA, *sodium-free* has fewer than 5 mg of sodium per serving, *very low-sodium* has 35 or fewer per serving, and *low-sodium* has 140 or fewer per serving.

To rank foods by concentrations of specific nutrients, visit: www.nutritiondata.com/tools/nutrient-search

Ironically, a great way of getting rid of bloating (besides *reducing* your sodium intake and *increasing* your potassium intake) is to drink *more* water. If you don't drink enough fluids, your body will compensate by releasing the hormone vasopressin, which triggers your body to retain fluids by reducing urination.

Why are many foods high in sodium?

Besides enhancing taste, salt is used as a food preservative. According to the FDA, "Salt is considered antibacterial because it restricts bacterial growth in many foods. It preserves foods by lowering the amount of 'free' water molecules in foods. Bacteria need moisture in order to thrive, so without enough 'free' water, they cannot grow well in foods that contain salt."

Be careful when buying bread products

While many weight-loss plans banish all breads, some bread products are desirable because many people would be lost if they were told that they could no longer eat sandwiches.

Almost all real-life dieters agree that 100% whole-wheat and 100% whole-grain bread products are acceptable. For many people, a zero-carbohydrate lettuce burger sans bun is no way to live.

As a compromise, some dieters opt for open-faced sandwiches, meaning that they use only the bottom piece of bread on their sandwich. And some people make a mini-sandwich by using one piece of bread folded over. These modifications add up to a big reduction in calories over the long-term.

The refining process generally removes some of the nutritious portions of the grains. When you buy *100% whole-grain* or *100% whole-wheat* bread products, make sure that *whole-wheat* or *whole-grain* is the first ingredient listed on the label.

Bread that has three to five grams of fiber per slice, and three grams of protein, will likely have 70 to 100 calories. Bread products vary in their slice thicknesses. Different slices have different caloric values.

Be informed and discerning—read nutrition labels.

When wheat bread *isn't* wheat bread

When bread's labeling says *wheat bread, whole-grain, whole-wheat, whole-grain blends,* or *made with whole grains,* this can mean that it may be only 1% wheat, or has but a trace of whole grains. And *enriched* is usually a sign that some sort of processing has gone on.

If the label doesn't say *100% whole-wheat,* or *100% whole-grain,* the labeling was probably designed to try to mislead you. And make sure the word *whole* is included, because the claim *100% wheat,* for example, is meaningless.

If the first or second ingredient listed is *wheat flour,* this doesn't necessarily mean *whole-wheat.* And the terms *multi-grain, seven-grain, harvest grain, stone-ground,* or *cracked wheat* don't tell you if the grains are whole or refined.

Read food labels, be informed and discerning, and make your purchasing decisions accordingly.

Watch out for certain cereals

Some cereals have more *total* sugar than a bowl of candy. In fact, some breakfast cereals contain four or five different types of sugars—which may include sugar (probably sucrose), high-fructose corn syrup, brown sugar, molasses, and honey. And many cereals are loaded with hydrogenated oil.

Avoid pseudo cereals like those. Instead, look for ones that are low in sugar, but high in protein and fiber, and made with natural ingredients.

Be informed and discerning—read nutrition labels.

And consider making oatmeal (porridge) your breakfast staple, as Stuart and Brad's wife have for many years.

Even accurate food labels can be misleading

While the list of ingredients on a food's nutrition label must be listed in the order of significance, even an accurate label can be misleading.

Let's look at the example of the breakfast cereal that contains five different types of sugars. While they are all sugar, when they are listed *separately* each will be placed much further down the list than if they were grouped as a single entry. And chances are that none of the individual sugars will be listed among the first two or three most predominant ingredients. This disguises the total quantity of sugar contained in the cereal.

For example, while the label may indicate that the cereal contains only 10 or 12 grams of sugar per serving (the refined, white sugar, or sucrose), the true amount of added sugar may be one-third to one-half of the total ingredients *when all types of sugars are considered.*

Understanding the new *Nutrition Facts* label

The new Nutrition Facts label makes it easier for people to know what's in the food they eat. Comparing these labels will help you to know which foods have lower fat or fewer calories, which foods make healthy snacks, and which are acceptable for special diets. And if you're a parent, use the new label to make informed food choices that will benefit your entire family.

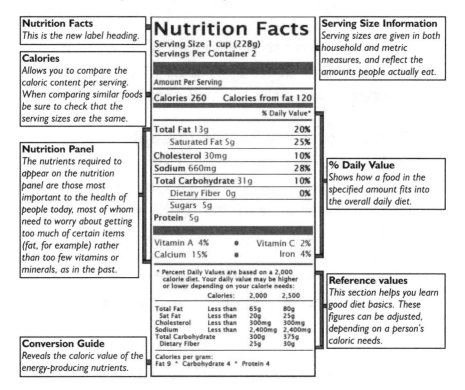

Nutrition Facts
This is the new label heading.

Calories
Allows you to compare the caloric content per serving. When comparing similar foods be sure to check that the serving sizes are the same.

Nutrition Panel
The nutrients required to appear on the nutrition panel are those most important to the health of people today, most of whom need to worry about getting too much of certain items (fat, for example) rather than too few vitamins or minerals, as in the past.

Conversion Guide
Reveals the caloric value of the energy-producing nutrients.

Serving Size Information
Serving sizes are given in both household and metric measures, and reflect the amounts people actually eat.

% Daily Value
Shows how a food in the specified amount fits into the overall daily diet.

Reference values
This section helps you learn good diet basics. These figures can be adjusted, depending on a person's caloric needs.

Nutrition Facts

Serving Size 1 cup (228g)
Servings Per Container 2

Amount Per Serving

Calories 260   Calories from fat 120

% Daily Value*

Total Fat 13g	**20%**
Saturated Fat 5g	**25%**
Cholesterol 30mg	**10%**
Sodium 660mg	**28%**
Total Carbohydrate 31g	**10%**
Dietary Fiber 0g	**0%**
Sugars 5g	
Protein 5g	

Vitamin A 4%	•	Vitamin C 2%
Calcium 15%	•	Iron 4%

* Percent Daily Values are based on a 2,000 calorie diet. Your daily value may be higher or lower depending on your calorie needs:

		Calories:	2,000	2,500
Total Fat	Less than		65g	80g
Sat Fat	Less than		20g	25g
Cholesterol	Less than		300mg	300mg
Sodium	Less than		2,400mg	2,400mg
Total Carbohydrate			300g	375g
Dietary Fiber			25g	30g

Calories per gram:
Fat 9 * Carbohydrate 4 * Protein 4

Information as provided by the USDA Food and Nutrition Service at http://www.fns.usda.gov/tn/parents/nutritionlabel.html

For much more detailed information on how to understand and use a Nutrition Facts label, visit www.cfsan.fda.gov/~dms/foodlab.html

Did you know that you can lose weight while eating ordinary foods like burgers, fries, tacos, and steak?

By showcasing what real people eat to lose weight and keep it off, this chapter gives you ideas so that you can enjoy your favorite foods while you lose weight.

When you've read this chapter you'll be able to create your own menus.

16

Real-life recipes for tasty meals

These recipes provide examples of how you can eat normal foods while on a weight-loss plan. These meals are what Brad ate during his weight-loss, and what he eats now while keeping the weight off.

Margarine caveat

Most butters and margarines add excessive calories; and margarine, generally, is unhealthy. But Brad found a great tasting "margarine" — Smart Beat Smart Squeeze™ nonfat margarine spread, that's only five calories per serving. Other "lowfat" margarines and butters can be as high as 35 to 50 calories or more per serving. The extra calories make a big difference over the long-term. He still uses Smart Squeeze™ everyday, in very small amounts. It's an important part of his success because he can prepare tasty meals that are still low in calories. And although it's called a margarine, and it's processed, it has no fat, and no trans fats, so it doesn't have the unhealthy constituents that most margarines have. Brad also uses I Can't Believe It's Not Butter!® Original Buttery Spray, which has zero calories per serving.

Hamburgers

Make your own hamburgers with 96%-lean ground beef and cook them on a grease-draining grill, or on an outdoor gas grill. Add a slice of fat-free cheese, and lettuce, if you desire, and serve on a fluffy 100% whole-wheat bun. Each quarter-pound (four-ounce) burger will provide approximately 300 calories, 32 grams of protein, 22 grams of carbohydrates, and 10 grams of fat. Use organic or sugar-free ketchup.

Burgers can also be made from ground turkey breast.

The illusionary big burger

Make your food appear larger via optical illusion. Brad tricks himself into thinking he's eating huge hamburgers. He makes his quarter-pound patties narrower, but thicker. He also mounds up some lettuce, and tops the burger with an extra-fluffy bun. His hamburgers appear huge, but, in reality, they are smaller and have fewer calories than the thicker, wider burgers he used to prepare. See how you can make your own four-ounce hamburger patty appear thicker.

Sandwiches

Lean turkey breast, chicken breast, or roast beef sandwiches, served on 100% whole-wheat bread with a dollop of fat-free mayonnaise, some fat-free cheese, and lettuce, can be enjoyed on a regular basis. Choose the most select, wholesome cuts of deli meats. And don't be afraid of an occasional peanut butter and jelly sandwich. Use all-natural peanut butter, and sugar-free or all-natural jams or jelly. Each sandwich will provide approximately 300 to 400 calories, depending on the ingredients.

Teriyaki chicken strips

Get some chicken breasts, trim off the fat, slice them into thin strips or nuggets, and bake them—depending on thickness—at 350 to 400 degrees for 15 to 25 minutes. You can also prepare a similar delicacy on the outdoor grill. Many marinades are loaded with high-fructose corn syrup. Avoid them. Check nutrition labels. Stick to organic or sugar-free sauces for the marinade.

Homemade fries

Slice some potatoes into small wedges, and bake them at 375 degrees for 30 minutes. Add a little organic or sugar-free ketchup, and vinegar, and you'll swear that you're eating "carnival fries."

Ninety-six-percent-lean sloppy joes

Mix two pounds of ultra-lean ground sirloin with three-quarters of a can of sloppy joe mix. The key is to go light on the mix, to avoid unnecessary calories. Serve on a 100% whole-wheat bun. Each sandwich will provide approximately 300 calories, 32 grams of protein, 20 grams of carbohydrates, and 10 grams of fat. And the leftovers will provide sandwiches for several days.

The sloppy joes can also be made from ground turkey breast.

Tacos and burritos

As long as you use 100% whole-wheat shells, and keep the portion sizes in check, these can be enjoyed on a regular basis. Begin by stir-frying—with extra virgin olive oil—diced filet mignon, chicken breast, or lean beef. Warm the taco shell in the microwave or on the skillet, and enjoy your taco or burrito with fillings like shredded fat-free cheese, fat-free sour cream, and shredded lettuce. Each taco or burrito will provide approximately 300 to 400 calories depending on the ingredients.

Lean filet mignon and New York strip steak

Select a lean cut, trim off all visible fat, and keep your portion sizes in check. A lean six-ounce filet will have approximately 370 calories, 47 grams of protein, and 18 grams of fat, while a lean six-ounce New York strip steak will have approximately 340 calories, 49 grams of protein, and 14 grams of fat. Sirloin may be the leanest of the more economical cuts.

Tasty 200- to 400-calorie mini-meals

These tasty mini-meals provide examples of what you can eat while you adhere to the required portion size per sitting. Some of them are more nutritious than others, but all will help you to lose weight when eaten within the overall plan promoted in this book.

You may eat the mini-meals at any time you want. For instance, Brad sometimes has scrambled eggs for dinner. And you can modify any meal by substituting different meats, breads, vegetables and fruits.

For quick, easy meals, many of these mini-meals can be pre-cooked in large batches, and reheated, or prepared in single-serving sizes.

And you can also get more elaborate and creative with your meal preparation when you have the time.

Review the caloric content of any food at www.calorieking.com.

Portion sizes and calories per serving can vary greatly from brand to brand. For example, two slices of 100% whole-wheat bread may be cut into different thicknesses, and this can cause a variance of hundreds of calories. Be mindful of this when you assemble your mini-meals, and double check the caloric content for your particular brand and serving size. If a brand is mentioned, then it's a brand that Brad has tried, and recommends as tasty and nutritious.

Breakfast

Scrambled eggs with diced Canadian bacon, and toast

Two slices of 100% whole-wheat bread

Dollop of Smart Squeeze™ nonfat margarine

Two whole eggs scrambled

Thin slice of Canadian bacon, diced

Approximately 400 calories

> *Brad uses Canadian bacon because it's leaner than other cuts. Commonly known by that name in the US, it's also called back bacon or Irish bacon.*

All-natural waffles with a glass of milk

Sixteen ounces of skim milk

Two Kashi® Go Lean® all-natural frozen waffles

Dollop of Smart Squeeze™ nonfat margarine

Dollop of organic syrup

Approximately 380 calories

Breakfast burrito

A 100% whole-wheat tortilla shell

Two whole eggs scrambled

Quarter cup of fat-free, shredded cheese

Diced Canadian bacon

Approximately 400 calories

Egg substitute ham-cheese omelet with English muffin

Four ounces of Egg Beaters® egg substitute

Thin slice of lean ham diced into small pieces

Slice of all-natural, fat-free cheese diced into small pieces

Eighth of a teaspoon ground black pepper

PAM® No-Stick cooking spray or extra virgin olive oil

Thomas'® 100% whole-wheat English muffin

Dollop of Smart Squeeze™ nonfat margarine

Approximately 250 to 300 calories

Cereal and milk

Half cup of Post® grape-nuts cereal

Sixteen ounces of skim milk

Approximately 380 calories

Canadian bacon bagel with cheese and glass of milk

Thomas'® 100% whole-wheat mini bagel

Slice of Canadian bacon

Slice of fat-free cheese

Twelve ounces of skim milk

Approximately 370 calories

Sunny-side-up eggs, and toast

Two slices of 100% whole-wheat bread

Dollop of Smart Squeeze™ nonfat margarine

Two whole eggs cooked sunny side up with extra virgin olive oil

Approximately 275 to 300 calories

Oatmeal and milk

A packet Kashi® Heart to Heart™ oatmeal

Sixteen ounces of skim milk

Approximately 330 calories

Lunch or dinner

Peanut butter and jelly sandwich

Two slices of 100% whole-wheat bread

Two tablespoons of all-natural peanut butter

A tablespoon of all-natural jam

Approximately 350 calories

Roast beef sub

A 100% whole-wheat roll

Four ounces of lean roast beef

Two lettuce leaves

A tablespoon of fat-free mayonnaise

Approximately 320 calories

Tuna salad sandwich

Two slices of 100% whole-wheat bread

A can of water packed light tuna

A tablespoon fat-free mayonnaise

Approximately 235 calories

Ninety-six-percent-lean, quarter-pound hamburger

A 100% whole-wheat bun

Quarter pound of 96%-lean, ground sirloin

Dollop of organic ketchup

Approximately 310 calories

Whole-wheat spaghetti, with a glass of milk

One and three-quarters ounces of 100% whole-wheat spaghetti

Dollop of organic spaghetti sauce

Sixteen ounces of skim milk

Approximately 400 calories

Pork and black bean chili

Four ounces of lean, diced pork tenderloin

A cup of rinsed black beans

Fifteen ounces of diced tomatoes

Quarter cup of finely sliced red onion

One tablespoon of fat-free sour cream

Two tablespoons of minced garlic

One-and-a-half teaspoons of chili powder

Approximately 185 calories

Turkey breast sandwich with apple

A medium apple

Two slices of 100% whole-wheat bread

Four ounces of lean turkey breast

Two lettuce leaves

A tablespoon of fat-free mayonnaise

Approximately 350 calories

Turkey burger

A 100% whole-wheat bun

Quarter pound of lean ground turkey

Dollop of organic ketchup

Approximately 300 calories

Chicken and brown rice medley

Four ounces of lean, diced chicken breast

A cup (cooked) of whole-grain brown rice

Dollop of Smart Squeeze™ nonfat margarine

Approximately 320 calories

Swedish meatball hoagie, with lean, ground turkey breast

A packet McCormick® Swedish meatball mix (follow the instructions on the packet)

A pound of lean, ground turkey breast (or 96%-lean, ground sirloin)

An egg

A 100% whole-wheat hoagie bun

Approximately 200 calories per four-ounce serving for meatballs alone

Approximately 350 calories, served on a 100% whole-wheat hoagie bun

Chicken breast, and potato

Four ounces of lean chicken breast

A medium potato

Quarter cup of fat-free, shredded cheese

A tablespoon of fat-free sour cream

Approximately 300 calories

The big chicken salad

Two cups of salad greens or lettuce

Four ounces of lean, diced chicken breast

Quarter cup of fat-free, shredded cheese

Two tablespoons of low-calorie balsamic vinaigrette dressing (or a salad dressing of your choice)

Approximately 225 to 250 calories

Chili made with lean, ground turkey breast

A packet McCormick® chili mix

A pound of lean, ground turkey breast (or 96%-lean, ground sirloin)

Sixteen ounces of tomato sauce or spaghetti sauce

(Look for organic or low fat/sugar varieties)

Sixteen-ounce can of kidney beans

Approximately 200 to 250 total calories per four-ounce serving

Chicken burrito

A 100% whole-wheat tortilla shell

Four ounces of lean, diced chicken breast

Quarter cup of fat-free, shredded cheese

A tablespoon of fat-free, sour cream

Approximately 375 calories

Pork barbecue wrap

A 100% whole-wheat tortilla shell

Four ounces of lean, diced pork tenderloin

Quarter cup of fat-free, shredded cheese

A tablespoon of barbeque sauce

A tablespoon of fat-free, sour cream

Approximately 375 calories

Turkey tortilla panini

A 100% whole-wheat tortilla shell

Four ounces of lean, diced turkey breast

Quarter cup of fat-free, shredded cheese

Quarter cup of roasted red pepper strips

Quarter cup of finely sliced red onion

Approximately 375 calories

Shrimp with brown rice

Four ounces of shelled shrimp cooked to your liking

(Flavor with garlic or other seasoning)

A cup (cooked) of brown rice

Dollop of Smart Squeeze™ nonfat margarine

Approximately 200 calories

Catfish sandwich

Four ounces of baked catfish

(Can be pre-cooked in larger batches)

Two slices of 100% whole-wheat bread, or a 100% whole-wheat bun

A tablespoon of fat-free mayonnaise

Approximately 275 to 300 calories

Seared salmon with wild rice

Five-ounce piece of salmon

(Sear salmon two-and-a-half minutes per side on hot frying pan with extra virgin olive oil)

A cup (cooked) of wild rice

Dollop of Smart Squeeze™ nonfat margarine

Approximately 350 calories

Grilled snapper with whipped potatoes

Four ounces of grilled snapper

(Can be pre-cooked in larger batches)

A medium potato whipped with fork

(Can be pre-cooked in larger batches and whipped with mixer)

Dollop of Smart Squeeze™ nonfat margarine

Approximately 290 calories

Snacks

Glass of milk

Sixteen ounces of skim milk

Approximately 180 calories

Yogurt

Six-ounce Yoplait® Light single-serving yogurt

Approximately 170 calories

Glass of milk with handful of peanuts

Sixteen ounces of skim milk

An ounce of peanuts without shells

Approximately 350 calories

Bars

E-fit foods® 3BAR® all-natural energy bar (210 calories)

Kashi® all-natural crunchy protein and fiber bar (180 calories)

Kashi® TLC™ crunchy granola bar (180 calories)

Clif® Builders® natural protein bar (270 calories)

The caloric values of bars vary greatly by brand and portion size. Check the nutrition labels.

All-natural quick snacks

Peanuts, dry roasted, without shells, an ounce (170 calories)

Almonds, dry roasted, an ounce (169 calories)

Cashews, dry roasted, an ounce (163 calories)

Pistachios, dry roasted, an ounce (162 calories)

Banana, medium (105 calories)

Apple, medium (81 calories)

Orange, medium (62 calories)

Seedless grapes, a cup (58 calories)

Raisins, dried, half cup (109 calories)

Peach, medium (37 calories)

Strawberries, a cup (45 calories)

Pear, medium (98 calories)

Kiwi, medium (46 calories)

Dates, five medium (114 calories)

Tangerine, medium (37 calories)

Baby carrots, three ounces (30 calories)

Low-calorie toppings and condiments

Heinz® sugar-free ketchup, a tablespoon (5 calories)

Smart Squeeze™ nonfat margarine spread, a tablespoon (5 calories)

Kraft® Miracle Whip nonfat dressing, a tablespoon (15 calories)

Kraft® fat-free cheese singles, a slice (30 calories)

Up Country Organics® Balsamic Vinaigrette dressing, two tablespoons (5 calories)

French's® classic yellow mustard, a teaspoon (0 calories)

Generally, obese people are less active than lean people, and this is a major factor behind their heavier weights.

Based on the activities that real people utilized to help them to lose weight and keep it off, this chapter will give you ideas on how to get moving.

17

Get moving

To lose weight, you *must* use up more calories than you take in. Don't be a couch potato.

But, in many cases, becoming more active isn't merely about applying some willpower and organization. There's often a physiological explanation for inactivity.

For example, consistent fatigue can devastate your ability to lose weight and keep it off. It's a very common problem among overweight people.

If you suffer from consistent fatigue, acknowledge its seriousness, discover the cause, and *put it right*.

If you haven't already, please study Chapter 8 to see if there are physiological problems that explain why you may find it so difficult to be active. Treating the problems could transform your ability to be active in general, and to be a regular exerciser.

Researchers at Missouri University concluded that periods of four hours or more of inactivity caused a near shutdown of an enzyme that controls the metabolism of fat. And with this enzyme shut down, the subjects in the study stored fat in lieu of using it for energy. But breaking the extended period of inactivity—by taking a walk, or by standing—kept this enzyme much more active.

No matter how busy you may be, there really *is* time to be more active. But you don't have to go to a gym.

When you go shopping, return your cart to the cart corral.

Go window-shopping.

Take a walk during your lunch break.

Organize a co-worker lunch-time walking group.

Walk around when you're making a cell phone conversation.

When you converse with someone, combine it with a walk.

Take an after-dinner walk.

Wash and wax your car.

Clean your garage.

Clean your house.

If you have a lawn, mow it with a push mower.

Rake leaves, pull out weeds, plant a garden.

Walk your dog. If you don't have a dog, borrow a neighbor's, or volunteer at a local animal shelter.

Do chores that you've been putting off.

Stand at social events.

Park farther from your destination each time you use your car.

Use the stairs whenever possible.

A tale of a more active life

According to a study conducted at the University of North Carolina at Wilmington, people who begin a sedentary office job gain an average of 16 pounds of fat in their first eight months.

Let's suppose Brad didn't have his current sedentary career. What if he was a full-time personal trainer, or a landscape laborer? These are strenuous careers, and he would be constantly on his feet and using his hands.

By being active—rather than sitting and typing into a computer—he could burn 1,000 additional calories a day. So, all other things being the same, Brad could routinely burn an additional 5,000 to 7,000 calories a week from such a change in his activity level.

Are obese women less active?

A study published in the journal *Obesity* concluded that obese women, generally, are less active than lean women, and this is a major cause for their heavier weight.

According to the study, on a daily average, obese women stood two hours less and sat two-and-a-half hours more than normal-weight women. And the study noted that lean women burned an additional 315 calories a day because of this.

By spending two to three more hours on their feet—by standing, working, cleaning, or walking—obese women could burn the caloric equivalent of about 32 pounds of fat a year.

Simple activities can burn *many* calories

Here are the approximate calories that an illustrative 200-pound man and 150-pound woman would burn during 30-minute bouts of various activities:

	200-pound man	*150-pound woman*
Running, 11 mph	645	550
Cycling, 20 mph	575	490
Jogging, 9 mph	540	460
Walking, 5 mph	285	245
Walking, 3 mph	120	100
Walking, 2 mph	90	75
Tennis	250	215

Golf (carrying clubs)	*160*	*140*
Weeding/gardening	*140*	*120*
House cleaning	*110*	*90*

Look at one or more energy expenditure counters on the internet, to get a feel for the calories burned from various activities at your bodyweight and gender. (Most counters are for *food*, however, not activity. "Calorie calculators" or "activity calorie counters" may be more accurate terms.)

For example, comparing the same activity and duration, it will take more energy to move a 300-pound body than a 150-pound one. And, generally, men burn more calories per minute than women, even if they have the same weight, because of the men's greater muscle mass percentage.

Let's look at the big picture for one of the illustrations—the 200-pound man. For example, the addition of a three-mph, 30-minute daily walk could burn an additional 43,000 or so calories in a year, which would be the energy value of about 12 pounds of fat. As he becomes fitter he could increase the pace. A five-mph, 30-minute walk would burn more than twice as many calories, which, over 12 months, would be the energy value of about 30 pounds of fat.

Couple this increased energy *output* with a daily *input* reduction of 100, 200, or 300 or more calories, and you'll see how simple it is to lose 50 to100 pounds in year without upending your life.

Small daily changes can amount to huge changes over time.

Total calories burned vs. net calories burned, *clarification*

When you see an approximation of calories burned—in this book and other publications, and on the internet—these figures (unless otherwise noted) are for *total calories* burned during the specified activities.

But not all of these calories are burned from the actual activities or exercises themselves. The figures are for *all* of the calories your body burns during a *period* of activity or exercise, and *includes* the calories burned by your basal metabolism, and for food processing, that *you would still burn even if you were totally inactive.*

To get the precise number of calories burned from the actual activity or exercise *alone*, you must subtract your resting caloric consumption, which may be around 70 to 80 calories per hour for a 200-pound man, and perhaps 50 to 60 calories for a 150-pound woman. After subtracting this resting caloric consumption you would get the *net calories* burned, which would be what you actually burned directly from the activity or exercise.

The more your heart rate and oxygen consumption are boosted, the greater the net calories burned.

But don't be overly concerned about the difference between net calories and total calories.

Be aware of the difference but, because so few people or publications refer to net calories burned, you can still continue to work in *total calories* even though they are not as precise as net calories when assessing the caloric output from the activity or exercise *alone*.

The much bigger concern is *caloric output in general.* Boost yours through activity and exercise, as explained in this book.

And always remember that even walking slowly is much better for caloric consumption than sitting down, or lying on the couch. Get moving!

Little daily activities are NEAT

Performing little activities—like tapping your foot, gently swaying in your chair, or twirling your hair—on and off throughout the day can also have a big impact over time.

The scientific community (per research from the Mayo Clinic) refers to these little daily activities by the acronym NEAT—non-exercise activity thermogenesis.

Research by the Mayo clinic, via their NEAT Levine Lab, suggests that some slim people may be so because they are much more active in their daily activities, or NEAT. According to the study, little activities can add up to big differences in caloric expenditure. They can burn up to 20 extra calories per hour, or about 350 each day. And that alone could add up to the equivalent of 30 to 40 pounds of fat in a year.

Another form of NEAT is gum chewing. Chewing sugarless gum burns some calories, and fends off cravings. A study by the *New England Journal of Medicine* suggests that you can burn the energy equivalent of 11 pounds of fat a year by aggressive gum chewing. But be respectful to those in your surroundings, and chew your gum in a courteous manner.

Some people use a mini-cycle peddling device under their desk so they can peddle while they work.

Some mothers play with their children at the playground instead of sitting on the bench and merely watching.

Some people get out their chairs every hour on the hour and take a walk for a few minutes.

And some people even watch television while standing in front of it.

Brad read about an office of health-conscious workers who have their computers on counter-level tables. They stand while working at their computers, rather than sit. And their boss takes this concept a step farther. His counter-level table is above a slow-moving treadmill. He walks while he works.

And some people who work at home, or in private, tap their toes, or sway and nod their head to music.

Any little daily activity is almost always better than nothing. Be creative and come up with some fun things to keep yourself active.

To become aware of the effect of these little daily activities, some dieters strap on calorie-counting devices (such as a bodybugg®) to help measure the calories they burn during the day.

But whether any additional activity translates to weight-loss depends on other factors.

If you were previously in energy *balance*—that is, you took in through food and drink what you used up through basal metabolism, food digestion, and activity

and exercise—the *additional* activity *would* lead to weight-loss. But if you were previously in caloric *surplus*, unless the additional activity uses up *in excess* of that energy surplus, you won't lose weight. And if you *increase* your caloric intake as you increase your activity level, you may *gain* weight.

But remember that, in many cases, becoming more active isn't merely about applying some willpower and organization. There's often a physiological explanation for inactivity.

For example, consistent fatigue can devastate your ability to lose weight and keep it off. It's a very common problem among overweight people.

If you suffer from consistent fatigue, acknowledge its seriousness, discover the cause, and *put it right*.

If you haven't already, please study Chapter 8 to see if there are physiological problems that explain why you may find it so difficult to be active. Treating the problems could transform your ability to be active in general, and to be a regular exerciser.

This chapter sets the record straight on the benefits of exercise, and the misconceptions of exercise.

18

The truth about exercise

You don't *have to* exercise in order to lose weight, and you don't *have to* exercise in order to keep the weight off. *But, when done correctly, exercise will help you to lose weight and keep it off, although you don't have to go to a gym.*

Even just walking, and no other form of exercise, can make a huge difference *if* you set about it as we describe in this book.

You don't have to exercise in order to be healthy; but, when done correctly, exercise will help you to be healthier, fitter and more robust. *And the healthier, fitter and more robust you are, the better equipped you'll be for everything you do, including losing weight and keeping it off.*

Be wary of exercise fanatics

You don't *have to* exercise fanatically in order to lose weight and get in good physical condition. Excessive exercising does more harm than good.

Stuart has written several books on exercise, and for 15 years he published and edited a magazine on exercise.

He knows that most people who start an exercise program don't stick with it because they follow excessive, inappropriate or unenjoyable routines, and do too much too soon, and burn out.

Exercise can even be harmful. Because of ignorance or foolishness, many people have damaged their bodies through exercise.

Brad is an example of this type of foolishness. The nasty calf injuries he sustained in 2003 and 2004—when he dive-bombed into a vigorous exercise program—foiled his weight-loss aspirations for many months. He got frustrated, gave up, and regained weight. He probably would have made faster progress if he'd simply stuck to low-impact exercise like brisk walking, or using a low-impact machine such as a stair-stepper, or a spin bike.

No exercise program will do you any good unless you stick with it for the long haul. But you'll never stick with an exercise program for the long haul if you dislike it, get injured by it, burn out on it, or never make much if any progress on it.

The ideal progression of exercise

The ideal exercise regimen includes strength training (from lifting weights), cardiorespiratory training, and flexibility work. It's what Brad and Stuart do, *but it's not realistic for most people, especially those starting out on a weight-loss plan.*

There is, however, another component of an exercise plan, and the *easiest* one to perform—low-intensity exercise specifically for increasing energy output, with walking being the prime option. Walking can be done *immediately*, by almost *anyone, anywhere,* without cost or special equipment, and it suits any level of fitness. And if you do enough of it, it makes weight-loss *much* easier.

Never mind about the ideal exercise plan, at least not for now. Just get started on the minimum plan—*walking*.

With walking as your sole form of exercise, in combination with the dietary plan recommended in this book, you can strip yourself of all your excess fat. Many people, whose only exercise at the time was walking, have lost hundreds of pounds.

And even if your exercise regimen never graduates past walking, that's still valuable. More exercise would be better, but only if you do it willingly, and safely.

Don't make the classic mistake of taking on more exercise than you can handle to begin with, and sooner or later packing it all in.

Many weight-loss plans expect you to be gung-ho right out of the gate, in an effort to lose weight rapidly. This is dangerous guidance, and a recipe for failure.

High-intensity exercise has worked wonders for people who are already physically fit, especially youngsters, but it's not advised for out-of-shape people.

Start with *a little* exercise, add to it *gradually*, and as you improve your physical conditioning and see and feel the benefits, you're likely to acquire an increased interest in exercise, and take on *a bit more* exercise, and then *a bit more still*, and so on.

Wean yourself onto exercise by following the gradual progression of stages that's promoted in this book.

What everyone needs to do for weight-loss

Start with:

Walking, for weight-loss only, as explained in Chapter 19

Then progress to:

Advanced walking, *and other matters*, for increased weight-loss *and* for fitness, as explained in Chapter 20

Optional but highly recommended methods of advanced weight-loss training

Start with:

Advanced walking, *and other matters* (Chapter 20), *plus* **home strength training** as explained in Chapter 21

Then progress to:

Advanced walking, *and other matters* (Chapter 20), *plus* **home strength training** (Chapter 21), *plus* **home flexibility training** as explained in Chapter 22

The truth on age and exercise

The older you are, the more important it is that you exercise. You can add life to your years, and probably years to your life, but you must exercise safely and effectively, or otherwise the results will be injury, frustration, and failure.

The older you are, the more urgent it is not to make mistakes, and the more knowledgeable you need to be. "Use it or lose it, but don't abuse it." This applies to all ages, but especially to older people.

The older you are, the greater the need for training consistency. A young person can lay off training for a few months, and then return to previous fitness levels quickly; but it takes longer for an older person, and the chance of incurring problems is usually greater.

More and more seniors are enjoying their golden years while participating in sports and healthy activities. In fact, at the park where Brad regularly walks, inline skates, jogs, or bicycles, he frequently sees men and women—well into their golden years— walking, inline skating, jogging, and bicycling, too.

When Brad was jogging at the park last year, a lady who was about 80 years old blew past him on her inline skates.

It's never too late to start exercising. You're never too old to be fit.

Older people often have some body parts that have restricted ranges of motion. Although ranges of motion can usually be improved, limitations will remain for some people. Some exercises may need to be modified, or even avoided.

The truth on strength training

Here's why we highly recommend strength training:

Strength training is the single most productive form of exercise, for men and women. It builds strength, develops muscle, improves overall fitness, improves posture, slows the effects of aging, increases resistance to injury, and transforms physical appearance.

And it produces many invisible physiological benefits. For example, it can improve blood test results, reduce resting blood pressure, increase resting energy consumption (because of increased muscle mass), help control body fat, and improve cardiovascular efficiency.

Some scientists believe that safe, progressive, and consistent strength training may offer more health benefits than cardio exercise alone, or any other *single* exercise modality. (Cardio— short for cardiovascular exercise—is any activity that produces a sufficiently elevated heart rate to produce breathlessness for a sustained period. But it can't be done for long periods because its intensity is too high for such durations.)

According to some reports, there's typically a loss of about 1% of muscle mass a year from about age 50 *unless* strength training is employed to prevent the loss of muscle tissue.

There can even be a substantial loss of muscle before middle age. Strength training is important for young people, too.

Loss of muscle has many negative consequences, including strength decline, reduced caloric requirements, postural deterioration, reduced fitness, increased tendency to gain body fat, weakened resistance to injury, and deterioration in appearance.

According to research from the University of Pittsburgh Medical Center, you'll burn about 100 fewer calories a day at age 35, and 200 fewer at 45, as compared to age 25, *unless* you exercise appropriately to prevent the decline. If you don't exercise, you could gain 8 to 12 pounds of fat a year (provided you don't adjust your caloric intake to compensate).

Strength training also applies stress on the skeleton, which builds stronger, denser bones that are less likely to fracture during accidents. Strength training also builds or maintains the strong muscles required for dynamic balance, to help reduce the incidence of some accidents.

One of the functions of the muscular system is to maintain good posture. A steady contraction of the postural muscles—including the back, thighs, neck, shoulders, and abdominals—keeps the body in position. When these muscles lose strength, posture suffers. Strong postural muscles are critical.

Strong muscles produce health benefits that reduce the impact of aging. Strength training helps you to stay young for your years.

But strength training alone isn't enough. Without a supple body, for example, muscles lose some of their elasticity and ability to function properly, and tendons, ligaments and joint capsules become brittle. Tissues in general become more susceptible to injury, and the body ages at an accelerated rate.

The truth on flexibility training

Here's why we highly recommend flexibility training:

A supple body isn't valuable merely to help with the performance of an exercise program, although that in itself is important. Without a supple body, movements in general become restricted, there's reduced resilience or give in the body to withstand sudden movements safely, dynamic balance is impaired, posture is negatively affected, the loose connective tissue of the body loses its lubricating properties, and aging is accelerated. (Loose connective tissue fills the spaces between muscle and nervous tissue, and between bone and cartilage, tendons and ligaments, and joints and joint capsules.)

Insufficiently flexible muscles are also involved in physical problems such as chronic pain or discomfort in the knees and lower back.

As a result of stretching, the connective tissue in and around the muscle is expanded, including the connective tissue that surrounds the bundles of muscle fibers, and the wrappings of individual fibers. Nerves also respond positively to stretching.

Stretching elongates *muscles*, not tendons or ligaments. Tendons and ligaments are almost *inelastic*. Muscles need to be lengthened only a little in order to produce significant improvement in a joint's range of motion.

After a few months of regular stretching you may increase your flexibility substantially. Thereafter you'll need to keep stretching in order to maintain your improved flexibility.

When Brad was trying to heal a calf injury, part of his doctor-ordered rehab was stretching the muscle to keep it from repairing in a shortened, more injury-prone condition. He now stretches every day, thoroughly. And he now enjoys his exercise program without injuries. Brad was never an advocate of stretching until he realized from this experience how valuable it is.

Further benefits from exercise

Strength training together with cardiovascular exercise produces further health benefits, including increased high-density lipoprotein (the "good cholesterol"), reduced blood pressure, reduced risk of diabetes, reduced incidence of various cancers, reduced incidence of Alzheimer's disease, and reduced likelihood of depression.

The heart is a muscle. It can be trained for greater strength and endurance. The potential benefits are extensive—a more efficient and thus healthier cardiovascular system (heart, lungs, and blood vessels), and other internal health benefits.

The fountain of youth

The combination of strength training, stretching, cardiovascular work, healthy nutrition, and a healthy lifestyle is the closest we can get to the fountain of youth, but the exercise must be safe, and effective.

Time and effort put into a good exercise program aren't expenditures. They are investments in your health and well-being.

Brad's once wheelchair-ridden mother reversed serious health problems at age 75 by adopting healthy nutrition, and following an exercise program.

And Brad's aunt and uncle recently began an exercise program in their mid 70s. It made them look fabulous for their ages, and feel a quarter of a century younger.

Heart age reversal

Washington University did a study of overweight people in their fifties and sixties, published in a 2008 issue of the *American Journal of Physiology*. Those who took a brisk 45- to 60-minute daily walk during the one-year study lost an average of 22 pounds, and developed the heart efficiency of a 30 or 40 year-old.

Regardless of your age, you must get a doctor's clearance before starting an exercise program. Even minimal exercise may be harmful for someone in poor condition.

The joy of the benefits of exercise

It's possible to be supple, fit and vigorous throughout your life—to be in your "prime" lifelong, including during your senior years—*provided* you look after yourself properly.

Imagine the boost to your productivity, usefulness, and enjoyment of life that *sustained* vigor will produce.

The joy of exercise

Train properly using activities you like and you'll experience the *exercise high*. Your workouts will become an essential part of your life—and they will make you look, function and feel better.

Done properly, exercise isn't drudgery. It's a blessing, and a joy.

Women . . . "But we don't want big muscles"

Many women are unwilling to strength train because they think it will develop big muscles. This concern is unfounded, and prevents them from obtaining the benefits that strength training produces.

Few women can develop big muscles even if they wanted to. Women are limited in strength and muscular size because of their hormones. They lack the large quantities of testosterone that produce many of the male characteristics. Furthermore, women generally have wider hips and narrower shoulders than men, have a higher body-fat percentage, and carry most of their fat around their hips and thighs.

A tiny number of women have narrow hips, above-average testosterone production, longer muscle bellies than are typical for women, and little body fat. These women, when highly trained, and when enhanced by bodybuilding drugs, may obtain the extreme development of some competitive female bodybuilders. But for the huge majority of women, the development of big muscles is impossible.

Women should train for strength and muscle. Even a little additional muscle can improve appearance greatly, and yield substantial health benefits.

Brad's 47-year-old wife lifts weights with fervor three times a week. And she loves the way her strength-training workouts make her look and feel.

Strength training for weight-loss, fitness, and health

Brad used low- to moderate-intensity jogging (coupled with a little weight lifting) as his exercise combination of choice for his final weight-loss triumph, but this wasn't always the case.

There were many times when he lost a lot of weight while doing *no* jogging or running. When he was competing in powerlifting, in college, Brad repeatedly lost 30 to 50 pounds to get down to a weight-class limit of 165.25 pounds (because he regained his weight and got fat once a contest was over).

All he did for exercise back then was walking to class *and* the intensive powerlifting workouts. He burned many calories during the workouts, and burned additional calories around the clock as a result of the extra muscle he built.

But this was over 20 years ago, and Brad enjoyed lifting weights at that point of life. When he lost his weight during 2005 and 2006, the jogging he did then worked well, too. Although both forms of exercise worked well for weight-loss, the excessive outdoor jogging took a toll on Brad's joints, and produced many injuries.

Now, Brad is once again working out with weights in lieu of excessive endurance work. And he now looks and feels even better than he did after his 2006 jogging-assisted triumph.

Many dieters place exaggerated importance on endurance work, which can be catabolic in nature, and break down muscle tissue. Consider how many dieters—men and women—become thin but scrawny. If they had built some muscle they would look better, and improve their health.

Generally, people end up doing what they enjoy for exercise, fitness or recreation. Some people like walking, others like jogging. Some like Pilates, others like yoga. Some like fitness DVDs. Some like dancing. Some play basketball. Some like a treadmill, stair-stepper, or spin bike. And some hike, or ride bicycles outdoors. *But whatever you do, make sure it's safe. You can't make progress if you're injured.*

But many men and women of all ages strength train. Both President Obama and Mrs. Obama strength train for fitness, and are advocates of its benefits. If they can make time for it, so can you. Follow their lead, and give it a try.

Powerlifting is a strength sport consisting of three lifts: the squat (where you squat with a barbell over your shoulders), the bench press (where you lie supine on a bench and lower the barbell to your chest and press it to arm's length), and the deadlift (where you lift a barbell from the floor until you're standing upright with your arms hanging vertically). Competitors are allowed three attempts at each lift, and their best effort at each contributes to their three-lift total.

Be leery of exercise gadgets

There have been many TV commercials for wacky exercise gadgets.

But there's no gadget that's going to magically speed up fat burning or muscle-gain compared with sensible training with conventional equipment.

Brad bought one of the push-up gizmos with rotating handles a few years ago, and followed the program. While he eventually could perform 100 consecutive push-ups, he never became ripped as a result of the gadget.

"Getting ripped" is the result of many factors, especially genetics.

Much of the exercise-equipment industry is full of lies and deception, along with fake testimonials provided by paid actors or models who claim that the gadget got them ripped.

But some of the muscle-building gadgets do provide alternatives to a gym membership, or to having multiple pieces of equipment around the home. But while some of them can provide constructive workouts if used properly, they can't get you ripped.

If you plan to buy exercise equipment, do some research via consumer websites, and make educated purchases.

Beware of abdominal gadgets

In an industry that preys on the gullible, many ab training gizmos may be the biggest rip-offs. Some of their ads are comical.

There's no device that, by itself, will give you defined abs in 8 to 12 weeks, or in any other time period.

The February 2008 issue of *Consumer Reports* noted that most of the "amazing results" depicted in infomercials are footnoted as "not typical," or stem from an overall "system" that includes a strict diet, and, in numerous cases, supplementary exercise. And *Consumer Reports* clearly notes that it would take a 165-pound person up to nine months to lose just a single pound of fat by *solely* utilizing the gadget under the recommended workout guidelines.

And from their tests, *Consumer Reports* found that most of the ab machines usually won't generate any better results that ordinary crunches performed correctly on the floor.

Don't fall victim to myths of abdominal training

Many myths of training the abs are perpetuated by companies and individuals who prey on ignorance. Here are seven:

Myth #1

Twisting movements will pare fat from the sides of your waist.

Go to most gyms and at some point you'll probably find people with a light bar across their shoulders, twisting from side to side. They do this under the mistaken belief that they will whittle away the fat on their waists. Some people have been doing this for years, without success. The twisting may, however, cause back problems.

Myth #2

Lots of ab work will pare fat from the front of your waist.

As with Myth #1, muscle and fat are different types of tissue. It's physiologically impossible to whittle away fat through working the muscle beneath the fat. Fat reduction in a specific spot of the body, through exercise, is impossible.

You could do three hours of abdominal work daily, but if your food intake and activity level don't combine to yield an overall energy deficit, you'll never reduce the fat around your waist. On the other hand, you could do no abdominal work, but if you're in sustained caloric deficit you'll draw on your energy stores and thus reduce your body fat.

Whether you do abdominal work is irrelevant in determining the amount of fat around your waist. But to build strong, well-developed abdominals, ab work is essential.

Myth #3

The abs need high reps.

To strengthen and develop the abdominals—which is all that ab work can do—keep the reps moderate and effort levels high, use sufficient resistance to make each set challenging, and gradually add resistance as you develop strength. Treat your abdominals like any other muscle.

Myth #4

The abs need daily work.

Although the abdominal muscles may tolerate more frequent work than most other body parts, they can be overtrained. Excessive training frequency for these muscles is connected to the mistaken belief that a lot of exercise for them will help reduce waist fat levels. Train your abdominals only two, or, at most, three times a week.

Myth #5

Everyone can develop a six-pack if they train and diet correctly.

Some people are genetically more likely to lay down fat on their waists than others. A few people may be lean throughout their bodies yet still have a layer of fat on their waists, whereas some others may achieve six-packs but have a thick layer of fat elsewhere on their bodies. The near-perfect bodies you see in advertising belong to genetically gifted specimens who have the natural ability to achieve lean waists.

Myth #6

Gadgets are needed to train the abs.

Some gadgets, properly used, do target the abdominals. There's nothing, however, a gadget can help you do that crunches can't, provided the crunches are done correctly. But many of the gadgets are ineffective and poorly made, and some are dangerous. Don't be misled by hype. Stick to crunches, which don't require special equipment, but do them well.

Myth #7

Electronic muscle stimulation is the easy way to great abs.

Electronic stimulation of muscles is a way to make people think they can exercise effectively without moving. There's some legitimate use for electro-muscle stimulation in physical therapy, but for healthy people it's a joke compared with proper resistance training.

Even if the electronic gadgets stimulated muscle like regular progressive resistance training does, you would still need to lose the fat to see your abdominals. No electronic stimulation will remove the fat that covers muscle.

Why aren't you exercising?

According to CNN.com/health, seven out of ten Americans abstain from exercise and do nothing for fitness, and only one in seven Americans exercises enough.

Many people consider regular exercise to be an essential part of their lives. And once you find activities you enjoy, and experience the benefits from exercise, you'll want to keep exercising.

Brad and Stuart don't work out because they have to; they work out because they want to. And they *make* time for it even though they have very busy lives.

Make haste slowly

Your body has tremendous abilities to adapt to and prosper from exercise *provided* you start out comfortably, and increase the demands *gradually*.

This applies to all forms of physical training—walking, strength training, stretching, and cardio work.

Make exercise *fun*

Many people view exercise as boring, and some people are intimidated by the word "exercise" because it suggests something unenjoyable. If that applies to you, instead of "exercise," substitute "activity," "sport," or "recreation." And adopt the attitude that you're doing activities you *enjoy*, to get your heart pumping in a rewarding way, to improve your health and appearance.

To stick with the plan, you must select exercise and activities that are *safe*, and that you *enjoy*. For instance, Brad's 47-year-old wife enjoys jogging, lifting weights, and speed walking with her dogs. She also enjoys using fitness DVDs.

The exercise-in-front-of-the-TV business—including fitness DVDs and videos, television programs, and internet sites—is a multi-billion-dollar industry.

There are some video games that have been helping people become active. Two of the more popular are Wii Fit™ and Wii Sport™. With Wii Fit™ you can use virtual personal trainers and engage in physical fitness programs. And with Wii Sport™ you can box or bowl, or play tennis, golf, or baseball. These games have helped sedate people to become active. Some senior centers even have Wii™ bowling leagues.

Whatever activity you *enjoy*, and that's *safe*, is fine by us as an alternative to walking as your minimum exercise plan. Just apply the same progression strategy to it as we recommend, in the next chapter, for walking.

How much do ultra-fit celebrities exercise?

It seems that whenever celebrities lose weight, they appear on the cover of magazines and are regarded as weight-loss experts. Some of these "experts" get major book deals. Ironically, despite the hype, they do nothing out of the ordinary.

Besides eating properly and possessing terrific genetics, most fit-appearing celebrities exercise their butts off. And they may have their own chefs, nutritionists, personal trainers, some surgical assistance, and even drug or hormone "supplementation."

Examine the workouts that some of these celebrities perform, and you'll see what it takes to look buff. You can't get lean and fit by lying on the couch all day—you *must* exercise.

Have you noticed how much weight some celebrities lose when they compete on the "Dancing with the Stars" television show? They bust their butts on the dance floor for several hours a day, and the results speak for themselves.

Health is wealth

Never take good health for granted. It needs to be worked at. Take all possible actions to preserve good health—for your sake *and* those who depend on you.

Stuart remembers a friend who worked at the factory in Cyprus where he had his books printed for several years. This friend dropped dead from a heart attack, in front of his young children. He was just 36 years old, but had neglected his health extensively.

His premature death robbed him of his most productive years, traumatized his family, and left a financial mess.

The greatest benefits from exercise

During his youth, Stuart was obsessed with bodybuilding. He sought muscle and strength primarily for aesthetic reasons, and he mistakenly thought that exercising was for young people only. Today—age 51 at the time of writing—he still has aesthetic concerns, and he still enjoys working out, but his primary motivation for exercising is *health*.

The health-related benefits from exercise should be the primary motivation for you to exercise.

There must be an investment of time in an exercise program, but the benefits are so huge that you should *make* the time to exercise. It's a myth, however, that it's necessary to have to do a great deal of exercise.

Stuart's exercise program, for example, is modest, but effective in keeping him fit, supple and vigorous—two well-designed, 90-minute workouts each week (weights and hard cardio), and a one-hour, full-body routine of yoga postures twice a week.

And he keeps himself active out of the gym, with walking, garden work, domestic chores, and daily golf practice.

Did you know that walking a mile can burn about the same number of calories as running it?

Many real-life dieters whose only exercise was walking have lost hundreds of pounds of fat. This chapter explains how they did it.

19

Walk on to weight-loss

Gut-busting exercise is *not* necessary for weight-loss. In fact, extreme exercising *harms* many people's chance of weight-loss success because of the dislike of exercise that that approach produces, and the injuries it often causes.

The mere thought of the supposed need to exercise very hard has killed many people's weight-loss aspirations because they can't follow that sort of regimen. And when people hate the exercise they do, it can even produce a negative stress response that prevents weight-loss.

Brad interviewed many dieters whose only exercise was walking, yet they achieved outstanding weight-loss success. Many of them lost *hundreds* of pounds.

If you currently do no walking other than that around your home, at your place of work, and to and from your car, start your exercise program by walking for just 10 minutes each day.

Walk at a leisurely pace—*take it easy*. Add a couple of minutes every few days. *Gradually* do more and more, so that after a couple of weeks (or longer if you need to progress more slowly) you're walking for *half an hour* each day, still at a *leisurely* pace.

Then continue the progression so that after a further few weeks (or longer, if you need to progress more slowly) you're walking for *an hour* each day, still at a *leisurely* pace.

But if you currently already do some regular outdoor walking, start your exercise program by walking outdoors for an *additional* 20 to 30 minutes each day, at a *leisurely* pace. Then add a couple of minutes every few days. *Gradually* do more and more, so that after a few weeks (or longer, if required) you're walking for an hour each day, still at a *leisurely* pace.

Don't feel intimidated by an hour a day of walking

Even if you feel that an hour of walking each day is a lot, and you're not up to it, start off with just a few minutes, and give yourself time to build up your physical conditioning. Sooner or later you'll find an hour of walking to be an easily performed part of your daily routine.

Your body is wonderfully adaptive *provided* you increase the demands on it *gradually*, and you're *patient*.

The one hour of walking doesn't have to be performed in one continuous segment. Spread it out, if you prefer. You could, for example, walk during breaks at work, have a group walk at lunchtime, and an after-dinner walk (perhaps with a partner for company, or a dog, or both).

Although he's now at his target weight, Brad still walks his dogs for 30 to 45 minutes almost every nice-weather evening, and most weekend days. This is in addition to a session of jogging or lifting weights every weekday morning, and walking a lot during the course of his everyday activities.

Build walking into your daily routine. For example, don't drive all the way to a destination—walk the final leg, and gradually increase that distance. Walk to and from your local shops rather than drive. And when you use a bus, get off one stop early and walk the rest of the way, or take the bus from a stop farther away than you usually embark from. Even mowing the lawn, and shopping, are walking.

No matter how you do it, or where, build up until you get in the one-hour total of walking *every day*. It really isn't as difficult as you may think *if* you accumulate a few minutes here and there throughout the day.

Are you sitting on your butt for 17 hours a day?

If you sleep for 7 hours a day, for example, you're awake for 17. Even if you accumulate an hour of moving around on your feet, you'd still be on your butt for 16 hours a day. So, working an hour of walking into your daily schedule shouldn't be deemed overly challenging.

Don't forget about the study that concluded that obese women sat two-and-a-half hours more each day than normal-weight women. This is a major cause for their heavier weight.

And according to a study by the Mayo Clinic, normal-weight people walk an average of 3.5 miles a day more than obese people.

How to implement the walking

Your feet must be properly supported so that you don't develop physical problems as you build up your walking. But provided you have good shoes, and build up your distance and pace *gradually*, you won't have any problems. If you don't already have good walking shoes, invest in a pair.

We recommend that you go to a specialty store where you can get a proper fitting by a trained professional. This should include analysis of your foot profile, and your gait.

Fix the time or times of day when you walk. For most people, a "fitting it in" approach doesn't work over the long-term. It's too easy to skip a walk because "something cropped up, and I didn't have time." But when you've *fixed* 5:00 pm, or 7:30 am, or 8:30 pm, or whatever time is practical for you, immediately that time comes around, *go for the walk*. If you prefer multiple short walks each day rather than a single longer one, fix several times each day.

Go walking straight out of the exit door of where you are at the time—home, work, or wherever—so that it's most convenient. But by all means drive somewhere to take some of your walks if you have the time, but that's not as convenient as doing it straight out of the front door into the local neighborhood.

Even if it's cold or snowy, don't let that stop you or serve as an excuse. Brad read about a man who lives in northern Minnesota who *still* walks or exercises outside year-round, *even* in the snow. Just dress to accommodate whatever elements you may encounter, and take the appropriate safety precautions.

Walk with company, if possible. Studies have shown that if you walk with someone, you're more likely to stick to it.

If you're by yourself, take an iPod or another music player, or take a self-help motivational recording to listen to, for example, to keep you company and make the walk more enjoyable.

But walking with just your own thoughts for company can be enjoyable. You'll always have problems to find solutions to, and projects to plan, for example. You could make walking your thinking and planning time.

Some famous authors used to walk a great deal, in part to help them think out what they were going to write next—Charles Darwin and Charles Dickens, for example.

Why the big deal about walking for weight-loss?

Walking a mile at a leisurely pace can burn approximately 70 calories, and is a great form of exercise for beginners, and *much* better than sitting all day, or lying on a couch. But even at "just" 70 calories a mile, the calories quickly add up.

It's much easier to walk a mile at a leisurely pace than it is to run it. Which are you more likely to do on a daily basis, walk at a leisurely pace, or run vigorously?

As a pure calorie-burning activity that can be done almost effortlessly on a regular basis, leisurely paced walking is the way to go. When something is almost effortless, you'll not have physical difficulty doing it.

If you increase your distance *gradually* (still at a leisurely pace), so that sooner or later you cover four miles more each day than you would from your normal activities, that's about 280 extra calories each day, or about 1,960 each week, or about 102,000 each year.

And 102,000 calories is the approximate value of 29 pounds of fat. Over four years, that's equivalent to about 116 pounds of fat—*from just four miles of leisurely walking each day*, which would take about an hour once you've developed a basic level of conditioning.

And these calories burned will increase as you gradually pick up your pace in the coming weeks and months. Eventually you may be able to walk at a *sustained brisk pace,* and this may burn around as many calories as running, which is about 100 calories a mile. At that rate, the caloric equivalent of 40 pounds of fat could be burned over a year using the aforementioned four-miles-per-day example.

But remember that the precise calories burned per mile is affected by your pace, body size and composition, and other factors.

Now you should see the great value of walking as a part of a weight-loss plan. Make it a mainstay of your weight-loss plan, and then keep it as a mainstay in your keep-the-weight-off plan.

Alternatives to walking

At least some of the time, you may prefer bicycling, in-line skating, spinning, aerobics, hiking, dancing, swimming, badminton, active games with your children, in-front-of-television exercise with a DVD for instruction, or other activities.

Do whatever you want *provided* it's safe, easy to perform, and enjoyable. Walking can satisfy all those requirements, and is also convenient, with zero cost (unless you use a treadmill).

Even if you prefer an activity or activities other than walking, *still work up to an hour a day, every day.*

Use a pedometer to ramp up the mileage

Set a target of eventually doing a *minimum* of 10,000 steps a day—about five miles—from the walking you do from your everyday activities *and* the additional walking for the primary purpose of burning extra calories. Use a pedometer to track your progress. The 10,000 steps do *not* have to be done in one continuous segment, but can be accumulated throughout the day.

A pedometer is a portable device that counts each step a person takes by detecting the motion of the hips. It's calibrated to the user's stride length, and can be set to read in kilometers or miles.

Pedometers are inexpensive, with basic units costing as little as $20. People who wear a pedometer are likely to walk more than people who don't. The mere awareness of wearing one is enough to make people walk more.

Some people have inter-office pedometer contests to see who can walk the farthest in a day or week, for example. And contests can have the same effect within a family. This can make the use of the device even more effective, and a lot more fun.

Once you reach the daily goal of 10,000 steps, your level of fitness will enable you to make a *new* goal to add *more* steps. On a few days each week you may set a goal to reach 10,000 steps *as well as* the extra hour of walking. This may seem like a great deal of walking, but if you think about it, it's only two or three hours on your feet per day. Some of the dieters Brad researched accomplish this seemingly huge feat several times a week, as routine.

Brad used to think that achieving a goal like this was impossible, but inspired by some real-life dieters he now does this on a regular basis as he strives to be less and less of a couch potato. He walks 10, 15 or 30 minutes here and there each day, and usually takes a longer walk with his dogs most evenings and weekends. Brad rarely walks in one continuous hour-long segment.

Including his 45-minute, slow-paced morning jog, his structured walks, and that he's on his feet as much as possible throughout the day, Brad routinely tallies 14,000, 16,000 and even 20,000 steps a day. Although he has a sedentary career, he *still* finds time for plenty of daily movement.

The little daily movements monitored via a pedometer can add up to many miles accumulated throughout each day.

The value of a home treadmill

Some people may feel too self-conscious to walk outdoors *until* they've lost a lot of weight. If you get yourself a home treadmill you can make walking super convenient, albeit after you've made the investment in the required equipment.

With a home treadmill you can walk while watching the television, listening to music, or holding a conversation. And you have climate control and some other advantages over walking outdoors. Of course, you could do some of your walking outdoors, and some of it indoors, depending on your preference, and the weather.

If you wear a pedometer as you use a treadmill, you'll see how easy it is to clock up many thousands of steps in the comfort of your home. Get into a routine of using a treadmill. *Fix* the times when you're due to use it, and stick to the routine.

Perhaps, for example, there's a half-hour soap you watch each day. Watch it as you walk on your treadmill.

Perhaps you watch the news for half an hour each evening. Watch it while you walk on your treadmill. If he can't walk outside, Brad always watches the evening news while walking on his treadmill.

Perhaps you watch a sports bulletin for half an hour each evening. Watch it while you walk on your treadmill.

When you buy a treadmill, invest in a high-quality piece of equipment—perhaps a used one in good condition—or you'll end up spending more money over the long-term. Brad's treadmill is 17 years old and still going strong. It should have an adjustable incline, and a belt that *yields*, to reduce impact forces.

There are alternatives to a treadmill. An elliptical machine, sometimes called a cross-trainer, has a blend of features from a treadmill, stepper and ski machine. It produces zero impact forces. And stationary cycling, and skiing, climbing and rowing machines produce zero or minimal impact forces.

But before you consider buying a machine, try one or more of them for a few sessions—not just one bout of a few minutes. Do this at a local gym—go for a few single-session visits, when a membership isn't required. Discover which type of machine you prefer most. Before one of them can become your staple for home exercising, you *must* like it. You must enjoy what you're doing if you're to stick with it over the long-term.

HONOR your exercise program.

HONOR your dedication to your weight-loss plan.

HONOR your commitment to your health and well-being.

No matter whether you're walking or doing an alternative activity, and no matter how you do it or where, build up to a leisurely one hour of it every day. When you've done that for 30 consecutive days, you're ready to progress to the next chapter.

Many real-life dieters achieved tremendous weight-loss success, *and dramatically improved their fitness*, without graduating beyond higher-intensity walking.

And higher-intensity walking can strengthen your heart just like running can, but without the risk of injury that running produces for many people.

This chapter will show you how higher-intensity walking produces benefits *beyond* burning calories alone. *And* it also explains other forms of exercise, and their weight-loss benefits.

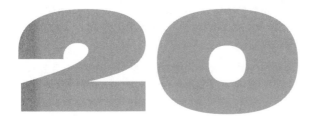

Advanced walking, *and other matters*, for increased weight-loss *and* for fitness

To make walking more demanding—for increased fitness benefits, to get more calorie burning in your daily hour of walking, and make an even greater contribution to your weight-loss and health plan—*crank up your effort.*

But never push yourself so hard that you kill your enthusiasm for exercise. Different people have different tolerance levels, and degrees of enthusiasm. Progress at a pace that works *for you*.

Advanced walking

Over a few weeks (or longer, if required), increase your pace of walking from leisurely, to *brisk* but not exhausting. Stick with an hour of walking—one continuous stretch, or several shorter stretches. And progress *gradually*.

Move at a brisk but not exhausting pace for a minute, then return to your normal leisurely pace for a few minutes, then again move at the brisk clip for a minute, and so on. Gradually increase the length of the brisk stretches, and reduce the length of the leisurely stretches. Eventually, perform the entire hour at a brisk but not exhausting pace.

As you increase your physical conditioning, and reduce your weight, you'll find it easier to maintain a brisk pace, and you may be able to make the brisk pace brisker without any apparent increase in required effort.

A pace you may find impossible to maintain for more than a few minutes now, you may be able to maintain for a whole hour after a few months, or perhaps after just a few weeks, depending on your rate of progress.

Your body is wonderfully adaptive *provided* you increase the demands on it gradually, and you're *patient*.

Many of the tenacious middle-aged women that Brad researched eventually worked up to an hour or even 90 minutes of low- to moderate-intensity exercise several times a week, if not six or seven times a week. Some of them spread the 60 to 90 minutes of daily exercise into multiple short sessions.

These ladies worked up to this level over several months, and they started with just a little slow-paced walking.

One woman performed 10 to 15 minutes of continuous moderate-intensity exercise several times a day rather than a single, longer but lower-intensity session. And that contributed to her loss of 80 pounds in just over a year.

How much exercise is best for weight-loss?

As much as you can perform consistently, which means it must be safe, and you must enjoy it.

Our minimum recommendation is one hour a day of walking.

An hour a day of walking—spread over one, two or more bouts—*but done every day, year after year,* is much better than an initial burst of enthusiasm that manifests in a two-hour gym workout four days a week, and two hours of vigorous walking on each of the other three days, but then after two months the gym is given up, and the walks hardly ever happen.

Doing too much, and then burning out and giving it all up, is a classic error of exercising.

Start off with a little exercise, then add to it as your physical conditioning improves, and your enthusiasm increases.

Government-recommended physical activity guidelines

How much exercise does the United States federal government say is best for weight-loss?

According to the physical activity guidelines released in 2008 by the US federal government, "people who want to lose a substantial (more than 5% of bodyweight) amount of weight, and people who are trying to keep a significant amount of weight off once it has been lost, need a high amount of physical activity unless they also reduce their caloric intake. Many people need to do more than 300 minutes of moderate-intensity activity a week to meet weight-control goals."

And anything less than this "may not be enough for most people to realize any type of significant weight-loss results."

Three hundred minutes equates to about 60 minutes of exercise performed five days a week.

But if you really want to lose weight, the government recommendation is that you should eventually do more than the 300 minutes of weekly moderate-intensity activity. This should be 420 weekly minutes, or even more for many of you.

Feedback from our real-life dieters confirms that 400 or even 500 minutes of weekly exercise isn't difficult to achieve *if* you make it part of your lifestyle. But no matter how many weekly minutes you eventually clock up, *you must enjoy what you're doing if you're to stick with it over the long-term.*

The workout that never was

One of Brad's best-ever workouts wasn't actually a training session. A few years ago he took a two-day vacation to New York City. There were so many things he wanted to see and do that he was on his feet about 14 hours a day, for two consecutive days. He walked at least 30 miles because he was zipping along. He was exhausted after this "workout," and his legs were sore for days. But because he was already used to a lot of daily brisk walking, he didn't suffer any blisters or stress fractures.

Walking can produce a terrific workout beyond burning calories alone, *if* you do enough of it at a sufficient level of effort.

The bottom line for weight-loss

It's possible to do no exercise whatsoever and yet still lose weight *provided* you eat very little. It's also possible to lose weight while consuming lots of food *provided* you do a great deal of activity and exercise. And it's also possible to be hugely active and burn lots of calories and yet still *gain* weight if you consume more calories than you need in order to maintain your bodyweight.

Find the right balance for you. For most people, it's moderate caloric intake *and* moderate activity and exercise. If you want to eat a lot more and yet still lose weight, you must be far more active in order to burn more calories, which isn't practical for most people.

No matter how much or how little you exercise, in order to lose fat *you still have to expend more calories than you take in.*

As an illustration, assume that the intake that maintains your bodyweight, without any allowance for exercise, is 1,800 calories. If you average that number each day and walk *briskly* (not merely leisurely) for four miles a day, that will take you about 400 calories a day into a *deficit* that will oblige your body to draw on its energy reserves (body fat) to make up the 400 shortfall.

That daily deficit would add up to 2,800 each week, or about 145,000 each year. And 145,000 calories is the approximate value of 40 pounds of body fat. Over four years, that's equivalent to about 160 pounds of fat.

There are two huge benefits from exercising. The first is that you can eat more food and yet still lose weight, which produces more satisfaction from eating, and a

greater supply of nutrients. The second is that exercise, provided that it's safe and you enjoy it, is good for your physical and mental well-being.

Higher-intensity walking for accelerated weight-loss

Once you can walk at a brisk but not exhausting pace for an hour, *increase its intensity*. For example, during some walks, include a hill or some undulating terrain. Some people wear a weighted vest or backpack to add resistance so that walking on even terrain can be made more demanding.

Include walks up flights of stairs as some of your hour-a-day of exercise. Start off with just a minute, and *gradually* build up to a few minutes at a comfortable pace. Then make some of it two steps at a time going up, but one step at a time going down.

Build up *gradually* so that eventually you can do a couple of minutes of continuous two-steps-at-a-time stair climbing—but without rushing the pace. You could use the elevator to return to ground level. Then not only will you get calorie burning benefits from your regular walking, you'll also get heart and lower-body strengthening benefits from the bursts of stair climbing.

An excellent way of increasing the intensity is "interval training." Walk at a slow-to-moderate pace to warm up, then walk at a brisk but not exhausting pace and interject 30- to 60-second periods of fast, exhausting walking. Alternatively, using a treadmill, you could walk at a steady pace but on a sufficient *incline* for the higher-intensity bursts.

After each higher-intensity interval, walk at your normal, comfortably brisk level for a few minutes—this is the recovery interval. Allow your breathing to recover, and then crank up the effort level for another vigorous 30 to 60 seconds. Repeat this pattern as often as you can.

Walking is a good activity in general, and brisk walking is even better. But interval walking, and walking uphill and up flights of stairs, or on a treadmill set at an incline and used at a brisk pace, can be sufficiently demanding that it's no longer walking per se, but cardiovascular exercise that gives your heart and circulatory system an excellent workout, to strengthen your heart and give your health a boost.

These higher-intensity variations of walking can produce the same effect on your heart as running but *without* the risk of injury that running produces for many people. Many people, especially heavy people, shouldn't run, or even jog, because the stress on their joints and backs is so great that injury is almost inevitable.

Many of the heavier or more elderly dieters Brad interviewed achieved all of their weight-loss success—*and* their dramatically improved levels of fitness—while never graduating past higher-intensity walking. Anything more demanding than vigorous walking put too much stress on their joints.

An inspiring "interval training" success story

In the late 1970s, when Brad was a teenager, he had a neighbor who was morbidly obese but wanted to lose weight and improve her health. Although she was well over 200 pounds at a height of about five-foot four-inches, and in her late 40s, she was determined to succeed. She started by walking around the house a bit more, and doing more household chores.

She also bought a stationary bicycle, and used it with passion. She knew that she couldn't run or jog, but she really felt the need to get her heart pumping.

Every afternoon, Brad and his friends would walk by the room where she rode the bicycle, and she was eventually seen to pump away at a remarkable clip.

She rode it everyday for 20 to 30 minutes, and after just several weeks she was doing stout cardio workouts that made her breathe heavily, and sweat profusely.

She couldn't pump away feverously for 20 or 30 minutes continuously, but she sped up for a short period, slowed down to regain her breath, and sped up again when she was ready. This is what high-intensity interval training is. And an obese, middle-aged lady performed this type of exercise without a hitch.

This type of cardio training—coupled with normal walking throughout the day, and reduced caloric intake—created a fat-loss of nearly 70 pounds over about a year. She looked and felt great.

And she enjoyed her workouts. They were rewarding, and she looked forward to them. Consistent, on-going exercise was one of the major reasons she was able to maintain her weight-loss over the long-term. And she still looks and feels great over 30 years later.

Even very heavy people can *gradually* gravitate to moderate- to high-intensity cardio training *provided* the exercise is low impact. It can be performed on a variety of machines (which you can also buy for your home)—treadmills, spin cycles, ellipticals, ski machines, or rowers, for example. And these fun, rewarding activities can be done in addition to ordinary walking.

Higher-intensity exercise *may not be for you*

Higher-intensity exercise is *not* for everybody. Nor is it imperative for weight-loss. And for many people it's not fun.

But for some people, higher-intensity exercise *is* fun. And it can accelerate fat-loss once you've progressed to the level of fitness necessary to accomplish this type of exercise. But before you start on it, get the approval from your doctor.

Sweat, huff and puff! And set personal goals—for example, achieve your best time on a three-mile walk, again and again; and make a new best distance from a one-hour walk, again and again.

Do the best that *you* can, even if you feel that your current level of fitness is embarrassing, or sub-par. Personal competition makes the journey more fun.

But *don't* rush into higher-intensity exercise. Remember how Brad blew out his shoulder and his calf when he rushed into a vigorous workout regimen? This set him back several months.

Always build up your training regimen *gradually*, over a period of time.

Some people who lost an extraordinary amount of weight on extreme weight-loss television shows ultimately exercised several hours a day in an intensive manner. While most of them were so heavy at first that intensive exercise was almost impossible, all contestants persevered and eventually were able to perform tough workouts that would be demanding for even conditioned athletes.

They may have had personal trainers continuously barking in their ears, but they still persevered.

While Stuart and Brad are against the excessively fast weight-loss illustrated on these television shows, and the extreme measures used, the examples of how very unfit people can become fit, through gradual progression, is valuable.

Exercise first thing each day

When you do *low-* or *moderate*-intensity exercise in a fasted or semi-fasted state—before you eat breakfast—your body may derive more of its fuel from your stored body fat than it would at another time. A study by the School of Sport and Exercise Sciences, University of Birmingham, entitled "Optimizing fat oxidation through exercise and diet," supports this assertion.

During your overnight fast, your levels of glycogen decline due to the provision of glucose for bodily functions that occur while you sleep. So, when you wake in the morning, you have depleted glycogen stores and lower blood sugar levels. When your primary fuel source (glycogen) is low, your body taps into its reserve fuel—body fat. This creates the ideal environment for burning fat during low- or moderate-intensity exercise.

If you do the exercise immediately after eating a meal, you'll still burn fat, but you'll burn less of it because you'll also use some of the carbohydrate you just ate.

When you exercise in a fasted or semi-fasted state, your body releases a fat-fighting agent called epinephrine, which attaches to your fat cells and permits fat to be burned as fuel.

To maximize this effect, some people have found it best to wait 30 to 45 minutes after the workout to have their first meal—shower, get dressed, and *then* eat.

But, according to an article published by *The New York Times*, although studies found conclusive evidence that exercising on an empty stomach burns more body fat, the subjects became fatigued much faster, and stopped exercising about 30 minutes earlier. So, it's best not to do *intensive* exercise—hard weight lifting, or hard cardio—on an empty stomach first thing in the morning.

And the consensus from real-life dieters is that it's easier to stay in a routine if you exercise—at least the low- to moderate-intensity type—first thing in the morning, rather than in the evening.

But if you can do your exercise only at other times, that's still fine. Do what fits into *your* schedule.

Start your day an hour earlier

People who blow off exercising until the evening usually blow it off entirely. Eventually, excuse after excuse gets the better of them.

If you find it easier to exercise in the morning—at least the low- to moderate-intensity type—start your day an hour earlier. (Brad's wife gets up every weekday morning at 5:15, to exercise.)

But go to bed an hour earlier to compensate. Many people, if not most adults, are already deficient in sleep, so getting up an hour earlier but without going to bed an hour earlier to compensate, would contribute to increased sleep deficiency.

As made clear in Chapter 8, sleeping in sufficient quantity and quality is a *major* component of good health *and* weight control, but not fully appreciated by most people.

High-intensity interval training (HIIT)

This is popular among exercise enthusiasts. It's an upgrading of "interval training," to make it more rigorous, formal, and effective for weight-loss and increased fitness benefits. Brad utilized HIIT during his final triumph. This is a form of *hard* cardio work, where breathlessness and a greatly elevated heart rate are produced.

Research from the University of New South Wales found that overweight women who followed a 20-minute HIIT routine lost three times more fat over the 15 weeks of the study than did those who exercised at a consistent pace for 40-minute routines.

The HIIT was rigorous, used a stationary bike, and required a non-stop rotation of 20-second periods for 20 minutes whereby an 8-second sprint was followed by 12 seconds of light cycling. So, 8 seconds flat out, 12 seconds easy, 8 seconds flat out, 12 seconds easy, and so on, for 20 minutes.

The scientists believe that this format would also work for walking, swimming, running, and rowing.

Other types of interval training that use longer work and rest periods are not as effective for weight-loss.

The research claims that intermittent bursts cause the adrenal glands to produce high levels of catecholamines—hormones that allow more fat to be burned by the exercising muscles. The resulting increase in fat oxidation causes greater weight-loss.

Furthermore, research from several prominent universities has concluded that subjects who incorporated HIIT lost more weight (as much as four times more) during the studies than those who worked out longer but without the high-intensity intervals.

And some women say that HIIT is the one type of exercise that helped reduce the stubborn fat around their butts (when, of course, combined with a proper eating plan).

Many fitness trainers believe that more benefit can be realized if you engage in several short, intensive workouts a day (incorporating HIIT) rather than one longer but easier session. For example, do three harder 20-minute sessions rather than a single not-so-hard 60-minute one.

Critics argue, however, that it's difficult for most people to find the inclination to exercise once a day, let alone two or three times. Do what fits into your schedule, but the "two-a-day" or "three-a-day" HIIT regimen can help to work wonders.

Exercise *care*

To get the most from an increased intensity of walking, and cardio in general, *you must not get injured.*

Only once you're close to or at your goal weight should you even consider *gradually* working into running, and then only if you're suited to it because you have a good gait, perhaps used to run well when you were a teenager, have no structural problems, and only if you run on a treadmill with a yielding belt, and only if you wear quality running shoes designed to reduce impact forces.

Too little has been written about the dangers of running and jogging. For some people, running is a terrific activity. But most people aren't well suited to running, or even jogging, and the alternative of walking—including some use of higher-intensity walking for cardio work—is much safer.

But even people who are suited to jogging and running can be overzealous, and rush their progress. Brad, for example, spent several months on the sideline with an injury that resulted from rushing his progress when jogging.

Alternatives to intensive walking

For at least some of your higher-intensity exercise, you may prefer bicycling, spinning, or use of an elliptical machine, stairclimber or rower, or another activity that you can control as easily as walking.

Do whatever you want *provided* it's safe, easy to perform, and enjoyable. Walking can satisfy all those requirements, and is also convenient, with zero cost (unless you use a treadmill), which is why we highly recommend it.

Workout log or diary

Once you're at the more advanced level of exercising, you may want to maintain a workout log. It could contain things like day, date, time, and location of your workout. And you can record your reps, sets or poundages if you're lifting weights, and time and distance if you're walking. Intensity levels, and how you felt, can also be recorded. The log can help keep you organized, focused, and motivated. Examples of workout logs are available on the internet.

Turn on your afterburners

The "afterburn effect"—excess post-exercise oxygen consumption, or EPOC—may occur following an intensive workout, and you may burn more calories for a period of time than you would if you'd not exercised intensively. It does this by elevating your metabolism above its normal resting state. EPOC has been the focus of more than a dozen scientific studies published in prominent medical journals over the last two decades.

According to a 2003 study published in the *Journal of Sports Medicine*, the physiological mechanisms responsible for this elevated metabolism include the replenishment of oxygen stores, phosphagen (ATP-PC) resynthesis, lactate removal, and the increased ventilation, blood circulation, and body temperature above pre-exercise levels.

And according to a 2003 Norwegian study, for a few hours after an intensive cardiovascular workout, each hour you would burn 15% to 20% of the total calories used during the workout *additional* to whatever calories you would normally burn during that period. So, as an illustration, if you burned 400 calories during an intensive 30-minute workout, for several hours you may burn approximately 60 to 80 calories per hour purely from the afterburn effect.

Following the workout it may take several hours for your body to recover to its normal resting state, depending on the intensity and type of exercise you do.

Lifting weights intensively may provide the longest post-workout afterburn effect—up to 24 hours to 48 hours—due to elevated blood lactate, an increase in circulating catecholamines and anabolic hormones, and because the trained muscles are being "repaired."

And generally speaking, the more intensive your workout is, the greater (and longer) its afterburn effect is. A study conducted at Wayne State University concluded that an intensive full-body weight-lifting workout can elevate your metabolism for up to three days.

To take advantage of the afterburn effect, try to do at least some of your hardest workouts in the morning *after* you've eaten, *not* on an empty stomach—so that you have the energy to sustain an intensive workout. (Stuart does all of his intensive workouts in the morning, after breakfast.) Your metabolism may stay elevated for a period of several hours after the intensive exercise.

But if you do your cardio at night, for example, your elevated metabolism will plummet when you go to sleep.

The stress here is on "intensive." But for most people, the required intensity of exercise is unrealistic. Just do the best you can—but you may be surprised at what you can do *eventually*, if you make small, gradual increments of progression.

But despite decades of studies citing the effects of EPOC, new research published in the journal *Exercise and Sport Sciences Reviews* suggests that EPOC may not be as readily produced as we've been led to believe it is.

While their research concludes that people do burn more fat when they are cycling than when they are not, they have no greater ability to burn additional fat over the next 24 hours.

The study's authors do say, however, that they can't rule out that more intensive forms of exercise (like strength training, for example) could lead to a more lasting post-workout fat burn.

But even if irrefutable evidence proved that EPOC doesn't occur following any type of exercise—even intensive strength training—strength training, and exercise in general, should *still be done* because of the many benefits they irrefutably produce.

How can walking burn calories at about the same rate as running does?

Walking at a *sustained brisk pace*—once you've *gradually* built up to that level—creates a lot of inefficiency and internal "friction" relative to leisurely walking. This boosts heart rate and oxygen consumption, and produces a greater overall burn of calories. And *that's* when walking has the potential to burn around as many calories per mile as running—about 100.

Avoid a workout dungeon atmosphere

Place your treadmill, stationary cycle, or any other exercise equipment in an upbeat room with natural light and pleasant surroundings. You'll be more apt to exercise if you look forward to going into an attractive, welcoming environment rather than "a workout dungeon"—a dark, dreary basement, for example.

Some people put their exercise gear in front of the television in their family room, or media room.

Jogging caveat

Some people's pace of jogging is slower than what they could walk briskly. But walking produces lower impact forces, and is a safer motion. Rather than jog, with its higher impact forces and risk of injury than from walking, you're probably better off to walk very briskly (perhaps with a bag on your back for additional resistance), or walk at a slight incline on a treadmill. This especially applies to people who are overweight. The larger your mass, the greater the impact forces, everything else being equal.

Brad usually jogs at an 8- or 9-minute-per-mile pace on his 45-minute morning jaunts. His wife usually speed walks at a very brisk pace in lieu of jogging. But while jogging is still Brad's exercise of choice, and what he enjoys a great deal, for variety he also enjoys speed walking with his wife and dogs.

Brad used to adhere to intensity percentages of his maximum heart rate, and its associated "fat burning zones," but he has since abandoned that approach.

Brad needs to enjoy exercise if he's to continue doing it. And trying to monitor heart rates, and follow charts, took the fun out his workouts.

Your exercise routine must be enjoyable if you're to continue with it for the rest of your life.

Stuart never jogs, even though he's of normal weight. He either walks, or runs. If he wants to make his walking vigorous, he walks at a fast pace on the flat, or at a regular pace on a treadmill set at an incline. And when he runs, he does it at almost the maximum pace he can sustain for just five minutes (following warming up with brisk walking for five minutes or so). Then he cools down for about five minutes at a slow pace. This is a prescriptive form of hard cardio work called the *graded exercise protocol*.

Stuart runs, but only on a treadmill. If he ran outdoors he'd almost certainly sustain injuries. Although Stuart isn't heavy, and he is structurally suited to running, he still takes care to minimize impact forces. He runs indoors on a high-quality treadmill that has a yielding belt.

The graded exercise protocol

Through intensifying the cardio work, the duration needed for cardiorespiratory benefits is reduced. The GXP was first developed by Dr. Robert Otto, and then adapted and studied by Drs. Ralph N. Carpinelli, Lesley D. Fox, Richard A. Winett, and Janet R. Wojcik.

Stuart explains the GXP in detail in his book *Build Muscle, Lose Fat, Look Great*.

HONOR your exercise program.

HONOR your dedication to your weight-loss plan.

HONOR your commitment to your health and well-being.

Build up, as described, to the one hour of higher-intensity walking (or alternative activity) every day. When you've done that for 30 consecutive days, and if you want to further improve your fitness and your ability to lose weight and keep it off, add home strength training, as explained in the next chapter.

Wouldn't it be nice . . .

Brad used to look at a lean person and say to himself, "Man, wouldn't it be nice to look like that? I wish *I* had perfect genetics."

But that was before he understood the big picture of why, usually, fat people are fat, and lean people are lean. Although he analyzed hundreds of real-life dieters, he also analyzed many lean people. His conclusions may surprise you.

While there were a few exceptions, generally, the lean people are more active, and eat fewer calories. And they do this on a consistent basis, year after year.

Imagine, for instance, that you're a bit more active, to the tune of burning 300 additional calories a day, and that you skip, say, one dessert each day, which would cut about 300 calories. That's an energy shift of 600 calories a day, or about 18,000 calories a month (which is equivalent to about 5 pounds of fat), or 219,000 calories a year (which is equivalent to about 62 pounds of fat).

Little changes in your daily life can amount to huge changes over the long-term. That's why the lifestyle-reform, weight-loss and health model promoted in **WEIGHT-LOSS SALVATION** is comfortable and enjoyable to implement, and as a result is doable over the long-term, to produce the required weight-loss and then *keep it off.*

How would you like to enhance your metabolism so that you can burn more calories each day *without* doing any extra activity?

This chapter will show you how to make this a reality.

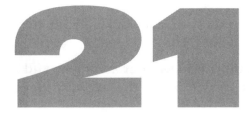

Home strength training, for increased weight-loss and fitness

As already noted, Brad interviewed many dieters whose only exercise was walking, yet they achieved outstanding weight-loss success. But when strength training is added, the benefits from the exercise program increase greatly.

Remember, strength training is the most productive single form of exercise, for men *and women*. It builds strength, develops muscle, strengthens bones, improves overall fitness, improves posture, increases resistance to injury, increases the body's energy expenditure, helps to control body fat, and transforms physical appearance. And there are other health benefits that further reduce the impact of aging. *Strength training plays a huge role in keeping you young for your years.*

No other *single* type of exercise produces all these benefits.

For such a small investment of time and effort, the return from strength training is huge.

But gut-busting, strength-training workouts at a gym *aren't* necessary. That type of training takes months, if not years to progress to, and isn't practical for most people.

For most dieters, a simple, *home* strength-training routine utilizing just five calisthenic exercises is all that's required.

The calisthenics don't require special apparatus, but use your bodyweight as resistance.

Don't lose heart if these exercises are very difficult to begin with. *Persist*.

If you follow the instructions you *will* get stronger, and that strength improvement will make the exercises less difficult to perform.

And as you lose weight, the exercises will become less difficult still to perform.

Eventually, you'll perform the exercises with ease.

To obtain the extensive health and appearance benefits that strength training produces, you must make substantial improvement in your strength level.

Never mind if you have to start at almost zero. Get started!

As you make slow, incremental progress you may surprise yourself with how much strength you can build. After a year or so of slow but steady progress, for example, you'll transform your strength level. You may then even be able to perform advanced versions of at least some of the calisthenics.

Bit by bit, progress is a cinch. But don't try to rush your progress. Progress at your own pace. *Make haste slowly*.

Remember . . . your body has tremendous abilities to adapt to and prosper from exercise *provided* you start out comfortably, and increase the demands *gradually*.

Exercise care

If you haven't exercised for a long time, and especially if you try to progress quickly, you'll probably experience muscular soreness for a day or two after exercising. A little muscular soreness is fine, but a severe degree isn't.

Severe muscular soreness causes discomfort, and can accompany injury or lead to injury. And you should never have discomfort in your spine or any other bony body part.

Provided you follow the guidelines given here, you'll avoid injury and stay clear of anything other than slight muscular soreness.

Don't hold your breath while exercising. Breathe freely. To prevent breath holding, *don't close your mouth*. Keep your mouth open—just slightly open will suffice—and your upper and lower teeth apart. It's usually when the lips are jammed together that problems with breath holding occur.

And don't close your eyes while you train.

"No pain, no gain" madness

Never do any exercise that hurts, don't train if you've hurt yourself, and never train through pain.

A little muscular discomfort, and some temporary general fatigue from a bout of exercise done correctly, are desirable, but pain isn't. Any sharp, stabbing, or sudden pain is a sign you've injured yourself.

Countless people have given up exercise because of having been hurt from following foolish advice. Those who live the "No pain, no gain" maxim usually regret it, sooner or later.

Exercise *at home*—as illustrated—by yourself, at your convenience, without any special equipment or clothing, and without the self-consciousness you may experience at a gym. And never mind how out of condition you may be to begin with. *Just get started.*

Technique of the five calisthenics

1. Crunch

This exercise primarily works the abdominal muscles.

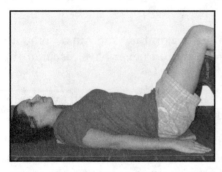 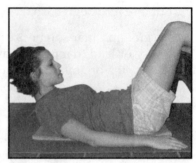

Get a chair, bench, box, or low table. Lie on your back on the floor, with a folded towel under your hips and back. Bend your knees and place your calves on the elevation. Keep your knees bent at about a right angle. Don't cross your ankles.

Rest your hands on the floor by your sides. Keep your arms and forearms relaxed, and feet immobile, then lift the tip of your lower back (sacrum and coccyx) slightly off the floor, press the rest of your lower back against the floor, and then take two seconds to roll your upper torso off the floor. Hold the top position for a second, then unfurl over a further two seconds. Once your upper back returns to the floor, again press your lower back against the floor, and initiate the next repetition, or rep.

Don't lift your entire torso off the floor—your lower back should retain contact with the floor throughout. Keep your chin *off* your chest during each rep, and keep your hands on the floor *and relaxed*.

Exhale during the ascent, and inhale during the descent; or, breathe freely and continuously throughout each rep. Keep your lips apart throughout each set. A set is a sequence of reps.

Never mind how many reps you can perform initially. Even if you can perform just one, persist, and as the weeks go by you'll gradually get stronger and be able to perform additional reps.

Once you can do 10 crunches in that manner, perform the exercise with your hands crossed on your chest, to increase the resistance.

Once you can perform 10 reps that way, place your fingers on your cheeks, forehead, or temples—but not behind your head or neck.

Once you can perform 10 reps that way, hold a sufficiently weighted object at your chest so that you can perform just 6 reps, and then over a few workouts, or as long as is required, progress to 10 reps again. Then hold a little heavier weight on your chest, drop your reps, build up to 10 again, and so on. For easy handling, get someone to place the weighted object into your hands at your chest once you're in position to start the exercise.

Again, don't try to rush your progress. Progress at your own pace. *Make haste slowly.*

Why sit-ups with straight knees are dangerous

Especially in days gone by, school students and youngsters elsewhere were urged by instructors to perform quick-fire sit-ups with straight knees, and hands interlocked behind their heads or necks. That technique can be harmful even for youngsters, and is potentially harmful for most adults. Avoid it.

Relative to sit-ups, crunches as described here are safe because the knees are bent, hips are flexed, and the lower back is properly positioned. As a result, your abdominal muscles pull you up and forward, and your hip flexors help as synergists (not prime movers) to keep your pelvis stabilized at the crucial moment the crunch is initiated by your abdominal muscles.

But in sit-ups with straight knees, the hip flexors are the prime movers as they first pull the lower back into a more arched position (curved to the *front*), and *then* they pull the torso up and forward. It's this initial pull on the lumbar arch that feels uncomfortable, and commonly creates problems.

Perform crunches, not sit-ups with straight knees.

2. Floor back extension

This exercise primarily works the lower back, mid back, buttocks, and rear thighs.

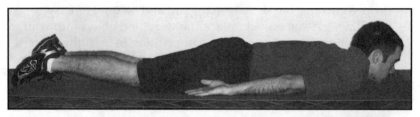

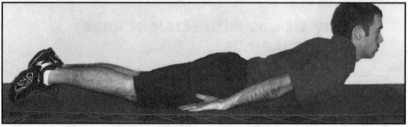

Lie prone (face downward) on the floor. Lift your head so that your chin clears the floor. Rest the back of your hands on the floor by your sides, and keep your feet together. Without using your hands to assist, slowly and smoothly lift your torso off the floor. Lift your torso until most of your rib cage just clears the floor. Hold the raised position for two seconds, then lower over a further two seconds. Repeat. Perform six reps, then rest a minute.

Now for the work set. While raising your torso, simultaneously lift your feet while keeping your knees straight or almost straight, with your toes pointed. Smoothly and slowly lift your feet until your knees just clear the floor. At that point, most of your rib cage should also just clear the floor, as illustrated below. At the top of each rep, hold for two seconds. Lower over a further two seconds.

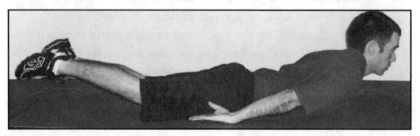

Exhale during the ascent, and inhale during the descent; or, just breathe freely and continuously throughout each rep without holding your breath.

If this full technique is too difficult, for the moment, do the best you can, and gradually increase the range of motion from week to week, strength permitting.

Never mind how many reps you can perform initially. Even if you can perform just one, persist, and as the weeks go by you'll gradually get stronger and be able to perform additional reps.

Once you can perform 10 full reps, increase the resistance. Cross your forearms and keep them against your chest for the duration of each set.

When you can do 10 full reps in that manner, increase the resistance further—keep your arms straight out in front.

Then to increase resistance further still, hold an object in your outstretched hands.

Whenever you get your full 10 reps, increase the resistance a tad at your next workout. But keep the reps smooth and controlled at all times.

If you have a history of back problems, this exercise may irritate your spine. But provided the exercise is performed with smooth technique, without an exaggerated arch, and is introduced in a careful manner, it will be safe and valuable for most people.

If you experience any negative reaction to this exercise—during performance, or afterward—drop it from your schedule, and seek professional help to find and correct the cause of the problem.

Again, don't try to rush your progress. Progress at your own pace. *Make haste slowly.*

3. Freehand squat

This exercise primarily works the thighs and buttocks.

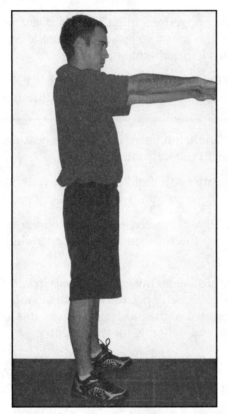 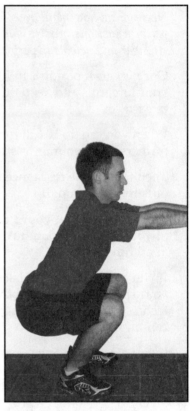

Stand with your heels about hip-width apart, and toes pointed out somewhat. If you imagine you're standing on a large clock face, with your feet being the outside ends of the hands of the clock, your feet would be positioned at about five-to-one. Tinker with the precise width of your feet, and degree of flare, to find what's the most comfortable and efficient for you.

Until you get a feel for the freehand squat, hold a sturdy object to help with balance. Once you're at ease with your balance, raise your arms out in front, and keep them there during the set. Don't look down—keep your eyes looking forward.

While standing, pull your shoulders back and stick your chest out, take a deep breath, then squat down slowly as if you were sitting onto a chair. Take two to three seconds for the descent.

Squat down as far as is comfortable for you, ideally to where your upper thighs are about parallel with the floor, then immediately but slowly ascend. Take two to three seconds for the ascent, and exhale on the ascent. While standing, pull your shoulders back once more, stick your chest out, take a deep breath, and immediately but slowly descend into the next rep.

As a beginner, you may only be able to go down to where your upper thighs are at about a 45-degree angle with the floor, but over your first few workouts (or as long as is required) gradually descend lower and lower until you're at the depth where your upper thighs are about parallel with the floor.

As you descend and ascend, don't allow your knees to buckle in. Keep them pointing in the same direction as your feet.

If balance is a problem, you may find it impossible to keep your heels flat on the floor. Wear shoes with a normal heel rather than do the squats barefoot. Regular practice of a good stretching routine should increase your flexibility, which in turn should help your squatting technique.

At first, however, descend in the squat only as far as you can without your heels coming off the floor. Eventually, you should be able to descend deeper while keeping your heels on the floor.

Perform one set of a comfortable number of reps—take it very easy to begin with. And rather than focus on building up your rep count, work on gradually increasing your depth of descent if you can't initially do the required range of motion. Then once your range of motion is good, and your heels stay on the floor throughout, focus on building up your reps.

As an illustration, perhaps to begin with you can perform just six half squats to a depth where your thighs are approximately 45 degrees to the floor. But over a few weeks you gradually progress to six *full-depth* squats where your thighs are parallel to the floor. Thereafter, you add one or two reps each week, and about two months later you can perform 20 full-depth squats.

Once you can perform those 20 squats, still target more reps each week. Eventually you may be able to perform 50, or even over 100. That may sound formidable now, but get started, plug away, and build up the reps *gradually*.

Once you can perform 20 continuous full-depth squats, add the wall squat to your workout. Finish each workout with it. Don't do it immediately after the squats. Your thighs should be rested when you start the wall squat.

Wall squat

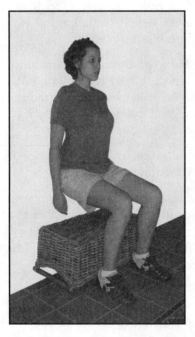

Stand with your heels about 18 inches from a wall. Without moving your heels, rest your back against the wall. Squat until your thighs are approximately parallel to the floor, with your back supported against the wall. Hold that position for time. There's no movement. And don't use any assistance from your hands.

Depending on your height and the length of your thighs and legs, you may need to stand a little closer or farther from the wall. Find the position that has your shins approximately vertical while you're holding the parallel squat position, according to what's comfortable for your knees.

You must wear non-slip shoes, and stand on a non-slip surface. And you must have a box or something similar immediately beneath you so that if you can't get up, you can gently sit onto the support, rest, and then stand.

The wall squat is done for time—you may be able to hold the parallel position for only a few seconds to start. Add a couple of seconds each week or workout. Eventually you'll be able to hold the wall squat for a minute, and later on you'll be able to hold it for longer still.

And remember that as your bodyweight decreases, you'll have less weight to lift and hold, which will make your progress easier in the squats and wall squat.

Again, don't try to rush your progress. Progress at your own pace. *Make haste slowly.*

4. Push-up

This exercise primarily works the chest, triceps, and shoulders.

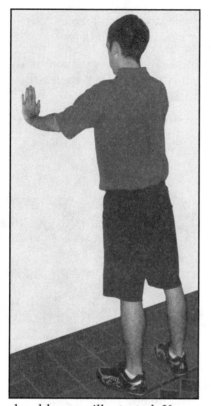

The higher your torso is relative to your feet, the *less* stressful the push-up is. Conversely, the higher your feet are relative to your torso, the *more* stressful the push-up is.

Here's a graduation of push-ups, from easiest to hardest. Start at the level that enables you to perform six reps without a struggle. Stay at that level until you can perform 10 reps, then graduate to the next level, drop your reps, and gradually build your reps up to 10 again, and so on.

For the wall push-up, wear non-slip shoes, and stand on a non-slip surface about two feet from a wall. Place your hands on the wall at about the height of the middle of your chest, and a little wider than your shoulders, as illustrated. Keep your back straight—don't sag— and *carefully* bend at your elbows until your forehead *brushes* the wall, then push back to the starting position. Take about two seconds for the descent, a second for the pause at the wall, and a further two seconds for the return phase. Your elbows should stay roughly lined up in the same plane as your wrists—don't allow your elbows to flare out.

Try to add reps, from workout to workout, or week to week, depending on your rate of progress. Once you can perform 10 in this manner, try the desk push-up.

Perform the push-up with your hands on the edge of a desk (which lowers your torso, relative to the wall push-up). Position your feet so that the edge of the desk touches your *lower* chest at the bottom of each rep. Your hands should be placed on the desk a little wider than the width of your shoulders. Maintain a rigid, straight line between your shoulders and heels. And, again, your elbows should stay roughly lined up in the same plane as your wrists. Follow the same controlled rep speed as during the wall push-up.

Once you've mastered the desk push-up and can perform 10 reps, progress to the box or low-table push-up (which lowers your torso, relative to the desk push-up), as illustrated below.

Place your hands on *stable* boxes or a low table—position the boxes or low table against a wall, for stability. Then follow the same guidelines as for the desk push-up.

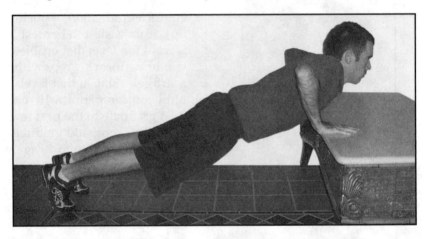

Once you can perform 10 reps of the box or low-table push-up, you may be ready for the regular floor push-up. But if you can't do at least six full reps of the regular floor push-up, do the modified floor version, or stick with the box push-up but use lower boxes in order to increase the resistance you push.

For the regular push-up, lie on the floor, face down. Place your hands at the sides of your chest, palms flat on the floor, two to three inches away from your rib cage. Spread your fingers and keep all digits other than your thumbs pointing forward. Keep your elbows approximately above your wrists at all times. And keep your eyes directed at the floor. Balance yourself on your hands and toes. See the top photograph on the next page.

Keep a rigid, straight line between your shoulders and heels, and slowly push until your elbows are straight. Take two to three seconds for the ascent, and exhale during it. At the top position, take a deep breath while sticking your chest out, and immediately yet slowly descend, over a further two to three seconds. Maintain the rigid, straight line between your shoulders and heels. Brush the floor with your chest, pause for a second without relaxing, then slowly push up and exhale during the ascent.

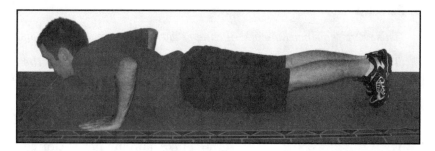

For the modified floor push-up (see below), use your knees as the fulcrum. Adopt the same starting position as for the regular push-up, but balance yourself on your hands and knees, as well as your toes. Place a folded towel beneath your knees, for comfort. Keep a rigid, straight line between your shoulders and knees. Other than the different fulcrum point, the modified floor push-up is the same as the regular version.

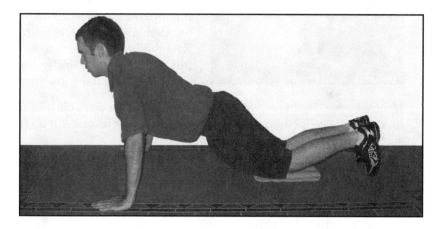

When you can perform at least 12 modified floor push-ups, graduate to the regular floor push-up.

Eventually, especially when you're at or near to your target weight, you may require more resistance than what even the regular floor push-up provides. Once you can perform 10 regular floor push-ups, elevate your feet by a few inches to increase resistance. This will probably reduce your reps. Gradually build up the reps to 10 (over perhaps a few weeks), then raise the height of the box by two inches, drop your reps, build back to 10, elevate your feet a little more, and so on.

Again, don't try to rush your progress. Progress at your own pace. *Make haste slowly.*

5. Pull-up

This exercise primarily works the upper back, biceps, and abdominals.

This movement is the trickiest of the five calisthenics, and the one you may find the hardest to perform. If it's too difficult, leave it until after you've lost a lot of weight, then try it again.

Here's a graduation of the pull-up, starting with the least stressful.

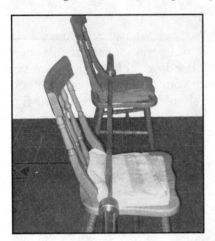

Take a broom handle, or substitute, and use it as your bar. Put two benches or boxes side-by-side about three feet apart. Their height should be about 15 inches. (A pair of chairs could substitute.) Much lower and you won't be able to fit into position properly. Much higher and the exercise will be too demanding to start with. Rest the bar across the tops, but put a folded towel under each end to prevent bar movement.

If, however, you do require a greater range of motion, elevate the bar a couple of inches on the chairs, benches, or boxes. *But do it in such a way that the bar stays securely in position.*

WARNING: The bar must be strong enough to take your weight, and the benches, boxes or chairs must be stable and strong. *The bar must not break, and the supports must not slip.*

Sit on the floor and slide under the bar, face up. The bar should be above your chest. Grab the bar with your palms facing away from you, a little wider than shoulder-width apart, and your forearms roughly perpendicular to the floor. Fine-tune this arrangement to find the most comfortable set-up for you. Your elbows will be bent at the bottom position because the range of motion for this exercise is short. Keep your knees straight. Your butt acts as the pivot point, *not* your feet. See the top photographs on the next page.

Take two to three seconds to pull your chest to the bar—or as near as possible. Hold for a second, then take two to three seconds to lower yourself. Once your back has touched the floor, pause for a second, then ascend again over two to three seconds.

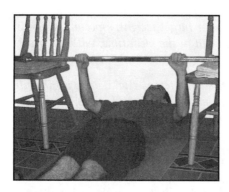 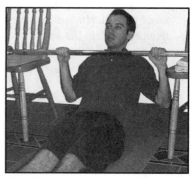

Exhale during the ascent, and inhale during the descent; or, breathe freely and continuously throughout each rep.

The range of motion will be determined by the height of the supports, your torso depth, and your arm and forearm lengths.

Once you can perform 10 full reps over this range of motion, use your *feet* as the pivot point, not your butt—see below. This greatly increases the difficulty. To minimize the increase in difficulty, bend your knees fully, and draw your feet *as close to your butt as possible*. The starting position has your feet, butt, and back on the floor. As you pull yourself up, only your feet retain contact with the floor.

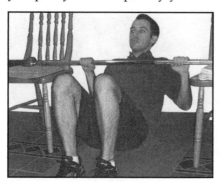 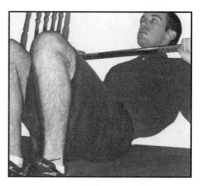

You're unlikely to be able to perform 10 full reps at the new pivot point. Perform as many as you can, no matter how few, and even include a few partial reps at the end of the set of full reps. Over time, build up to 10 full reps.

Now move your feet an inch farther away. A small change in your feet positioning—your pivot point—can make a substantial difference to the difficulty of the exercise. Once you can perform 10 reps at that level of difficulty, move your feet an inch farther away, and so on.

You may find it especially difficult to progress to using your feet as the pivot point until you're near to your target weight, especially if you're a woman. But do the best that you can in the meantime, with the pivot point of your butt.

Even if you can perform no more than a few partial reps to begin with, that's fine. Just work to increase that performance. Later on you'll be able to do a few full reps. Then later on still you may be able to perform 10 reps. Provided you register some progress each month, you'll be on track.

Once you're able to do pull-ups with your feet as the pivot point and your knees not bent substantially, you may be ready to do a few of them while suspended vertically from an overhead bar — for example, while out for a walk, use the monkey bars or jungle-gym at a children's playground. Alternatively, securely fix a bar somewhere at home well above your height.

Again, don't try to rush your progress. Progress at your own pace. *Make haste slowly.*

Weekly schedule for the calisthenics

It's easy to overtrain on strength training. Excessive frequency of strength training has undermined if not ruined the progress of many people.

Two workouts a week where you challenge yourself to make a little progress each week are sufficient. You need the three or four days between workouts for full recuperation.

Of course, if the exercise is leisurely, you won't need much recuperation time because you won't be stimulating any muscle growth and strength increase. But for strength training to be effective, it *must* be demanding *and* progressive.

Fix your workout days and times. For most people, a "fitting it in" approach doesn't work over the long-term. It's too easy to skip a workout because "something cropped up, and I didn't have time."

But when you *fix* Mondays and Thursdays at 6:00 pm, or Tuesdays at 6:00 pm and Saturdays at 10:00 am, as examples, or any other two evenly-spaced workout days that are practical for you, *as soon as workout time comes around, train.* Allow nothing to interfere.

Perform the five exercises as a circuit. Complete one set of the first exercise, rest for a minute or so, then move to the next exercise, and so on.

To begin with, however, take it easy at each workout. Don't push yourself hard on any exercise. *Gradually* increase your effort level over the first few weeks. Thereafter, train hard, and do your best to register a little progress each week on each exercise.

Perform just a single circuit at each workout for the first three weeks. Then perform two circuits at each workout for the next three weeks—take two or three minutes rest between circuits.

If you're really keen, you could progress to a maximum of three circuits at each workout. *But always keep in mind that quality of strength-training exercise is more important than quantity.*

Rather than do four or more circuits at a workout, increase your effort level and do just two or three.

And it's better that you do just two or three high-effort strength-training circuits *and* the mini stretching routine given in the next chapter, rather than four or more strength-training circuits but no stretching.

Mental focus

Treat your training time as sacrosanct. Make each set perfect— perfect technique, perfect control, and perfect concentration. This is possible *provided* you keep your mind on *one set at a time.*

The instant you're in your training location, switch off from non-training matters. Ideally, train during quiet times when there are few if any distractions.

Protect and respect your privacy while you train.

HONOR your exercise program.

HONOR your dedication to your weight-loss plan.

HONOR your commitment to your health and well-being.

Record keeping

In a notebook, record *precisely* the reps for each set, any exercise set-up changes, and any weight used. An accurate training logbook is essential so that you know exactly what you did last workout, and thus what you need to exceed next time in order to notch up progress. Don't try to rely solely on your memory for record keeping.

How strength training builds muscle

Training of sufficient intensity is the catalyst for stronger and bigger muscles. The "breaking down" of muscle tissue through training stimulates your body to repair it *and* build a little extra tissue. The "little extra tissue" is called *overcompensation*, and it accumulates to produce bigger muscles.

Proper strength training provides only the *stimulus* for muscle growth. You must provide a few days of rest between workouts to *permit* your body to repair the muscle "damage," *and* overcompensate. Only then should you deliver another bout of growth stimulation.

If you train too often, you won't give your body enough time to repair the "broken-down" muscle tissue and build the overcompensation tissue.

Recovery time between workouts is only part of the anabolic environment. You must also provide a healthy, nutrient-rich diet—that's the source of the raw materials for muscle growth.

When you've done the home strength training twice a week for a couple of months—in addition to the advanced walking—you'll be ready to add some home flexibility training, as explained in the next chapter. But if you want to start stretching earlier, by all means do so.

Then later on—but perhaps not for a year or more—you may want to seek much greater strength and fitness, and further increase your ability to lose weight and keep it off. At that point you may be interested in progressing to gym training in addition to the advanced walking, and the home stretching routine. Gym training would involve hard cardio exercise, and the use of machines, barbells and dumbbells for strength training.

If you plan to start working out a gym, you'll need to know precisely what to do. For safe, practical and effective information on how to train at a gym, you may want to check out Stuart's book **Build Muscle, Lose Fat, Look Great**. At 638 pages, and with nearly 400 photographs, it's thorough.

Many dieters never fully realize the importance of flexible muscles until after they sustain injuries. For example, Brad was never an advocate of stretching until *after* he injured his inflexible calves.

He now stretches regularly, and enjoys his exercise program without injuries.

But stretching produces many valuable benefits *in addition* to helping to prevent injuries.

This chapter explains how you can start to get your share of the benefits from increased flexibility.

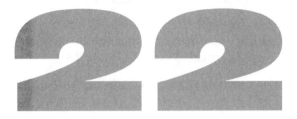

The 10-minute home stretching routine, for increased weight-loss and fitness

"How will stretching help me to lose weight and keep it off?" you may ask.

Without a supple body your muscles lose some of their elasticity and ability to function properly, and your tendons, ligaments, and joint capsules become brittle. Your tissues in general become more susceptible to injury, and your body ages at an accelerated rate.

By being supple you'll stay young for your years, and you'll be better equipped for being an active, vigorous person. And *that* will directly help you to lose weight and keep it off. Furthermore, if done properly, stretching is enjoyable and invigorating.

When you combine walking and advanced walking, other enjoyable exercise, strength training, and stretching—all of which can be done without having to visit a gym—you'll have a terrific exercise program for helping you to lose weight and keep it lost. And while the loss of weight will produce many health benefits, the exercise program will yield numerous *additional* health benefits.

As noted earlier, the combination of strength training, stretching, cardiovascular work, healthy nutrition, and a healthy lifestyle is the closest we can get to the fountain of youth.

Don't lose heart if these stretches are difficult to begin with. *Persist.*

If you follow the instructions you *will* improve your flexibility, and that will make the stretches less difficult.

Eventually, you'll perform the stretches with ease.

Never mind if you have to start at almost zero. Get started!

As you make slow, incremental progress you may surprise yourself with how much flexibility you can develop. After a few months of slow but steady progress, for example, you'll transform your flexibility.

Bit by bit, progress is a cinch. But don't try to rush your progress. Progress at your own pace. *Make haste slowly.*

Your body has tremendous abilities to adapt to and prosper from stretching *provided* you start out comfortably, and increase the demands from the stretching *gradually*.

Weekly schedule for the stretching

Stretch twice a week, immediately after your home strength training. This has two big benefits. First, you strength train and stretch in the same session, for simplicity and efficiency. Second, because of the strength training, your muscles and tendons will be warm, and many of your joints will be lubricated with synovial fluid. This will help you to develop flexibility more quickly, and decrease the chance of injury.

Many dieters stretch in front of the television while watching a specific program, such as the evening news.

Stretch on a safe, comfortable surface. A non-slip yoga mat on top of a carpet is perfect, and what Stuart uses. Bare feet on the mat provide better grip than feet in socks. Stretch in a warm room, and keep yourself covered.

This routine, with three reps for each stretch (or three for *each side* for two of the stretches), can be completed in just 10 minutes or so.

After a few months of following this routine you're likely to increase your flexibility substantially. Thereafter, keep stretching in order to maintain your improved flexibility.

The routine has just five stretches: four primary directional motions—forward bend, back bend, side bend, and twist—and a calf stretch. The back bend, side bend, and twist have the potential to be invigorating—they are Stuart's favorite stretches.

How to stretch

Done correctly, stretching is safe. Follow the instructions carefully. Don't try to rush your progress. Never force a stretch. Never bounce while stretching. And avoid holding your breath—breathe freely. Keep your lips and teeth slightly apart.

Never move immediately into your current full level of flexibility for a given stretch. Move there in stages. Do two progressive warm-up reps, and then a single rep at your current maximum flexibility. Hold each rep for at least 20 seconds.

You should feel only *slight* discomfort as you stretch. As you hold each rep of a stretch, you should feel the muscular tension diminish. Depending on the stretch, and the individual, you may need to hold a stretch for 30 or so seconds before you feel this slackening. The easing of tension is the signal to relax for a few seconds, then move further into the stretch in order to make the muscle(s) feel tight again. If you don't feel the tension diminishing even after a hold of about 30 seconds, let the stretch go for a few seconds, then slowly move into the next rep.

Never force yourself to feel pain, but you must feel tension during each stretch. Never have anyone force you into a stretch. And never be in a hurry.

Some days you'll be less flexible than others, so don't expect to stretch equally well every session.

Two of the stretches are performed on the floor. Be careful how you get up from the floor, so that you don't irritate your lower back. Don't sit up with straight knees. While on your back, bend your knees, roll to one side and, using your hands for assistance, push into a sitting position.

You may find that muscles of one limb or one side of your torso are less flexible than those of the opposite limb or side. If so, perform an additional rep of each relevant stretch for the less flexible side. Be patient, and persistent. Over time this should yield symmetrical left-right flexibility *unless* there are restrictions that require treatment from a professional therapist.

Warning — pre-workout stretching

Many people think that they need to stretch *thoroughly* before any type of workout—for example, outdoor walk, treadmill walk, jog, or strength training—or before any recreational sport.

Such stretching can do more harm than good. It often causes pre-workout irritation to muscles and tendons that leads to injury during the workout proper. Or, the actual stretching can cause injury itself. And this risk is increased if the stretching is done first thing in the morning, before the body is physiologically fully ready for exercise.

By all means do a *little, very gentle* stretching prior to any other form of exercise, or recreational sport, to *carefully* loosen up any area that isn't at its *usual* flexibility, *but nothing more than that.*

An ideal time to stretch is *after* a strength-training workout, as already recommended. Then your body is warmed up *internally*.

Even if you're in a warm environment, that doesn't mean that your muscles and tendons are ready to be stretched. A high ambient temperature doesn't necessarily correlate to internal preparedness for stretching or any other type of exercise.

HONOR your exercise program.

HONOR your dedication to your weight-loss plan.

HONOR your commitment to your health and well-being.

Technique of the five stretches

1. Calf stretch

This stretch—specifically for the gastrocnemius muscle (the largest member of the calf group)—is very important. Supple gastrocnemius muscles are required for correct joint position and stride length when walking and running. Many leg muscle injuries arise primarily as a result of tight gastrocnemius muscles.

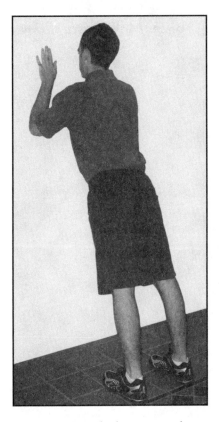

Stand at arm's length from a support such as a door frame, post, or wall. Stand upright, at ease, with straight knees and relaxed thighs. By bending at your wrists, elbows and ankles, lean forward just sufficiently so that you feel a little tension in your calves. Hold that position until the tension eases. Return to the starting position for a few seconds. Then lean forward again until you feel tension, and hold that position until the tension eases. Again return to the upright starting position for a few seconds. Repeat for a third rep. *Keep your heels on the floor throughout the reps.*

As the weeks go by you'll gradually be able to lean farther forward before you feel the required tension in your calves.

Once you reach the stage where your head touches the wall, change your starting set-up. With your heels close together, place the balls of your feet on a book or board about half an inch thick, and *keep your heels on the floor.* See the illustration on the next page.

The elevation will reduce how far you need to lean forward before you feel the required tension in your calves. Then progress as before, by leaning farther forward as your flexibility increases.

If you feel tension behind your knees, you're overstretching or rushing the stretch, and you should ease back.

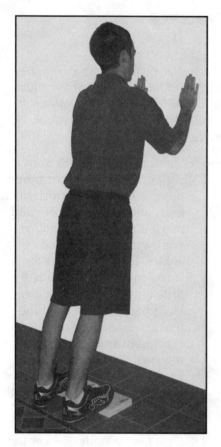

This stretch is for your calf muscles, not your Achilles tendons. As noted already, tendons are almost inelastic.

Develop symmetrical flexibility.

Don't try to rush your progress. Progress in flexibility at your own pace. *Make haste slowly.*

2. Forward bend

This modified forward bend is done lying, for control and safety. It stretches the hamstrings—the three muscles at the rear of the thighs.

Lie on your back on the floor with your heels against a wall, and knees bent sufficiently so that there's no tension in your hamstrings. (Have a small cushion under your head, for comfort.) Then move close enough to the wall so that you feel slight tension in your hamstrings. Hold this position until the tension eases, then relax, and repeat. This time, straighten your knees a little, to increase tension. Then relax and repeat once more.

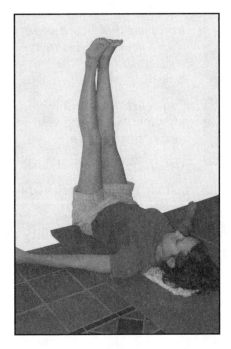

There should be no tension behind your knees—there's no hamstring muscle behind the knees. If there is tension behind your knees, reduce the tension until it's felt in your hamstrings.

Later, to increase tension further, move closer still to the wall.

When you can do this with your hips against the wall, and knees straight (as illustrated), but without tension in your hamstrings—which may take several weeks, or longer in some cases—you're ready for the more advanced version.

Dispense with the wall. Lie on your back on the floor, with your head on a small cushion. Bend your knees, but keep your feet flat on the floor. Bring one knee near to your chest, and then bring the other one there, too. Then straighten them both, until your legs are vertical, like they were when supported by a wall.

Use a towel, strap, or belt, and loop it stirrup-like over the *arches* of your feet. Then, *keep your back and shoulders pressed against the floor, knees straight, and toes above your heels.* Don't pull on the balls of your feet, because that would cause your calves to tighten, and mar the stretch for your hamstrings. Your calf muscles should be *relaxed.* See the illustration on the next page.

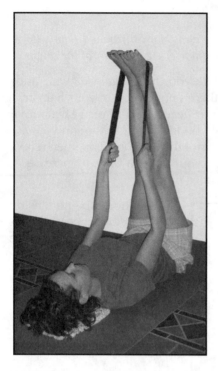

Gently pull the towel, strap or belt until you feel tension in your hamstrings. *Keep your knees straight.* Hold this position until the tension eases, then relax, and repeat. This time you should be able to pull a little farther, but still keep your knees straight. Hold this position until, again, the tension eases, then relax, and repeat once more.

Remember that if there's tension behind your knees, reduce the tension until it's felt in your hamstrings only.

To progress in flexibility, incrementally bring your legs nearer to your face.

Develop symmetrical flexibility.

This stretch will involve muscles you may not have stretched for a long time, and which may currently be tight.

Don't try to rush your progress. Progress in flexibility at your own pace. *Make haste slowly.*

3. Back bend

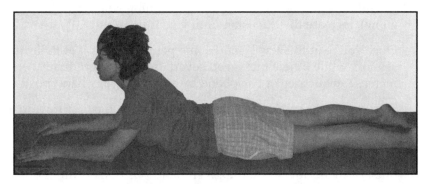

Lie face down with your arms and forearms outstretched—keep your forearms about shoulder-width apart. Lift your head and shoulders as you bring your arms toward you so that your elbows are bent and lined up with your chin. Keep your forearms flat on the floor as you arch your back as much *as is easy and comfortable.* Hold for about 20 seconds, then return to flat on the floor. Repeat.

If that's easy for you, and there's no negative reaction, progress to the next stage at your first session. But if the first stage was difficult, stick with it for as many sessions as you need until you can do it easily.

Now for the second stage, as shown below. With your head and shoulders off the floor, and your elbows again lined up with your chin, extend your elbows as you raise your chest off the floor as much as is comfortable. Hold for about 20 seconds, then return to the floor. Relax for a few seconds, then repeat and hold a little longer and a little higher. Then repeat one more time.

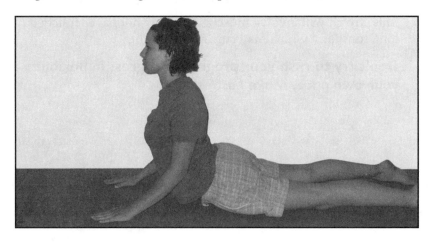

Next session, if you're not already fully extending your elbows (and extending your back as far as that positioning will comfortably allow), increase the extension until you are.

Once you're at this level—and some people can do it at their first session, while others may need several sessions—gradually increase the degree of back bend.by adjusting your hand position.

Start your next session with your hands an inch closer towards your torso, which will enable you to bend back a little more as you fully extend your elbows. Week by week, an inch at a time, start with your hands a little closer towards your torso. But you must *easily* be able to hold a given hand position at full elbow extension for at least 20 seconds before you graduate to the next hand position.

Shortly, you may be able to set up with your hands by the sides of your shoulders, prior to making a substantial back bend. But even then, don't move immediately into the full back extension—go there progressively, over several reps.

Later on you may be able to set up with your hands by the sides of your chest, prior to making a more substantial back bend.

At all times in the back bend, keep your head in a neutral position. *Don't arch your neck.*

This spine extension, provided it's not exaggerated, can be great therapy for back discomfort. It can also help to prevent back pain. This stretch can also help to maintain the natural curves of your spine, which tend to flatten with age.

Develop symmetrical flexibility.

This stretch will involve muscles you may not have stretched for a long time, and which may currently be tight.

Don't try to rush your progress. Progress in flexibility at your own pace. *Make haste slowly.*

4. Side bend

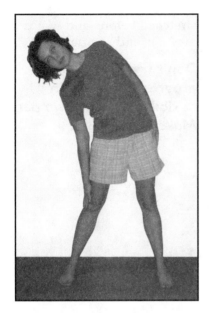

Stand with your feet wider than hip-width apart. With your hands resting on the sides of your thighs, slowly lean to your right. Your right hand must travel down your outer thigh towards, to, or beyond your right knee, depending on your flexibility and limb lengths. *You must maintain that firm contact with your hand, to control the stretch.* Your left hand will travel up your left thigh towards or to your left hip.

Descend only until you feel *a little* tension in your left side. Hold that position until the tension eases. Then return to the upright position, and do the same to the other side. Then repeat to the right side, but this time a little farther than the first time. Then do the same for the other side, and so on. Do three reps to each side.

All movement should be *lateral*. Don't lean forward, or backward.

From session to session, *gradually* increase your range of motion.

Eventually you'll be able to reach your outer calf muscle with your leading or lower hand, and thus have a substantial range of motion. When you can do that easily, place your higher hand on your chest. That will enable you to increase the stretch effect on your side.

After you've adapted to that over a few sessions (or longer), place your higher hand on your head, as illustrated on the next page.

The advanced version would have your higher hand outstretched in line with your torso, for maximum effect—see the bottom photograph on the next page.

Whatever you do for one side, do the same for the other. Develop symmetrical flexibility.

This isn't just a stretch. It will also strengthen your obliques (sides of your waist), and some of your spinal musculature.

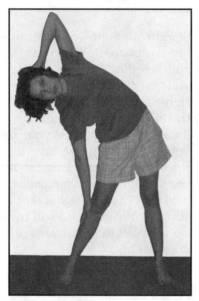

This stretch will involve muscles you may not have stretched before, and which may currently be tight.

Don't try to rush your progress. Progress in flexibility at your own pace. *Make haste slowly.*

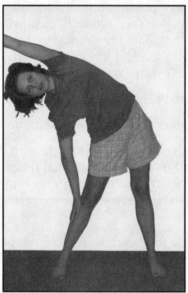

Photography credits

Thank you to Nicholas Charalambous and Korinna McRobert for posing for the exercise photographs.

5. Twist

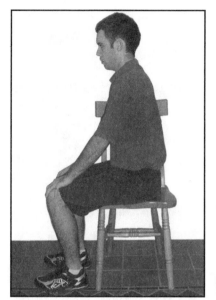 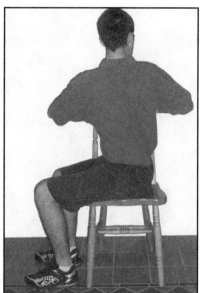

Sit *sideways* on a chair that doesn't have arms, with your right side against the back. Keep your knees bent at about a right angle, and feet flat on the floor about shoulder-width apart. Rotate to your right and grab the back of the chair with both hands. This is the starting position.

Gently rotate your torso and neck to your right. Stay upright— don't slouch—and keep your buttocks and thighs on the seat. Rotate to the point where you feel tension in your back, waist, and neck. Hold until the tension eases, then return to the starting position. Pause for a few seconds, and repeat to the same side. This time, rotate a little farther. Then repeat yet again.

Turn around and perform three reps for your other side.

Develop symmetrical flexibility.

This stretch will involve muscles you may not have stretched before, and which may currently be tight.

Don't try to rush your progress. Progress in flexibility at your own pace. *Make haste slowly.*

Although this is an introductory stretching routine, it will yield substantial benefits if properly implemented for long enough. But if you want to experience the full benefits that stretching offers, you'll need to follow a comprehensive routine.

This book has already given you hundreds of real-life weight-loss tips.

And this chapter will give you additional tips from real people who beat their battle with the bulge once and for all.

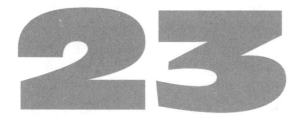

Additional weight-loss tips and tidbits

Although the following nuggets of guidance don't slot neatly into any of the other chapters, they will still enrich your knowledge. Act on them and you'll make your weight-loss easier.

Focus on the *big* picture

If you decide to cheat on occasion, or give in to cravings, don't fret. Just get back on track tomorrow.

There's no need to be a party pooper because you think that you aren't allowed to have fun on a weight-loss plan. You can attend an occasional party that may lead to a *moderate* overindulgence.

The key is to know what "on occasion" means.

"On occasion" doesn't mean weekly. An overindulgent night at a party once a week can easily kill your progress. One night off the rails will undo all the good work during the rest of the week. When Brad gorged once a week while on his wedding diet, his weight-loss stopped even though he was ultra-disciplined the rest of the time.

There will be times, such as during holidays, when you may put on a few pounds. Many real-life dieters do, but they get back into the groove the day after the holiday, and then are on track again.

Once again, *it's the big picture that matters.* A few days of splurging out of a year won't derail your long-term plan, but weekly splurging or binging will.

Always remember the basis of weight-loss—*you must use up more calories than you take in.* If you feel like eating excessive food at a party or some other event, ask yourself what your plan is for burning it off, *because if you don't burn it off it's going to be stored on you as fat.*

If you take in more calories than you use up, you *will* put on fat.

Busting through periods of stalled weight-loss

If you've stopped losing weight, don't panic, and don't give up. Plateaus are to be expected—your body always tries to adapt to what you do to it.

Especially when you hit a plateau, vary your caloric intake and perhaps some of your food choices, and vary your exercise programs and intensity. Then you'll bust through the plateau.

Losing fat is a complex process, and your body must occasionally regroup. Although some plateaus lasted for several weeks, Brad broke through them all.

You'll bust through your plateaus, too. *Be persistent.*

You won't lose weight every week. But you'll probably have great weeks as well as frustrating ones.

A plateau can be the result of muscle-gain, or water-weight-gain. You may have lost fat, but at the same time you may have added muscle. And as you gain more muscle, and maintain hydration, your muscles will retain more glycogen and hold more water. This won't show a positive result on the weighing scale, but it will in the way your clothes fit. Because of this, don't panic if the scale isn't budging.

A plateau can be caused by not periodically reducing caloric intake. It takes fewer calories to support a lighter weight. You'll need a reduction of approximately 70 daily calories for every 10 pounds you lose.

But don't panic and reduce your caloric intake too much, or you may trigger off the *starvation effect* reaction. Your body would then retain its fat because it will "think" that a famine is underway.

Try this trick: When you vary your calories every other day, be a bit more aggressive on your higher-calorie days, to try to boost your metabolism.

For example, when varying his calories, Brad tried to eat a little more on some of his higher-calorie days. When he was stuck at 201 pounds, he was at about 1,400 calories on his lower-calorie days, but he ramped up his higher-calorie days to 1,900 to 2,100, to help elevate his metabolism, and ward off the starvation effect. It worked.

Another plateau-busting trick is to keep your existing calories the same, but add one or two meals to your day.

To do this, make each meal a little smaller and spread your calories over seven or eight tiny meals a day. This may further boost your metabolism via diet-induced thermogenesis because your body has to work more to digest the additional meals.

Sometimes, a period of stalled weight-loss is due to carbohydrate intake that's too high or too low, or protein intake that's too high or too low.

Or, sometimes, it's the result of simple overeating. Perhaps some of your 200- to 400-calorie mini-meals have crept up to 500 or 600. Get your food journal back out, and monitor what you're eating.

The plateau may also be because you're burning fewer overall calories. Perhaps you've blown off too many exercise sessions.

Unless you're using up more calories than you're taking in, you're not going to lose weight.

A plateau can also be the result of medication such as prednisone, or of food intolerances or nutritional deficiencies. Consult your doctor to help you sort out any of these possible causes.

Eventually, however, you'll reach your true set point, which is your body's floor for how much weight you can realistically lose. Although your floor level can be misinterpreted as a plateau, it's a plateau that will never end.

Your weight-loss goal may have been unrealistic, and it may not be possible for you to be as slim as you desire—like a fabulously fit celebrity or athlete, for example.

When the snag releases

Think of a plateau as a snag, and when the snag releases, a change can happen quickly. Brad had five plateaus during his final weight-loss journey.

He'd been stuck at 202 pounds for three weeks, then stepped on the scale to find that he weighed 199 pounds. The three pounds seemingly evaporated overnight. Although he was stuck in a plateau, his body was undergoing internal processes that would lead to the snag releasing.

Later on he was stuck at 192 pounds for a while. Again, almost out of nowhere, he weighed in at 189 pounds as the snag released. He was also stuck at 181 pounds for a while, but then weighed in at 178 pounds—again, seemingly out of nowhere.

How to monitor your weight-loss progress

When people lose weight, those who try to rush the process will generally lose fat and *muscle*.

But remember, what you're trying to lose is body *fat*, not muscle.

You may have to use multiple methods to determine if you're losing body fat. As well as weighing yourself via a scale, monitor how your clothes fit, and also monitor pinch-points on your body.

Initially, you can usually tell if you're losing fat by the way your clothes fit—especially your pants.

Pinching fat between your thumb and forefinger at certain spots on your body is a good method of tracking fat-loss. (Alternatively, use fat calipers.) Pinch the fat under your skin to the depth of the muscle there. The pinch-points include the waist for men, and waist, hips, and thighs for women.

When monitoring your progress via the scale, use one that's calibrated—for accurate measurements.

Weigh yourself under the *same* conditions. Having a weigh-in, for example, after becoming temporarily dehydrated, will lead to frustration because at the next weigh-in you'll likely weigh more.

And inadvertent water retention can skew your results by creating the illusion that you gained fat.

Almost all successful dieters weigh themselves regularly to gauge their progress, and stay on track. Some weigh every day, some every week, and some every month.

Weighing yourself too often can be frustrating, however, because daily fluctuations in your body's water retention can produce misleading weight readings.

Brad weighed himself weekly during his final weight-loss journey, and he now weighs himself monthly during his maintenance phase. He trusts the way his pants fit as a reliable week-to-week indicator.

But while it's still a trusted staple for many people, weighing yourself via the scale can still be a poor barometer for your overall progress because there's usually no consideration given to body *composition* and whether you've gained (or lost) muscle mass.

For example, crash diets can cause you to lose a lot of weight via the scale, but much of it isn't body fat but muscle and superfluous water weight. Although Brad lost 57 pounds via the scale during his wedding diet, roughly 10 to 15 of it was muscle tissue, and the rest was a combination of fat and temporary water weight.

But when Brad was stuck at his 181-pound plateau for a few weeks he was lifting weights intensively. He may have lost fat while he gained muscle, and produced a "zero pounds lost" net effect.

Another marker of overall progress, and health benefits, is waist circumference reduction. Intra-abdominal fat is associated with diabetes, cancers, and heart disease. And seeing a gradually decreasing waist girth should be satisfying aesthetically, too.

See if your doctor can perform a regular body composition test via accurate body fat measuring equipment. With this, you'll discover what sort of weight you're losing.

Although, via the scale, Brad lost "only" 102 pounds on his final weight-loss journey, a body composition test calculated that he lost 114 pounds of fat because he put on approximately 12 pounds of muscle tissue.

Variety keeps you fresh

Vary the exercises you do, but always choose *safe* ones you enjoy.

Come up with a list of nutritious foods that you enjoy eating, and vary your meals somewhat from day to day.

If you crave something, have *a little* of it.

Eating a variety of foods may help you to get more pleasure out of your meals. And you must enjoy your new lifestyle if you're to stick with it.

Vary your entertainment when you use a stationary bike or treadmill, for example, or walk outdoors. A portable MP3 Player, DVD player, or cable television, can keep you entertained so that you don't get bored during your indoor exercise.

Remember that your body naturally tries to adapt to anything you do. It will adapt to the same routine of lifting weights, and the same routine of walking. Your body will become more efficient. A workout that used to be taxing, will become easier to accomplish. This is why you must push yourself with new goals, and different workouts.

Find a support group

It's easier to succeed when you have a support group.

Let your roommates, officemates, family, or partner know what you're trying to do, and why. Ask friends and family for their support, and ask them not to parade any fattening food around you. If your friends and family care about you, they'll understand, and cooperate.

Many of Brad's officemates abandoned processed food when they saw that he had lost a ton of weight.

Find a weight-loss buddy who has similar struggles and goals— someone who can go through this with you.

But make sure that your buddy isn't going to be a partner in crime for cheating, or a nag. Look for someone who can empathize, and support you.

And find a partner who doesn't make food a focus when socializing. Go for a bike ride or a walk together, for example, rather than go out for pizza, beer, or chicken wings.

Belonging to weight-loss support groups that have meetings can be helpful because they offer emotional encouragement. According to a University of Missouri study, women who joined a weight-loss group lost three times as much weight as those who joined a gym.

Some people also belong to exercise groups such as walking, jogging, bicycling, yoga, Pilates, spinning, and basketball.

And enlist some professional help, too. Many of the dieters that Brad interviewed enlisted registered dieticians, personal trainers, and even psychologists to help them deal with the problems that were thwarting their results. *Sometimes, you can't do it on your own.*

As Brad lost weight, many friends and family members climbed aboard his "weight-loss express," and began getting fit themselves. They saw Brad finally succeed, and it proved to them that weight-loss *is* possible. And as you succeed, your success will become contagious, too.

Use smaller plates, bowls and glasses

Many people naturally eat until they are full, but this is bad for weight-loss.

An easy way to trick yourself into thinking that you're full, is to consume a smaller meal that appears to be a larger one because it's heaped over a small plate or bowl.

Brad replaced all of his large plates and bowls with small ones. Do the same. After a while you won't notice the difference in the size of your crockery.

And skinny or small glasses can trick you into drinking less, too.

Another trick is to move your food from a large container or multi-serving box, into a small bowl or plate. This isn't just for presentation—people naturally eat more if the serving-size seems unlimited. For example, put microwave popcorn into a few smaller bowls instead of eating it out of the bag. You're likely to eat less.

Do you have an appetite for blue food?

The color of your crockery can make a difference. Upon the recommendation of their nutritionists, many real-life dieters use blue plates and bowls.

Blue may suppress appetite—a view supported by research from the International Color Research Institute.

According to the research, the premise to this theory is that blue only rarely exists as a natural color for food, and therefore humans don't have an appetite for blue food.

And when our ancestors were searching for food, blue was one of the colors of poisonous berries, so anything blue was avoided.

So, it seems logical that blue plates and bowls would be the least likely to stimulate your appetite.

One of the ladies Brad talked to took this theory to the extreme, and painted her kitchen blue. Some people use a blue light in their dining area, and some use a blue light bulb in their fridge to help reduce temptations.

Brush your teeth after every meal

Not only is brushing your teeth after each meal important for oral hygiene, it may keep you from snacking between meals. Brad's wife, and Stuart, are big advocates of this trick. They don't want to eat when their mouths have a freshly brushed feeling.

You can also gargle with mouthwash, or put a breath strip into your mouth if you get the urge to snack. The intense flavor in the breath fresheners can overwhelm your taste buds and fend off the craving.

Do obese people have more fat cells than slim people?

While most obese people don't necessarily have more fat cells than slim people, the globules within their fat cells hold more fat.

When you lose weight you don't get rid of fat cells, you merely shrink them. And according to a recent study by the Karolinska Institute—in Stockholm, Sweden—the body constantly replaces its dying fat cells, and holds the overall number constant. This study also shows that you're stuck with the number of fat cells you had when you became an adult.

Even ultra-ripped bodybuilders and athletes still have 3% to 8% body fat, and *plenty* of fat cells. While the fat cells aren't visible under their skin, they are still there. And these ripped individuals still possess several pounds of internal fat, which protects and insulates vital organs.

Is liposuction a solution for weight-loss?

Liposuction is cosmetic surgery that removes fat from specific areas of the body—such as the abdomen, thighs, buttocks, and upper arms—via a hollow tube and a suction device called a cannula.

But it's not an alternative to exercise and diet. Nor is it intended for *overall* body fat reduction.

Liposuction is a method of removing localized fat from areas that don't respond to diet and exercise. The best candidates for it are normal-weight people who have pockets of excess fat in certain areas. While the amount of fat removed varies, it's typically less than 10 pounds.

According to a study published in *Dermatologic Surgery*, the overall clinical complication rate was 0.7%—7 out of 1,000. But the surgery does have some sporadic risks via anesthesia, bleeding, and surgical complications.

Although it's a relatively safe procedure that's performed under local anesthesia, the recovery period can take several weeks, during which you would likely miss work. There's usually swelling and bruising, but these generally subside within a few weeks. And you would usually be required to wear a support garment for several weeks post-surgery.

Your skin may take up to six months to mold itself around the modified areas of your body—you could be left with extra folds of skin for a while. But some areas may not be elastic enough to mold to the modified areas, which means you may have to undergo another surgery—which can be expensive—to take a tuck or lift to fix the problem.

Although liposuction removes fat, if too much is removed, the skin can mold unnaturally to the underlying muscle and tissues, and create an irregular appearance. Furthermore, liposuction can't eliminate dimpling or cellulite.

And according to a study by the University of Colorado Health Sciences Center, the fat removal isn't permanent in all cases. Although the pockets of fat that are removed during liposuction are gone forever, that doesn't mean you won't develop new pockets of fat. Remember, according to the study by the Karolinska Institute in Stockholm, your body can replace fat cells over time.

So, if you don't maintain sound eating and exercise habits, your body fat may gravitate back to your troubled areas, whether it's your belly, butt, or saddlebag hips.

Your surgeon will discuss the pros and cons of liposuction with you, and you may also have to see a psychiatrist to make sure you're in the right frame of mind to undergo the procedure.

Liposuction is an expensive surgery that's usually not covered by health insurance.

Gastric-bypass surgery

For the super obese, the morbidly obese, or the clinically obese who are also suffering from serious obesity-related health problems, an option for losing weight may be gastric-bypass surgery, which is the most common form of bariatric surgery. Bariatric surgery refers to all surgical treatments for super obesity and morbid obesity.

You must be educated about the risks, benefits, and details of this surgery before you can determine if it's appropriate for you. It must be discussed with a surgeon who has extensive experience of it.

The most popular type of gastric-bypass surgery in the US is the Roux-en-Y (proximal) bypass. In this case, the surgeon sections off the stomach to reduce its size by well over 90%, then rearranges the upper part of the small intestine.

Patients must overhaul their eating habits for a lifelong commitment. They must learn to live on three-ounce meals, and get used to cutting their food into pea-sized morsels. And to replace nutrients no longer absorbed by their digestive tracts, they generally have to adhere to a regular supplement regimen complete with vitamins (including B$_{12}$), calcium, and nutrition shakes.

According to the American Society of Bariatric Surgery, 3 out of every 1,000 patients die from gastric-bypass surgery.

The main risk stems from having an abdominal operation. Severely obese patients are at a disadvantage when having this type of surgery.

Having an abdominal operation places a great deal of stress on the body. It creates an open wound, which can bleed or fail to heal, and it creates a potential for infection.

And the reaction of the body to an open wound of this magnitude can cause increased blood clotting, which can lead to a fatal pulmonary embolism.

And four in ten patients develop complications within the first six months, according to the US Agency for Healthcare Research and Quality (AHRQ). The complications include vomiting, diarrhea, infections, hernias, and respiratory failure.

Furthermore, up to 40% of gastric-bypass patients can suffer nutritional deficiency, which can result in anemia and osteoporosis. And research from the Mayo Clinic suggests that this may be responsible for making former patients' bones more brittle, which can make them much more susceptible to fractures.

And because gastric-bypass surgery rearranges the digestive tract, many patients experience gastrointestinal problems. A majority of people who have a gastric-bypass experience "dumping syndrome"—when sugary, undigested foods empty directly into the small intestine, causing nausea, vomiting, light-headedness, cramping, and gas.

A 2005 study by the *Journal of the American Medical Association* found that 20% of gastric-bypass patients were re-hospitalized the year after surgery, often for follow-up operations.

But while there are significant risks from this surgery, the benefits generally outweigh the risks for most candidates. In 2007, doctors performed 205,000 bariatric surgeries, and over 80% of them were performed on women.

Besides weight-loss, gastric-bypass surgery has also been shown to place type II diabetes in complete remission. Most patients return to normal blood pressure and cholesterol readings within a few months. And the surgery can eliminate sleep apnea, and help stave off many weight-related cancers.

A 2007 University of Utah study, which was published in the *New England Journal of Medicine*, found that gastric-bypass surgery patients were 56% less likely to die of coronary heart disease, 60% less likely to die of cancer, and 92% less likely to die of diabetes than obese people who didn't have the surgery.

And many patients see an improvement in exercise tolerance, and breathing ability, within the first few months after surgery. Patients who have barely been able to walk are able to participate in more activities, even exercise. And they experience relief from pain in their weight-bearing joints.

Furthermore, most patients end up much healthier, and generally lead fuller, more productive lives.

But gastric-bypass surgery isn't a quick fix, or even a permanent solution. After weight-loss surgery, your success will come *only* with a long-term commitment. Like with anyone who maintains weight-loss over the long-term, you have to stick with a healthy diet and exercise regimen for the rest of your life.

If you slack off on exercise, and eat more food, you'll regain the weight.

And if you continue to overfill your stomach by eating larger-than-recommended portions, you can stretch your minuscule stomach to twice its post-surgical size.

Although initial weight-loss can be dramatic—gastric-bypass patients typically shed around 70% of excess weight—a majority of patients gradually regain 20% to 25% of what they lost. And according to Lee Kaplan, M.D., director of the Massachusetts General Hospital Weight Center in Boston, fewer than 10% of patients ever achieve a normal BMI (18.5 to 24.9).

And you'll have to make regular appointments with your surgeon for several years. It's common for serious complications to develop when patients become complacent three to five years post-surgery.

Gastric-bypass surgery alternatives

The alternatives are gastric band surgery, and obesity implants.

Gastric-band surgery is a minimally invasive surgical approach that requires no intestinal re-routing, cutting, or stapling of the stomach wall or bowel. It appears to have fewer risks and side effects, with a much lower short-term mortality rate than gastric-bypass surgery. And it's often performed on an outpatient basis.

Gastric bands are offered by the manufacturers of two competing brands—Allergan, which makes the Lap-Band, and Johnson and Johnson, which makes the Realize Band. The band is an adjustable silicone belt that goes around the top of the stomach. It helps control hunger, to achieve a feeling of fullness sooner.

Obesity implants trick the nerve cells lining the stomach to release a chemical signal that tells the brain the stomach is full. Feeling a genuine sensation of fullness, the individual stops eating. This yields caloric restriction, and weight-loss.

But these medical procedures can be extremely expensive, and may not be covered by health insurance.

"Addiction transfer" as a result of gastric-bypass surgery

Gastric-bypass surgery has helped people to lose weight, but it can lead to the serious, post-surgery complication called "addiction transfer."

According to an article published in *Bariatric Times*, "There are millions of people who've had surgery who are dealing with this [addiction transfer] and want to bring it to light." They eventually transfer their addiction from food (which they can no longer overeat on) to another addiction such as alcohol, shopping, compulsive spending, compulsive gambling, smoking, or promiscuity—with alcohol being the most common.

Many former gastric-bypass patients have become alcoholics.

Because the issues behind their eating disorder hadn't been addressed—for example, child or marital abuse, rape, depression, or death of a loved one—their addiction to food was transferred to something else.

Most gastric-bypass surgery patients are emotional eaters. When they can no longer eat in that way, they are left with what to do with their emotions.

Help should be sought to discover and treat the root cause of eating disorders. This may require a psychiatrist, or a psychologist.

But not everyone who requires this sort of help has the courage to see a psychiatrist or a psychologist, and even those people who have the courage may not find the support they require merely from one-on-one counseling. Addiction can create feelings of isolation and worthlessness. And because of this, support groups have become alternative solutions for dealing with addictions.

Support groups for dealing with addictions

There are many support groups. Check the internet, or your local phone book, to find the chapters in your area. The groups include:

Alcoholics Anonymous (A.A.)

Food Addicts Anonymous (F.A.A.)

Food Addicts in Recovery Anonymous (F.A.)

Overeaters Anonymous (O.A.)

Gamblers Anonymous (G.A.)

Narcotics Anonymous (N.A.)

Sex Addicts Anonymous (S.A.A.)

Debtors Anonymous (D.A.)

Does the diet industry *really* want women to be slim?

Hollywood, models, and thin celebrities contribute to the pressure on women to be slim, which boosts sales of products sold by the diet industry.

Most women are sensible *until* the carrot of a new "miracle" diet plan, product or technique is dangled in front of them. Then many of them think they have found the weight-loss holy grail— regardless of how bizarre it may be, or the lack of research behind it. This is why most diet ads are targeted at women. Many women fall for these snake-oil pitches time and time again.

The diet industry feeds on the insecurity, guilt, yearning to be desired, and gullibility of many women. And it tries to persuade them to fall for a snake oil-pitch, buy a meal replacement, or order a whacky diet plan or exercise product.

Some of the plans and products that promise weight-loss may work over the short-term, but they rarely work over the long-term. And these quick fixes never address the women's underlying problems such as low self-esteem, insufficient knowledge about nutrition and exercise, and the probable presence of psychological and physiological problems.

But it seems that the diet industry doesn't really want women to be slim, because most slim women don't buy many if any diet products.

WOMEN (and men, too) . . . see how the diet industry is ripping you off, *and then cut your ties with it.*

Study this book, become an expert on weight-loss, take charge of your weight, and get in charge of your life.

Did you know that drinking plenty of *ice-cold* water may help you to lose weight?

This chapter explains how real people successfully incorporated beverages—including the alcoholic variety—in their weight-loss plans.

Brad and many dieters believe that drinking a lot of zero- and low-calorie fluids each day is one of the most important tactics to help them control their eating. *Without it, Brad doubts that he would have achieved his transformation.*

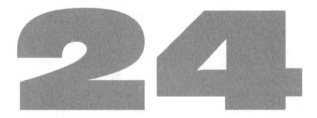

Drink up

While drinking plenty of water is a fundamental component of losing weight, the consumption of excess calories from beverages is one of the main reasons why so many people are overweight.

What should you be drinking to help you to lose weight?

Drink a lot of zero- and low-calorie fluids

Being properly hydrated is essential for your health. Regardless of its temperature, water replenishes your body's fluids, and helps to flush waste away. Sufficient water intake is required for your body's systems to operate effectively and efficiently. Proper hydration is critical for protein metabolism and muscle repair, as well as every other vital process in your body. And an adequate intake of water may reduce your risk of various cancers.

Proper hydration may even increase the neurotransmitters that signal fat release from your fat cells.

Drink a large glass of ice-cold water when you feel the slightest sensation of hunger, *and* when you feel the slightest sensation of thirst. According to research from Virginia Tech, drinking a pint of water before breakfast can reduce caloric intake at that meal by as much as 13%.

Have a glass of ice-cold water with each other meal, too. The water can help create the sensation of fullness, and cause you to eat less.

Many dieters have also discovered that drinking a large glass of water in the late evening greatly reduces nighttime hunger pangs.

And drinking plenty of ice-cold water may help you in other ways to lose weight. According to a study conducted in Germany, drinking *ice-cold* water may temporarily speed up your metabolism because additional energy is required for your body to heat the water up. And this may temporarily spike your metabolism to the point where you can burn a few dozen extra calories a day, depending on how much ice-cold water you drink. This may be worth a few pounds of fat-loss over a year. The German scientists found that drinking a pint of *ice-cold* water when you first roll out of bed may boost your metabolism for up to 90 minutes.

While some dieters drink more, and some drink less, Brad's research suggests that the typical minimum measure of how much water to have each day is the fluid-ounce equivalent of half of your bodyweight in pounds. For example, a 200-pound person may want to drink upwards of 100 fluid ounces a day—100 fluid ounces is about six pints, or three quarts.

But this water requirement includes almost all fluids consumed, not just pure water—for example, herbal teas, green tea and other zero- or low-calorie drinks, as well as milk and pure juices. *Most fluids are mostly water.* The water requirement is also dependent on climate. When the temperature is high, increase your fluid intake.

As noted earlier, Brad and his wife often mix up a gallon of ice-cold, sugar-free Kool-Aid® or Crystal Light®, which are five calories per serving. A recent study shows that women who drink flavored water, like Crystal Light®, consume 20% more water.

But if you don't like *ice-cold* water and other fluids, or you like them only during hot weather, drink them at the temperature you prefer. *Fluid intake is the priority.* The

temperature is a personal preference, although ice-cold fluids may provide benefits beyond hydration alone.

Stuart starts his day with a large drink of water, but he prefers hot water at that time, even during the summer. During the rest of the day he has hot and cold drinks.

Brad usually has 8 to 16 ounces (half to one pint) of ice-cold water with each meal. And he drinks water and low-calorie fluids between meals. Furthermore, each evening he drinks upwards of a quart of ice-cold water (most often flavored water), which fends off late-night eating.

While Brad drinks a lot of water and other fluids, many successful real-life dieters don't drink nearly this much, for a number of reasons. A lot of fluid consumption leads to a lot of urination, which may not be convenient (especially at work), so you must do what works for you—*but it's essential that you're properly hydrated.*

To be properly hydrated, remember our earlier guidance: Drink enough water over the course of the day to produce at least four *clear* urinations a day (in addition to colored ones). The quantity will vary relative to your activity level, and the climate you live in.

But many dieters do drink fluids *beyond what's required for proper hydration*. Drinking a lot of water and other fluids each day produces the sensation of fullness that can help reduce food consumption. Although it's an elementary concept, it's very effective in practice. *Many dieters consider it to be one of the most important tactics to help them control their eating. Without it, Brad doubts that he would have achieved his transformation.*

Watch your calorie-laden drinks

Drink skim milk instead of whole milk. Artificially flavored coffee drinks and fruit-juice drinks can be loaded with calories—have them only sparingly, if at all. And if you must drink soda, choose diet instead of regular.

Watch out for sports drinks. Many of these vitamin-enhanced drinks are essentially high-calorie, sugared water. They are tasty, but many are formulated for athletes, not couch potatoes.

Also be careful with your portion sizes when having nutritious drinks. A large glass of skim milk or pure orange juice with each meal unnecessarily adds to your daily caloric intake.

Eat an orange instead of orange juice—this can save you about 185 calories. The orange also has more fiber than the juice, which slows sugar infusion. And according to the *American Journal of Clinical Nutrition*, citrus fruits like oranges can increase abdominal fat oxidation.

Solid foods take longer for your body to digest, and thus they create more diet-induced thermogenesis.

Liquid calories don't satisfy your body like solid-food can, but they can easily add up to many calories, albeit perhaps with few nutrients.

For example, if you have a few sugar-laden sodas each day, by eliminating them you could lose 10 to 30 pounds of fat in a year. An average 20-ounce, non-diet soda contains 17 teaspoons of sugar.

Watch out for excessive calories, dietary sugars, or high-fructose corn syrup in anything you drink.

Many large, fast-food milkshakes have more than 1,000 calories. Some specialty shakes can exceed 2,000 calories. Brad used to drink them often, as a treat—no wonder he was so fat.

Americans are drinking themselves fat

Consumption of liquid calories has increased in tandem with the obesity epidemic. Studies by Bloomberg School researchers have linked the intake of sugar-sweetened beverages to the American obesity epidemic.

According to a study published in the April 1, 2009 issue of the *American Journal of Clinical Nutrition*, the reduction of liquid calories—especially sugar-sweetened beverages—can significantly help weight-loss.

In the study, researchers examined beverage consumption among adults, and found that weight-loss was positively associated with a reduction in liquid calories. It also found that liquid calories had a stronger impact on weight than solid-food calories.

According to the lead author of the study, "Our study supports policy recommendations and public health efforts to reduce intakes of liquid calories, particularly from sugar-sweetened beverages, in the general population."

And even 100%-pure fruit juices are loaded with calories due to an excessive concentration of fruit sugar. They are best avoided, or consumed in only very small quantities.

Alcoholic drinks as part of a weight-loss plan

Many people enjoy alcoholic drinks, and they want to know how they can enjoy some and yet still lose weight. They want to enjoy their lives without deprivation and sacrifice.

A 2006 survey conducted by Harris Interactive® states that 86% of adult Americans responsibly enjoy alcoholic drinks—that's about 176 million Americans.

Many weight-loss books and plans say *no* to alcohol of any kind, but that's not necessary. Brad and Stuart are moderate drinkers, yet both are lean. And there are many teetotalers who are overweight. Furthermore, strictly *in moderation*, alcoholic drinks can be good for you.

While red wine has long been known to provide numerous health benefits via its disease-fighting antioxidants and resveratrol content, recent studies have found that beer and other alcoholic drinks (in moderation, of course) may provide health benefits, too.

A study by the University of Scranton suggests that consuming two beers a day may reduce your risk of atherosclerosis. Japanese scientists have concluded that moderate beer drinking may help fight various cancers because of the polyphenol content from hops. Harvard scientists have discovered that people who drank two beers a day had a lower risk of heart attacks, and of type II diabetes.

Moderate beer consumption has also been shown to reduce the risk of Alzheimer's, reduce the formation of blood clots, suppress the inflammation that can lead to heart disease, and help build stronger bones because of the silicon contained in the beer's hops.

Scientists have also noted that beer has traces of the antioxidant xanthohumol, which may inhibit tumor growth. And according to research performed at Tufts University, minerals in beer can protect bone density.

Other studies have concluded that *moderate* alcohol consumption protects against diabetes, gallstones, and kidney cancer, as well as raises the levels of high-density lipoprotein—the "good cholesterol."

And research from the University of Florida found that *moderate* alcohol consumption can reduce the risk of heart disease by as much as 30% to 40%.

The key to the responsible consumption of alcoholic drinks is *moderation*.

"Moderation" for Americans is defined as no more than one drink a day for women or lighter-weight men, and no more than two drinks a day for other men. A drink, for Americans, is defined as a 12-ounce can or bottle of beer (or wine cooler), a 5-ounce glass of wine, or 1.5 ounces of 80-proof liquor.

An alternative view of "moderation" is the one used in the UK—*units*. To quote Dr. Jeffrey Tobias—a consultant specializing in cancer medicine at University College London Hospitals for over 20 years—from the website of the British Broadcasting Corporation, "The present [maximum] recommendations for alcohol are 21 units weekly for men, and 14 for women (a unit is a standard pub measure of wine or spirits, or a half pint of beer)."

But the units *aren't* cumulative. If a week's 21 units for a man are consumed over a weekend rather than seven days, for example, that would be harmful.

If you consume alcoholic drinks, have no more than three units a day if you're male, or two if you're female. Have them with meals or soon after eating (to slow the absorption of the alcohol into your system), not within three hours of bedtime (to avoid marring the quality of your sleep), and only when consumption doesn't put you or others at risk.

And don't drink and operate complicated machinery, including motor vehicles.

But remember that every drink you consume usually possesses at least 100 calories. And a night of binge drinking, along with excess eating that often accompanies or follows drinking, can easily negate a week's worth of progress with your weight-loss regimen.

And some of the umbrella drinks or large margaritas can contain 600 to 800 calories—with large amounts of sugar or high-fructose corn syrup. A few of those will ruin a week's worth of progress.

Alcohol can, however, suppress your body's ability to burn fat. A study published in the *New England Journal of Medicine* found that just three ounces of alcohol can slow your fat metabolism by about 30%, which means that while your body is burning alcohol, it's not burning fat.

And according to Adkins.com, alcohol is burned at a preferred rate by your body, meaning that your body will burn the alcohol first, and store your food calories as fat. Your body stops assimilating all other forms of calories until it squelches the alcohol from your system.

An occasional party or event may lead to the overconsumption of alcoholic drinks. While this isn't healthy, it's a reality. You may need a strategy for countering an occasional splurge.

To help counter some of these extra calories, stand while drinking, because standing burns twice as many calories as sitting. And play some bar games, or dance. Do something to stay more active.

And generally speaking, as their health progresses, people tend to cut back on excessive drinking because they have more pride in their health.

Dieters become the proverbial "lightweights" because the effects of alcohol seem to hit them harder once they make substantial progress with their health and weight-loss. This is due to the increased impact of alcohol because of decreased exposure to it and tolerance of it, and because a reduced quantity of food is usually consumed with the alcohol.

Drinking relaxes inhibitions and often leads to late-night overeating. As a diversion, have a balanced meal high in protein and fiber before you drink at the special event. This not only helps to control hunger, but slows the alcohol absorption and fends off the desire for late-night overeating. Don't go to a cocktail party on an empty stomach or you're asking for an alcohol-initiated food binge.

You don't have to refrain from these occasional social gatherings or parties, but keep your food portions to a minimum, and your food choices healthy. And quench your thirst with plenty of water before you start drinking the alcohol, so that you'll be less tempted to have the alcoholic drinks out of thirst.

But if you have overdone it the night before—*work it off*. Next morning, get up, drink some ice-cold water, and do some exercise.

Sweating profusely via a hard workout won't do anything to speed the removal of alcohol or waste from your body, but many people feel that the exercising offsets an occasional party by burning off at least some of the excess calories.

Heavy alcohol consumption is harmful

Avoid anything more than a *moderate* consumption of alcoholic drinks. Heavy alcohol consumption is harmful to the body in many ways, but moderate consumption may have health benefits (except for people for whom alcohol is harmful).

People who shouldn't consume alcoholic drinks include pregnant women, anyone who has had an alcohol problem in the past or has a family history of alcoholism, anyone with a condition that's irritated by alcohol, and anyone who takes medication that's incompatible with alcohol.

Alcohol is a cause of many fatal traffic accidents. And it's also a cause of many other preventable deaths, including many of those from liver disease, for example.

To quote Prof. David J. Hanson, Ph.D., of the State University of New York, Potsdam (www2.potsdam.edu/alcohol-info/), "All of the many health benefits of drinking apply only to moderate consumption—never to heavy drinking. To the contrary, heavy drinking is associated with reduced longevity and increased risk of a diversity of diseases."

The harm done by alcohol to your alertness and reflexes is exaggerated if you have a sleep debt. If you haven't slept well recently, you'll have a sleep debt.

To quote Dr. William C. Dement from *The Promise of Sleep*, "A fact little known by the public at large is that in nearly every accident linked to alcohol consumption, sleep debt almost certainly plays a major role." Even a small amount of alcohol can have a major sedating effect if it's consumed when there's a sleep debt.

Beer belly stereotypes

There have long been references to "beer bellies" on people who carry excess blubber around their midsection. And some people erroneously believe that beer encourages fat deposit in this area.

Fat accrues when caloric intake exceeds caloric expenditure on a sustained basis. A brochure put out by Anheuser-Busch—the largest brewing company in the United States—claims that where fat is deposited on the body may primarily be determined by gender and genetics, not by the type of food you eat or drink.

And according to BBC News, researchers in the Czech Republic (which has the highest per-capita alcohol consumption) studied tens of thousands of beer drinkers for decades and found no evidence that beer drinking yields a beer belly. These findings were substantiated by similar research from the Harvard University School of Public Health.

How many calories are in alcoholic drinks?

Here's a list of the caloric content of some popular alcoholic drinks, for common US-serving sizes.

Mixing a spirit, such as vodka or rum, with calorie-laden mixers such as orange juice or a pre-made concoction, will greatly increase the caloric content per serving.

Miller Genuine Draft 64	*12.0 oz.*	*64 calories*
Bud Light	*12.0 oz.*	*110*
Sam Adams Light	*12.0 oz.*	*124*
Gin (80 proof)	*1.5 oz.*	*96*
Rum (80 proof)	*1.5 oz.*	*97*
Vodka (80 proof)	*1.5 oz.*	*109*
Whiskey (80 proof)	*1.5 oz.*	*109*
Champagne	*5.0 oz.*	*96*
Wine (red)	*5.0 oz.*	*123*
Wine (white)	*5.0 oz.*	*120*

For additional drinks and their caloric content, visit www.calorieking.com.

While past studies have indicated that caffeine may have fat-burning effects, recent studies show that it may not.

This chapter explains the products that may assist weight-loss.

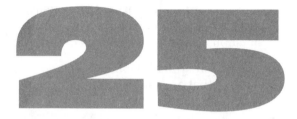

Weight-loss aids

While there are many dietary supplements that claim to provide weight-loss benefits, most are *not* backed by legitimate, unbiased scientific research conducted on human beings. And because of this, most of these products can't be trusted.

And some products may contribute such negligible benefits (maybe a fraction of one percent) that they aren't worth the cost.

Because of the abundance of scam products, this chapter provides comment on the few weight-loss aids that are backed by multiple sources of valid, unbiased science, or have conclusive research published in respected medical journals.

Contrary to what their ads may claim, even legitimate, non-prescription weight-loss aids help only a few percent *at best*. If you were to lose 100 pounds, approximately 98 of it would be from exercise and diet, and only 2 or so would be from the contribution of a weight-loss aid.

Supplements that may provide benefits

As noted in Chapter 12, omega-3 fatty acids, like the kind found in fish and fish oil, can trigger enzymes that may help to lower body fat. The University of Missouri-Columbia proposes that omega-3 fatty acids can stimulate fat oxidation in the liver. A study conducted by Australian scientists found that those people who took a two-gram dose before a workout lost 5% more body fat than those who didn't. And according to Harvard University, omega-3 fatty acids can help the body secrete leptin, a hormone that can raise the rate of metabolism and boost feelings of satiety.

Some vitamins and minerals may help with weight-loss. Vitamins are organic substances that are essential (in just small quantities) to the functioning of the body. They are found in minute quantities in natural foodstuffs, and they are sometimes produced synthetically.

There are two groups of vitamins: the fat-soluble, and the water-soluble. Vitamins A, D, E, and K are fat-soluble, while vitamin C and the vitamin B complex group are water-soluble.

Minerals are any of the inorganic elements—such as calcium, iron, magnesium, and potassium—that are essential to the functioning of the body, and are obtained from foods.

An Arizona State University study found that vitamin C plays a critical role in fat oxidation. Vitamin C may also improve your body's ability to fight fatigue, which will help you to be energetic. And chromium, selenium, calcium, and zinc provide a supporting role for weight-loss.

Because of the vital roles that vitamins and minerals play, we recommend that you take a daily multivitamin-mineral tablet—at the *minimum*, a simple, RDA-level store-brand. (RDA stands for US Recommended Dietary Allowances.) But make sure it has the USP symbol, as proof that it has been approved by the United States Pharmacopeia, and thoroughly tested.

And some research has shown that conjugated linoleic acid, or CLA, may help in a very small way to promote fat-loss.

Caffeine

Caffeine is a central nervous system stimulant, and a mild diuretic. Used in moderation, it has several benefits. It can improve concentration and cognitive functions by blocking adenosine, which slows brain functions. And by temporarily warding off drowsiness, it improves alertness and vigilance.

Caffeine improves athletic performance and stamina. This is why caffeine in high levels has been banned by the International Olympic Committee. Because of this effect you may be able to walk a little farther or faster, for example, and burn more calories. And this is why caffeine may be effective as a weight-loss aid.

While past studies have indicated that caffeine may have fat-burning effects, recent studies show that it may not.

According to the University of Michigan Health System, researchers once thought that caffeine improved endurance performance by stimulating a greater use of fat for energy, so that less glycogen was burned, but recent studies don't support this.

One of the recent studies—entitled "Caffeine ingestion does not alter carbohydrate or fat metabolism in human skeletal muscle during exercise"—was conducted by a collaboration of three major universities, and published in the *Journal of Physiology*. The study concluded that that caffeine ingestion stimulated the sympathetic nervous system but didn't alter fat metabolism.

Be careful how you obtain caffeine. Many coffee drinks, energy drinks, and caffeinated drinks can be high in calories and sugar, and this can be counter-productive to your weight-loss aspirations. Read the nutrition labels, or stick with black coffee or tea, with non-caloric sweeteners and, perhaps, skim milk in lieu of cream.

And use caffeine in moderation because too much can be harmful.

Green tea, and green tea extract

Green tea contains caffeine, as do other types of tea (provided they aren't decaffeinated), but because of the way that green tea is produced, it has a unique blend of beneficial properties.

Green tea has long been used as traditional medicine in areas such as China and Japan. And modern science has proven that many of the benefits claimed for green tea—such as reduced risk of cancer and cardiovascular disease, and improved cognitive

function—are real. Green tea is rich in polyphenols and other compounds that are thought to improve health. Some of these compounds are antioxidants.

We recommend that you have green tea daily— either drink it, like Stuart does, or have the extract in capsule form, as Brad does.

We're referring to pure green tea that's been processed by traditional methods. Ready-made green tea drinks, or processed green tea, for example, are no substitute for the real thing.

Green tea *extract* is especially rich in the properties that are good for health, and possibly helpful for weight-loss. But make sure that your green tea extract has EGCG (epigallocatechin-3-gallate)—*check the nutrition label.* It's this polyphenol that's mostly responsible for breaking down norepinephrine—the neurotransmitter for regulating your metabolic rate and fat burning—resulting in thermogenesis (the increase in caloric output).

British researchers showed that, during moderately intensive exercise, average fat oxidation rates were 17% higher after ingestion of green tea extract than after ingestion of a placebo. And research from Tufts University suggests that catechin polyphenols in green tea can activate the fat-burning mechanisms inside abdominal fat cells.

A 2007 study published in the journal *Obesity* found that drinking a mixture containing green tea catechin, caffeine and calcium three times a day, increased 24-hour energy expenditure by 4.6% in healthy, young, lean men and women.

Green tea extract capsules may work better than the liquid form due to increased absorption from capsules.

Brad and his wife take a green tea extract complex that has approximately 125 mg of EGCG per serving.

Some little-known nutrients may provide weight-loss benefits

According to a study published in the *Journal of Nutrition*, researchers from the University of Georgia discovered that a mix of two antioxidants—resveratrol and genistein—reduces fat cells' ability to store fat, and makes them self-destruct at a higher rate than normal. This combination may help your weight-loss *a little*.

Resveratrol can be obtained from grapes, raspberries, peanuts and blueberries, while genistein, which is a soy isoflavone, can be obtained at health-food stores. Red wine is rich in resveratrol, which is one of the reasons why, in moderation, red wine has health benefits.

According to the *Journal of Agricultural and Food Chemistry*, anthocyanin extract can help fat cells stimulate lipolysis—the breakdown of lipids to be burned as fuel instead of being stored as fat. Sources for anthocyanins include strawberries, cherries, raspberries, blueberries, blackberries, and red grapes.

And a study from Vanderbilt Medical Center has found that sulforaphane helps fat cells to release toxins that would otherwise lead to fat storage. So, by getting rid of those toxins, fat storage tendencies will be reduced. Cauliflower, Brussels sprouts, cabbage, and broccoli are good sources for this phytochemical.

What about FDA-approved weight-loss pills?

Your doctor can prescribe FDA-approved weight-control drugs. To qualify, you generally have to be obese *and* demonstrate that you've attempted to lose weight through traditional means.

But the pills may only help 5% to 10%, meaning that proper diet and exercise will *still* account for 90% to 95% of your results. There's no quick fix.

For example, according to a recent trial of a new drug seeking FDA approval, patients on the experimental obesity drug lost an average of 14.5 pounds—compared with 5.7 pounds for those on a placebo—after *52 weeks*. While this difference is deemed medically and statistically significant, 14.5 pounds lost in a year wouldn't make a compelling caption on a diet pill ad.

And the pill, which will be available via a doctor's prescription, created a fat-loss of only 8.8 pounds more than the placebo group. This means that one of the best weight-loss drugs will— by itself, unaided by diet and exercise—*create a fat-loss of only 8.8 pounds over a year*.

The next time you see an ad for a weight-loss pill that claims fast results, remember that one of the best pills that legitimate medical science has to offer will create a fat-loss of less than one pound *a month*. Any pitch that, by itself, claims a faster result than this is a lie—*snake oil*.

Is Alli™ your new ally?

Alli™ is an FDA-approved, over-the-counter, orlistat-based drug that prevents the absorption of fats from food intake, thus reducing overall caloric intake.

Intended for obese subjects, orlistat works by inhibiting an enzyme in the pancreas that's responsible for breaking down triglycerides in the intestine. Without the enzyme, fats are prevented from becoming absorbed, and may then be excreted from the body undigested. It's estimated that this drug blocks approximately 25% of all fat consumed.

The major side effects of this drug are excessive flatulence, and uncontrollable diarrhea, which can be painful, and embarrassing.

But don't expect a quick fix with this drug. According to a 2008 report posted on MayoClinic.com, Alli™ can help you lose some weight, but the loss likely won't be much. And even the manufacturer of the drug proclaims that the program requires a commitment to healthy eating habits to realize any of the drug's benefits.

Many people regain their weight once they stop taking it. And, taken regularly, Alli™ is expensive.

If you're considering trying a food supplement, or a weight-loss aid, first review it with your doctor to see if it's appropriate for you. And if it is appropriate, discuss the dosage that's right for you.

But always remember that the only proven means to substantial, sustainable fat-loss that experts unanimously agree on, *is proper diet and exercise.*

Brad has spent thousands of dollars testing various pills and potions that claimed to have "miraculous benefits," *but the anticipated miracles never materialized.*

When you begin your weight-loss program, the changes you make will influence your entire family.

By showcasing what real people do to get their children to adapt to a healthier lifestyle, this chapter will give you ideas so you can create your own at-home support group.

26

How to succeed with weight-loss if you have children

To succeed with a weight-loss plan over the long-term usually requires a support group. Why not make your support group your own family?

Many struggling dieters have said, "If it weren't for my children's junk food and fast food, losing weight would be much easier."

When you get your entire family on the same page, you can all live a healthier lifestyle, and help each other.

What about your children and their bad habits?

Some real-life examples will give you an idea of how others have dealt with this situation.

Two of Brad's friends—Tiffanie and Robert, a middle-aged mother and father who lost 26 and 53 pounds respectively—initially had difficulty getting their children to join the healthier lifestyle, because the children still wanted fast-food and non-nutritious snacks. But this was remedied when the children saw their parents eat well and exercise, and lose weight and have more energy.

The children eventually gave in—electively—and began to eat better, too. They were never pushed into anything; they adapted on their own as they mimicked their parents' healthy behavior.

Many dieters have used similar versions of this no-pressure, adaptation method.

Other friends of Brad's have set a healthy environment since their children were infants. They never had processed food in the house, and their children were raised on nutritious foods only.

But if you can't instill a healthy environment in your household, you may, at least initially, have to provide a compromise. If your children insist on having junk food, and you can't stop it, you may have to let them have it.

Give them their own zone—maybe a drawer, cabinet, or basement fridge—where they can stock their crud. And because it's their personal zone, you must stay out of it. But you get to have your own zone, too.

Set a great example with your own healthy eating, weight-loss, and much improved fitness, and you may win your children over to the better lifestyle.

The clean-your-plate mentality

Food choices aren't always an option for children. While Brad usually liked the food served in his household when he was a child, and he routinely enjoyed his second and third helpings, this wasn't always the case. His mom served the occasional meal that was unpleasant.

When he complained about the lousy-tasting meals, Brad's late father would say, "Son, you're *not* leaving the table *until you clean your plate."*

Brad had no choice but to accept this old-school "eat it or get in trouble" mentality. No wonder he has psychological problems when it comes to food.

Your children may put up a fight if you try to enforce healthier ways, but they may respond well if you implement the healthier lifestyle in a tactful, gradual way, without forcing it upon them.

The family as a team

When you begin your weight-loss program the changes you make will influence your entire family.

Children can be fickle. Just because you're on a diet doesn't mean that they want to be, too. They know what the word usually means—deprivation, no fun, and regimentation. If diets provide misery for adults, the children know that the diets will also provide misery for them. And if restrictive diets don't work for adults, why would they work for children?

If you begin a diet, but still bring home junk food and fast food for the rest of the family, you'll most likely fail to lose weight.

And your children will most likely fail on such a diet, too. They'll rebel if they are expected to make changes while other family members maintain their status quo.

Based on input from real-life dieters who have families, an effective way to lose weight and get healthy *is for the entire family to do it together, as a team.* But it has to be a long-term, healthier-lifestyle approach, not a mere diet for a finite period.

The family plan in real life

As a parent, set a good example because your children naturally look up to you for guidance. If you eat junk, they'll usually eat junk. But if you eat healthily, they may eventually eat healthily as well, although you shouldn't force this upon them.

As Brad's friends Robert and Tiffanie ate better, and exercised, and lost a lot of weight, they set an example in their household. Although they prepared more nutritious but still tasty home-cooked food for themselves, they never forced it on their children. They let them make their own choices. Eventually, however, the children saw that their parents were enjoying these home-cooked meals, and they didn't want to be left out.

The children sampled more of the nutritious meals, and eventually came to like them more than fast food and junk food. And they discovered that the nutritious food made them feel better, and gave them more energy without the highs and lows of their former sugar rushes.

Because the children made the food choices themselves, without coercion, they made nutritious eating a habit. And they became more active, too.

One of the children complained that her dad's exercise was taking time away from their quality time together. To solve this he invited her to take a jog with him. They eventually made it a regular fun family activity, along with their dog. And they now also ride bikes and inline skate together.

Childhood obesity's appalling statistics

According to the Centers for Disease Control and Prevention (CDC), based on data from 2003 and 2004, 16% of children 6 to 19 years of age were obese or overweight, and another 15% were considered "at risk" of becoming overweight. But because the most recent data was complied several years ago, the numbers today will probably be even worse.

And according to the CDC—also based on data from 2003 and 2004—over the past three decades the obesity rate has more than doubled for preschool children (2 to 5 years of age) and adolescents (12 to 19 years of age), and it has more than tripled for children who are 6 to 11 years of age. And again, today's figures are likely to be much worse still.

Overweight adolescents have a 70% chance of becoming overweight or obese adults; and this figure increases to 80% if one or more parent is overweight or obese.

For children born in the United States in 2000, the risk of being diagnosed with type II diabetes at some point in their lives is estimated to be about 30% for boys, and 40% for girls. And approximately 60% of obese children 5 to 10 years of age had at least one cardiovascular disease risk factor—such as elevated triglycerides, blood pressure, or total cholesterol—and 25% had two or more risk factors.

You won't succeed unless you give up excuses, get motivated, and commit to a healthy regimen.

This chapter will show you that excuses really are no excuse.

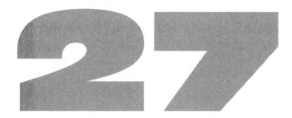

Excuses are no excuse

Most overweight people make lame excuses day after day for not sticking with a weight-loss plan. Brad used to.

Do your friends and acquaintances make excuse after excuse for not living a healthier lifestyle? Brad's used to.

But Brad changed his ways, and stopped being influenced by people who didn't support his goals and new lifestyle. That's why he transformed himself, *finally*. And so will you *if* you follow his example.

Top excuses for not living a healthier lifestyle

"I don't have enough time to exercise"

Everyone has the same 24 hours in each day. It's up to you to choose what you do with the time. President of the United States, Barack Obama—who is, arguably, the busiest person in the world—*makes* time for exercise, up to six short workouts a week. If he can make time to exercise, so can anyone.

Brad often worked 12 hours a day while he lost the final portion of his weight, but he still made time for daily exercise. Like a meeting or an appointment, he made it part of his day.

Combine exercise with something else. For example, a dieter Brad researched makes business calls while hiking or power walking.

If you have time to watch television, you have time to exercise. And you could combine them by exercising in front of the television.

On a blog written by a middle-aged lady who lost 200 pounds, Brad found this exchange:

"How do you find time to do so much walking and exercise?"

"I make the time by not watching so much television."

"I don't have the time to eat healthily"

How does eating healthily take more time than eating unhealthily? At least have an all-natural, meal-replacement bar, or a glass of milk, if you're pressed for time. Such meal-replacement bars are great pocket or purse foods.

Making a sandwich, or pre-preparing healthy foods in batches ahead of time and reheating single servings in a microwave, takes much less time than driving to a restaurant or fast-food joint.

"I don't have the time to eat"

No matter how busy you are, *make* time to eat on schedule. But if you keep your daytime meals simple, and if you've prepared some food in advance, little time is required for daytime eating. The "no time" excuse isn't valid.

And not eating during the day isn't good for working productivity anyway. Eating regularly and healthily during the day is *required* for your best working productivity.

Some people claim that they don't have time to eat anything during the day, and then return home to a large dinner late in the evening, and consume a majority of their daily caloric intake in a single binge session. Brad has witnessed some people gain over 100 pounds each by following this routine regularly.

"Healthy food has no taste"

Nutritious food can be tasty. Learn to prepare food better. There are many cookbooks that provide guidance on the creation of tasty and nutritious meals. Eventually, you may find that you dislike the taste of fast food and junk food.

"Dieting is too hard. I can't stick to it"

Don't make dieting hard. Just eat healthily 80% to 90% of the time, but enjoy your favorite foods and some occasional cheating in *small* quantities. A little cheating won't wreck a diet, but binging will.

Many successful dieters, like Brad, removed temptations from their lives. You'll be much less apt to gorge on a bag of chips if it isn't there in the first place. Eventually, Brad lost all desire for crud, and eliminated it from his life. He adapted, *and so will you.*

"I hate exercise"

Never mind "exercise." *Just start moving.*

Be kind to yourself. Show interest in your own fitness and well-being. Just as inactivity becomes a habit, so does activity. And as you become better at it, and feel better as a result, you'll be more inclined to keep being active.

For beginners, "exercise" can be as simple as walking a dog, grocery shopping, gardening, vigorous house chores, walking through a mall, going for walks with a partner, or even walking around the office during a lunch break.

Eventually, turn at least one activity you like into formal exercise.

"I'm too heavy to exercise"

Brad was too heavy to jog when he first started. But he began by walking, then graduated to jogging.

Just *get started*—walk.

If you watch extreme weight-loss television shows you can see people advance through the hierarchy of human locomotion. Be positive. Get started. Everyone can do something.

"I'm too old or sickly to exercise"

So was Brad's 75-year-old mother. But when she saw that Brad could get in better shape, she decided she could, too. She emerged from her wheelchair and began moving 10 feet via a walker. After a few months, she progressed to walking with the assistance of a cane. And after a few more months, she was cane-free, and could walk the length of a shopping mall. She even had the enthusiasm to participate in low-intensity water aerobics at a local health club.

"It's not my fault I'm overweight"

You *are* responsible for your actions, and you *are* responsible for the size of your body. Of course, people and circumstances can influence your actions, but *you* are the one who takes the actions.

Brad once blamed his wife for his weight-gain because she put him into situations that triggered his binge-eating problems. But she wasn't the one shoveling the food into his mouth—he was.

When you take full responsibility for your actions you'll have a much better chance of losing weight and changing your life for the better.

And don't be resistant to getting professional help if you feel you need it. It has helped millions of people to regain control over their lives, including control over their weight.

"Obesity runs in my family. I can't lose weight"

Does obesity run in your family because of genetics, or because of *conditioned behavior*? Many generations of families are obese because that's all they know. Everyone in these families overeats as conditioned behavior, and each person enables the others.

Do you eat together at fast-food restaurants, eat fried chicken together for dinner, devour delivered pizzas together, and snack together on junk food on a regular basis? And do you starve together and then binge together?

But even if your condition is genetic to some degree, you *still* have the ability to lose weight. It may take some medical intervention, but this is still no excuse.

"I don't care about my health"

Neither did Brad's late father, late mother-in-law, late father-in-law, and several dead middle-aged friends.

Don't assume that premature death won't happen to you.

Don't put your family and loved ones through preventable anguish. It's your responsibility to be healthy—for yourself, for your children, and for people who rely on you. *Take care of your health.*

You won't succeed with weight-loss unless you give up excuses, get some motivation, and get into a healthy lifestyle with commitment.

In just three or four weeks, a healthy lifestyle will become second nature. Just give it a chance.

Most people who succeed at weight-loss say the same thing—*once you get over the initial hump, you're almost home-free.*

This chapter summarizes what it took Brad nearly 30 years to learn, which means it also summarizes the fundamentals that the guidance of this book is based on.

The guidance of this book has already worked for Brad and the hundreds of successful dieters he interviewed. *And it will work for you, too.*

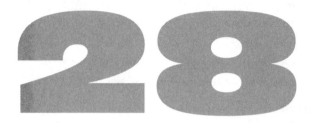

What *Young Brad* could have learned from *New Brad* to prevent decades of yo-yo dieting, *and how this can help you*

When Stuart asked Brad to write this chapter, he said, "Go back in time to when you were a 13- to 25-year-old, but retain the experiences and savvy you amassed during the many years since. Give your young self a summary of the guidance that, if followed, would have prevented the weight-related agony you went through.

"Then, because it's going to be read by people who *are* able to follow it, it *will* help those people, and that's the point of the assignment."

Here's the result of the assignment, in Brad's words:

How I lost control of my eating

Before I get to the assignment proper, you need to know how my eating got out of control in the first place.

By the time I graduated from high school I was already a veteran yo-yo dieter. I went on my first formal diet at age 11—for my breakfast and my lunch all I had for each was a half pint of low-fat milk. Throughout my teens my weight would fluctuate as much as 20 to 30 pounds, depending on whether or not I was active in a sport.

During my teens I experimented with self-created diets. On one of them I had no breakfast, and a mere pretzel rod for lunch.

But my eating problems really began to escalate when I went to college, in 1983. I was finally outside of parental supervision, and free to go wild.

I was exposed to a world of unlimited food-court processed food, binge drinking, and binge eating as a consequence of the excessive beer drinking. We were legally allowed to drink beer at age 18 then.

Since I already had the mind-set that second and third helpings were par for the course, I continued those eating patterns but in a more prolific way.

I became addicted to the food-court processed food, and the social elements attached to eating. Eating became a form of entertainment and social interaction. And it was extended with late-night-pizza eating after the taverns closed.

Those times were some of the most enjoyable of my life. I equated eating with comfort and happiness, much like I did during my childhood.

Nutritious options were few and far between at the campus-union food courts, so healthy eating was off the radar.

Although I didn't know it at the time, this caloric free-for-all launched my triggers for binge eating into overdrive.

I put on 40 pounds by winter break of my freshman year—a period of just over four months. Then to counter that I went on an ultra-severe crash diet and quickly lost 45 pounds, as I got trim for a spring break trip. But I put all the weight back on shortly thereafter.

This yo-yoing continued for the rest of my college years, and beyond. I either crash dieted or crash gorged, with seemingly no in-between. By the time I turned 25 I had lost and regained almost 300 pounds.

And by the time I turned 40, I had gained back over 600 pounds of previously lost weight.

Pinpointing my problem

Ironically, at college I majored in health education, and I was president of the University's Weightlifting and Exercise Association. I had a great deal of knowledge in the field of fitness, and I knew much about how to lose weight.

During my sophomore-through-senior years I was a powerlifter, and had to make weight for competitions. I would routinely lose 30 to 50 pounds to get down to my 165.25-pound weight class. That added fuel to my yo-yo dieting fire. I either crash-dieted to make weight, or I was a glutton.

Why would someone with extensive knowledge about health and fitness struggle with his own weight? *Today* it's easy to pinpoint my problem—lack of patience. That spawned my never-ending quest for the magic plan or pill that would yield the fast results.

At that time I was gullible. I believed the ads for fat burners, and the promises of fast results.

That's why I succumbed to the promises of the mega-hype program. If people really were losing 100 pounds in 12 weeks, why couldn't I? That's why I embarked on that program with such a gung-ho attitude.

It's time for New Brad to help Young Brad

New Brad would have stepped in, bopped Young Brad on the head, sat him down on the couch, and said, "The manufacturers of the mega-hype program are *lying* to you. The subject on the cover of the box did *not* lose 100 pounds of fat in 12 weeks. The before-and-after pictures are *bogus*, the testimonies are *lies*, the pills are *worthless*, and the program is a *sham*. You're being *duped* into buying a $125 exercise-and-nutrition pamphlet."

"Then how can they get away with this deceitfulness?" Young Brad asked, "Don't they have to tell the truth in ads?"

"No. Deceitful ads, and lying, are common in the weight-loss industry. Did you notice the 'results not typical' disclaimer in the fine print? This means that *one* person could have temporarily lost an enormous amount of weight through a brutally severe weight-loss boot camp, and the ads can loosely 'claim' the results.

"What they don't tell you is that most of their test subjects (if there were any) may have achieved only modest results, if any results. Stop being so gullible.

"It's unrealistic to lose more than one or two pounds of *fat* a week if you still want to have a life. You may be able to lose four or five pounds per week if you're dedicated to an ultra-strict diet, lift weights like a bodybuilder, and do a great deal of cardio twice a day.

"But you can't be 100% dedicated to a program like this and still have a life. You like to eat, party, and have fun. Do you think you can part with those things?

"If you follow this program you'll lose a ton of weight because the program is so severe. But when the program is over you'll revert to your old ways and put all the weight back on. This program has no chance for long-term success because it takes you too far from your comfort zone."

"Comfort zone? What's that?" asked Young Brad.

"Your normal life. If any plan takes you too far from your comfort zone, you'll fail every time."

"But I want to lose 50 pounds. I don't have the patience to ride out a weight-loss plan that will take over six months. I want results *now*," countered Young Brad.

"No you don't," argued New Brad, "you want results that are permanent. Some 95% or so of restrictive diets fail over the long-term. What's the point of losing a ton of weight over a few months but then put it all back on, and then perhaps some?"

"So how do I lose weight *and* keep it off?"

"Rather than go on a diet," said New Brad, "adopt a new, fresh outlook—the lifestyle-reform, weight-loss and health plan.

"Successful weight-loss plans that keep your weight off over the long-term must be based on behavior that you're already comfortable with. In fact, most successful real-life dieters say, 'The best diet is the one you don't know you're on.'

"You *must* enjoy the plan. Eat your favorite nutritious foods, just eat less of them, and prepare them in a healthy manner. *Enjoy* your exercise rather than treat it like a grueling, all-or-nothing boot camp. And it's okay to cheat a little every now and then. You can't be perfect 100% of the time.

"And *take your time*. If you try to lose more than two pounds of fat a week, you'll fail every time. If you want to lose 50 pounds, it had better take you at least six months, if not eight or even twelve.

"And if you don't listen to me now," argued New Brad, "you'll fail for many years before you finally try what I'm about to tell you. You'll go on to lose 50 pounds more than half a dozen times. And you'll put the weight back on every time.

"You'll fall for every stupid weight-loss pill and potion on the market. And you'll try every worthless fad diet, too. You'll waste thousands of dollars testing this worthless junk. Your friends will end up calling you 'the human guinea pig for failed diets.'

"You'll go on to weigh 266 pounds and wear 44-inch waist pants. If you think you're fat now, imagine yourself 50 pounds heavier.

"So, what do you want it to be? Lose 50 pounds the right way and be done with dieting? Or lose 50 pounds the wrong way—by following the mega-hype program, or some other crash diet— regain the weight, and then repeat that process over and over?"

"It's a no-brainer. Tell me exactly the *right* way"

"In a nutshell," explained New Brad, "here are the basic elements to apply if you're to lose weight the right way:

"Keep yourself active—I know you like jogging, bicycling, and lifting weights. Stop being such a couch potato. Over time, even simple daily activities like standing and moving around, rather than sitting, can amount to several lost pounds.

"You basically live off fast food and junk food. And you have late-night binges almost every weekend. Where do you think those thousands of excess calories end up if

you do nothing to burn them off? Don't eat anything two to three hours before bedtime.

"Eat some sort of nutritious mini-meal or snack every two to four hours. You can still enjoy burgers and sandwiches—just prepare them in a nutritious manner, and don't make them so big.

"And every time you eat, remind yourself that what you're eating is providing nourishment for your body. You're fueling a finely tuned 'machine.' Focus your eating primarily on nutrition, not primarily on convenience and entertainment.

"Stop trying to lose more than two pounds of fat a week. Take it one step at a time—day-by-day, week-by-week, month-by-month . . . one pound at a time. Take your time.

"And stop being gullible. Gimmicks, gadgets, supposed shortcuts, and pills and potions that claim to have miraculous benefits, aren't the answer for real weight-loss. Not a single person I interviewed attributed their weight-loss to any of that hokum.

"Enjoy the ride, and enjoy your life. Besides eating the foods you enjoy, and doing the exercise you enjoy, you're allowed to cheat a bit, *occasionally*. You can even enjoy some drinks. You can have a life while on a diet.

"And loosen up. Stop being all-or-nothing with your attitude to weight-loss. Take pleasure in the process because the new lifestyle-reform, weight-loss and health plan will grow on you, and eventually become your permanent lifestyle. And people who succeed with plans like this one, exercise and eat well because they want to, not because they feel they have to.

"Find new hobbies and interests to divert your energy away from food and eating.

"You're a compulsive overeater—you have an eating disorder, but don't panic. Millions of people have this disorder. It's one of the major reasons why you overeat, and binge. Deal with the disorder. Get help. Don't be in denial of the compulsive overeating.

"And never forget the most basic fundamental of weight-loss—*you must expend more calories than you take in, if you're to lose body fat.* This creates an energy imbalance or deficit in your body. You need to ingest fewer calories, and burn more calories.

"These are just the fundamentals, to get you started. There's much more to the overall plan. Start from here, and you'll spare yourself a life of continued yo-yo dieting, unremitting weight-loss failure, and the accompanying health problems."

Will *you* heed the advice?

Obviously, the point of this chapter isn't to help Young Brad—it's too late for that. The point is to help *you.*

WEIGHT-LOSS SALVATION provides all the guidance you need to lose weight, keep it lost, get healthy, and change your life.

And this guidance works just as well for women as it does for men—just make sure that your caloric intake is appropriate *for you*, and choose activities, interests and exercise that *you* enjoy.

Put the guidance to work, *and make yourself a weight-loss success story.*

Anyone can lose weight, *but keeping it off is another matter.*

This chapter will show you what it takes to maintain your weight-loss for the rest of your life.

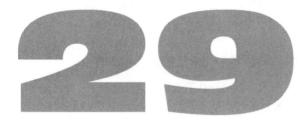

You've lost the weight . . . *now what?*

How do you maintain your weight-loss?

How do you preserve the new you?

First of all, *reward* the new you

Now that you've lost the weight, get rid of your "fat clothes." Indulge in new, fashionable "thin clothes."

As Brad went from 44-inch pants to 42, 40, 38, 36, 34, and, finally, a loose-fitting 32, he was thrilled to slip into the new, smaller pants and discard the "fat pants." You can experience the same sort of great fun yourself.

When they bought new clothes, some dieters jumped the gun and purchased pants or outfits that were a size (or several sizes) below what they actually wore at the time. That further motivated them to make the progress required to get into their new clothes.

Brad was so obsessed with wearing size-32 pants that he bought them prematurely. They looked painted-on for a while, but they eventually became loose and comfortable.

Take pride in your new appearance. Treat yourself to a spa treatment, massage, manicure, and a fabulous haircut. You earned it, and you deserve it. Spoil yourself.

But spoil yourself with fun things like the aforementioned, *not* food.

Don't blow it once you've met your goal

Remember, according to the Federal Trade Commission, restrictive diets have a 95% failure rate.

You must continue to follow the principles that created your weight-loss in the first place. The biggest mistake dieters who have lost a lot of weight make is to think that they've "crossed the finish line" and they are done. They mistakenly believe that they no longer have to eat sensibly, or exercise, once they are done with the program.

The healthier-lifestyle approach never ends. It has no finish line. But adjust your caloric intake and exercising so that you can comfortably maintain your ideal weight for the rest of your life.

Remember the time, effort and dedication you invested to get to the trim, new version of yourself. Don't let yourself down now that you you've done the hardest part. Stick with the program, and *enjoy* your new life.

The 100-pound regression

Here's an illustration of how over-zealous diets fail:

In 2007 Brad advised a local man, Tom, who had an obsessive goal to lose 100 pounds. Starting at a bodyweight of 304 pounds, Tom embarked on a fanatical dash to achieve his goal. His diet was overly strict, and his exercise program was overly vigorous.

The approach worked wonders, initially. He lost an average of three pounds a week, but Brad knew that Tom was destined to burn out with this over-zealous approach. Citing examples of his own failures, Brad repeatedly warned Tom that the fanatical approach was a recipe for long-term failure.

Tom reached his goal in eight months. In early 2008 he showed off his results, and triumphantly proclaimed, "I did it . . . I lost the 100 pounds. In fact, I lost 105 pounds. I now weigh 199!"

In March 2009 Brad saw Tom for the first time since the triumphant announcement. Brad was stunned by what he saw. Tom had put all the weight back on—because he hadn't acted on Brad's counsel.

Anyone can lose weight, *but keeping it off is another story.*

A way of life . . . *the maintenance phase*

Brad has maintained his weight-loss for well over three years. He was used to losing an average of 1.62 pounds of fat a week while he was shedding 114 pounds of fat, which is a better-than-typical pace. That rate of loss amounted to about 5,650 weekly calories. Because he currently keeps his activity levels high, and continues to eat in a nutritious manner, he can enjoy a relatively normal lifestyle and yet still break even bodyweight wise.

Maintaining your weight is much easier than losing weight. The maintenance phase—which will be the rest of your life—is a breeze, comparatively speaking.

Just don't stray from the general principles and guidelines that you utilized to realize your fabulous results. Don't revert to your "fat ways."

Make changes that you can live with forever, and follow through day after day, month after month, and year after year.

Although it may seem like a pipe dream now, the beneficial changes you'll make will quickly become second nature. And then you may wonder how you lived an unhealthy lifestyle in the first place.

Many studies prove that the people who sustain long-term weight-loss are those who maintain their activity levels, and continue to do some type of formal exercise. People who returned to their sedentary ways after they lost their weight were over twice as likely to regain that weight.

To illustrate this, say you were walking *briskly* (not merely leisurely) about three miles a day five days a week as part of your maintenance regimen. If you stopped that you'd reduce your energy output by about 1,500 calories a week. To avoid weight-gain you'd have to reduce your weekly caloric intake by 1,500. And if you didn't, you could regain about 20 pounds of fat in a year.

But don't be overly hard on yourself. It's acceptable to fluctuate a few pounds throughout the year. You can still enjoy holidays and special occasions, as well as life in general.

It's okay to make *occasional* mistakes. Focus on the big picture, not the small hills and valleys.

You can also make your goal weight *a range*. Brad wanted to weigh 165 pounds, but got down to 163. He knows that anything between 163 and 168 is good for him, and he allows himself to fluctuate over that range throughout the year.

How Stuart maintains his weight

Stuart varies his *daily* caloric intake and output somewhat—because of moderate day-to-day variation in quantity of food consumed, and in activity levels. But because he's consistent with his *weekly* figures, he maintains his weight effortlessly.

He knows the caloric intake that matches his caloric output, and he's consistent with matching the figures, for perfect balance. Thus, because he never consumes more weekly calories than he uses up, he can't gain weight.

If you do the same when you're in maintenance mode, you'll effortlessly maintain your weight, too.

Never forget the fundamental principle of weight-loss:

To lose weight you *must* establish an energy imbalance or deficit in your body.

So, the next time you overeat, what's your plan for burning the extra calories off?

And remember what will happen to the extra calories if you don't burn them off—*they will be stored as body fat.*

As silly as this may seem, some real-life dieters wrote themselves "goodbye fat self" letters to help bring closure to their former ways. If you feel that this may help you, be creative and have some fun with it.

Remember, if Brad, the "human guinea pig for failed diets," can achieve and maintain his big weight-loss, you can, too.

Good luck with *your* weight-loss. *And cheers to the new you!*

Did you ever dream of eating like a "normal" person?

When you've read this chapter you'll know that this dream can become reality.

30

How real people ate to *lose* weight, and how real people eat to *maintain* their healthy weights

Here's a summary of a typical day in Brad's life from when he was losing weight. And there's also a summary of a typical day of a real-life woman—Mary—when she was on her way to losing 80 pounds, which she has kept off for over six years.

There's also a summary of how Mary, Stuart, Brad's wife, and Brad eat as they *maintain* their weights.

These illustrations reflect what the guidance in **WEIGHT-LOSS SALVATION** teaches.

Although the guidance is personalized to each individual's lifestyle and preferences, the illustrations provide examples for you to draw on when you design your own daily schedule.

A typical day in Brad's life during his weight-loss

When people hear that Brad lost over 100 pounds in a single stretch, and kept it lost, they usually ask him, "How did you do it?"

Because what worked for Brad will also work for other people, here's a typical higher-calorie day during his transformation.

Your schedule may be different, you may not care for the foods and activities that Brad likes, and you may not be able to consume as many calories as he did, so revise the schedule to suit you.

6:30 am: He woke and drank a pint of ice-cold water.

6:50 am: After having warmed up, and stretched *gently*, Brad usually jogged on a treadmill for 30 minutes, or jogged outside for 45 minutes—depending on his mood and the weather. He drank another pint of ice-cold water after the workout.

7:45 am: He showered, groomed, and got dressed.

8:00 am: For breakfast he usually had two whole-grain, all-natural waffles with a pat of fat-free margarine and a dollop of sugar-free syrup, 12 ounces of skim milk, Canadian bacon, and a large glass of ice-cold water. This provided about 350 calories, 40 grams of carbohydrates, and 30 grams of protein. Instead of the waffles he sometimes had two scrambled eggs and a 100% whole-wheat bagel.

8:45 am: He arrived at his office and got some work done.

11:00 am: He usually ate a pre-prepared turkey breast, chicken breast, or lean roast beef sandwich on 100% whole-wheat bread, a small apple, and a large glass of ice-cold water. This mini-meal provided 300 to 350 calories, 40 grams of carbohydrates, and 25 grams of protein.

If he was pressed for time, instead of that mini-meal he would grab a "pocket meal" like an all-natural protein bar, an all-natural meal replacement bar, or a pint of skim milk.

1:00 pm: Brad usually left his office for a brisk walk. And he sometimes ate his 1:30 sandwich or "pocket meal" on this walk, to conserve time.

1:30 pm: He usually had a pre-prepared 96%-lean quarter-pound hamburger on a 100% whole-wheat bun, string beans or peas with pepper and fat-free margarine, and a large glass of ice-cold water. This mini-meal provided about 350 calories, 30 grams of carbohydrates, and 30 grams of protein.

3:30 pm: He usually had a meal-replacement drink or an all-natural meal replacement bar, and a large glass of ice-cold water. This snack provided 200 to 220 calories, 20 grams of carbohydrates, and 20 grams of protein.

6:00 pm: Brad left his office and went home.

6:30 pm: He usually ate chicken breast, a few peanuts, a small glass of skim milk, and a large glass of ice-cold water. This provided 200 to 300 calories, 10 to 20 grams of carbs, and 25 grams of protein.

7:00 pm: Time for his session of lifting weights in his home gym. It lasted about 30 minutes. (He didn't lift weights every day.)

7:45 pm: He usually chugged a small protein shake, a little turkey breast, and a large glass of ice-cold water. This provided 200 to 250 calories, no carbohydrates, and 25 grams of protein.

He always kept his carbohydrates to a minimum in the evening. Generally, however, it's good to have carbs immediately after a workout, to help with recuperation.

8:00 pm: He would spend quality time with his wife, and pets. He would sip on a pint or two of ice-cold water throughout the night, to give him a sensation of fullness and fend off the possibility of rogue nighttime snacking. And sometimes he had a 40- to 70-calorie snack during the evening via an all-natural, low-fat cheese stringer, a few peanuts, baby carrots, pickle spears, or some turkey breast.

11:00 pm: Bedtime. Brad tried to get about seven-and-a-half hours of sleep per night.

For this example of a higher-calorie day, he had 1,700 to 1,900 calories—about 150 to 180 grams of carbs, and 160 to 180 grams of complete protein—and drank about 100 ounces of ice-cold water.

Brad didn't obsessively count calories, or follow specific macro-nutrient ratios. But he was aware of what he ate, and always met his daily requirements, give or take a little. And he usually consumed 1,400 to 1,600 calories—and reduced carbohydrates—on non-weight-lifting or lower-calorie days. He varied his calories (and carbs) day-to-day. The reason his lower-calorie day was so low was that he was trying, partially, to follow the "seven-times-bodyweight caloric intake" approach that was popular at the time.

These numbers are based on an active, 200-pound man, and are cited as an example. Of course, smaller or larger male weight-loss subjects, and many women, will have to adjust their calories accordingly. For example, as Brad continued to lose weight on his way to 165 pounds, he gradually reduced his daily caloric intake by approximately 70 calories for every 10 pounds he lost.

How a woman lost 80 pounds and *kept it off*

The following is Mary's story—a real-life dieter who lost 80 pounds, and then kept it off for more than six years *and counting*. She was one of the many real-life female dieters who inspired Brad.

Her parents own a chain of sports-themed restaurants known for huge portion sizes, and Mary was raised on unhealthy, highly addictive food. And in her 20s she was stuck in a terrible marriage, with the misery that ensued.

Mary ate for comfort, to try to find solace. The restaurant-eating (as well as the near-nightly binge drinking) eventually became her sole source of entertainment and happiness. The more depressed she became, the more she ate and drank at her parents' restaurant. It was a debilitating downward spiral.

To try to alleviate her profound weight-gain, Mary went through a phase where she thought she ate "healthy." For dinner, she ate the restaurant's salads. But she eventually discovered that the dressing-soaked, topping-laden salads were not the answer, because she gained even more weight. At the time she didn't know that the salads' toppings were hugely calorific.

This horribly unhealthy lifestyle ultimately produced a weight of 225 pounds, on her five-foot six-inch frame.

After years of living this way, and after her terrible marriage ended in divorce, Mary decided to change her life. At 30 years of age it was time to lose weight, and get healthy. It was time to stop living on processed food, and booze. And it was time to start exercising.

Upon realizing how the food in her family's restaurant was prepared, and how fattening it was, she understood what she was doing to her body, and how many daily calories she was consuming. She made a commitment to do the *opposite* of what she had been doing previously.

Inspired by the organic food fervor of the early 2000s, Mary replaced the processed fare with a diet almost exclusively of organic foods. And she started exercising regularly, and quickly progressed to doing daily exercise that she enjoyed.

After 14 months Mary got her weight down to a healthy 145 pounds, which she has maintained to this day.

To make her story even more triumphant, she finally had the confidence to introduce herself to the man she had a long-time crush on, and they married in 2006.

Here's a summary of a typical day in her life as she lost the 80 pounds. You may not like the foods and activities that she does, so you may need to revise them to suit you.

For breakfast, Mary usually had all-natural, whole-grain cereal, and skim milk. Or, if she had the time, she prepared organic-egg omelets, or organic scrambled eggs with 100% whole-wheat toast. She also had coffee, a small glass of orange juice, and plenty of ice-cold water. When pressed for time, she grabbed some fresh organic fruit—an orange, for example. No matter how busy she was, she *always* had something for breakfast—but something *healthy*.

For lunch and dinner, Mary became known as the "organic salad queen." She pre-prepared batches of organic chicken breast, and made super-tasty salads flavored with a near-zero-calorie vinaigrette dressing and a variety of organic vegetables and spices. She kept them in sealed containers and ate them in a grazing fashion throughout the day. Although she was nibbling on these salads by the hour, each nibbling session was worth only a hundred or so calories. The grazing kept her hunger in check, and warded off cravings for the ever-present restaurant food.

Her snacks were anything that was organic and nutritious. And although she snacked all the time, she was taking in so few calories that they didn't add up to anything substantial.

Although Mary still enjoyed a few drinks at the weekends, for a reward, she never binged on beer like she used to, but enjoyed wine instead—in moderation, of course.

Mary is the dieter we mentioned in Chapter 20 who "performed 10 to 15 minutes of continuous moderate-intensity exercise two or three times a day."

She had been intimidated by the thought of "long and grueling" exercise sessions. To reduce the intimidation factor she performed a short session in the morning, another during her lunch break, and another in the evening. She used a spin bike or an elliptical machine. And she became more active in general by doing more household chores, some daily walking, and more window shopping at the mall.

Swapping unhealthy fare for healthy fare reduced her daily calories dramatically, as well as her fat, salt and sugar intake. And she had almost no high-fructose corn syrup in her diet.

Brad estimates that Mary averaged 1,200 to 1,500 calories a day. While she didn't count calories, her sustained reduction in daily intake, coupled with a much more active lifestyle, created a daily energy imbalance of about 650 calories, which created a fat-loss of about 1.3 pounds a week over the 14 months it took to reach her new weight.

She has maintained her new weight by adopting a lifestyle based on her weight-loss plan. Her new husband is a gourmet-level chef, and he cooks fabulous, healthy meals based on lean, organic meats, and organic fruits and vegetables. Together they adopted a healthy, organic-food-based lifestyle.

Mary eats a little more during her maintenance phase than when she was losing the weight—300 to 500 more calories a day. And she scaled back some of her exercise to make the long-term lifestyle even more manageable. She performs one or maybe two 10- to 15-minute moderate-intensity exercise sessions on each weekday, *and* she takes her dogs for twice-daily walks.

She monitors her weight every few weeks and, when necessary, adjusts her caloric intake, and exercise, to keep her weight at 145.

The new way of life she adopted is, in effect, the same lifestyle-reform, weight-loss and health plan this books promotes. While Mary based her new life on organic and whole foods, it's because she replaced "foods that man made" with "foods that nature made" that was the basis of her big daily caloric reduction. And this, coupled with a much more active lifestyle, created the daily energy imbalance that created her new self.

Follow Mary's lead—get off the crud, eat only nutritious foods, and get moving!

Organic and "clean" foods aren't necessarily any less calorific than "regular" grocery-store-bought meats, fruits and vegetables; and neither will they necessarily help you to lose weight any faster. But if you can afford them, and they help instill a sense that you're eating even healthier, by all means enjoy them.

Brad and most dieters don't eat many organic foods because, generally, they are too expensive. They usually eat healthy "regular" foods, and meats that are on sale. And that may be the most practical solution for you, too.

The solution to *"But I can't eat so few calories!"*

In this book you've read examples of people eating 1,200 to 1,800 calories a day. If you've been a big eater for a long time, a daily caloric intake under 2,000 may seem tiny.

Determining *your* daily caloric intake for weight-loss isn't an exact science. Many factors influence this number, especially your body size, body composition, and overall activity level. Some plans recommend higher daily intakes than others, and some recommend a caloric intake as simple as seven-times-bodyweight.

But once you've reached your goal weight you can consume substantially more calories than you did during the period of weight-loss. This will yield greater satisfaction but while still enabling you to maintain your new weight.

What worked for Brad and Mary may not work for you. You may need to consume fewer calories to lose weight, or you may be able to consume more than they did. And you may not want to lose weight as quickly as they did.

If you feel that consuming, for example, an average of 1,600 calories a day for a man, or 1,300 for a woman, will present too great a challenge, adjust your strategy. If you want to eat more—for example, an average of 2,000 calories a day—be more active than Brad and Mary were, or accept a slower pace of weight-loss.

Most people choose the slower pace of weight-loss. Of the hundreds of successful dieters who were researched for this book—and who maintained their weight-loss over the long-term—the average fat-loss was just under a pound a week, or 3.84 pounds a month. But that's still nearly 50 pounds of fat lost in a year.

Brad was aggressive and able to average 1.62 pounds of lost fat a week over the long-term. *But what if he had lost weight at the same pace as everyone else—an average of 0.96 pounds a week?* Provided his activity levels remained unchanged, he would have been able to eat significantly more than he actually did.

He would have been able to eat an average of 330 more calories each day. His higher-calorie days would have been a much more fulfilling 2,030 to 2,230, and his lower-calorie days would still be an ample 1,730 to

1,930 calories. And his Saturday treat day would have been a highly satisfying 2,500 calories.

The overall period to meet his weight-loss goal would have been longer—about 29 months instead of the near 19—but he still would have lost fat at the same average pace as everyone else.

And if Mary wanted lose weight at the same pace as our average dieter (0.96 pounds of fat lost per week), she would have been able to average roughly 200 more calories a day *provided* her activity levels stayed the same. And it would have taken her 21 months to reach her goal, instead of 14.

This slower pace is what most dieters find to be more enjoyable, and easier to adhere to over the long-term.

Many studies confirm that those people who try to rush their weight-loss end up failing over the long-term.

Even if you average a seemingly snail's-pace fat-loss of a single pound each week—but 52 pounds of lost fat in a year—you'd still make *terrific* progress. So, really, what's your hurry?

Do you resent slim, lean people?

Being overweight can be frustrating. For most of his life Brad resented slim people. He would look at a lean person and think to himself, "It must be nice being born with perfect genetics. I wish I could have been that lucky." Many dieters Brad interviewed shared versions of these sentiments.

But as Brad researched why people are slim, he came to another conclusion. A very few people are winners of life's genetic lottery for leanness, *but most lean people are that way because of their lifestyle and eating habits.*

He brought up this topic with Stuart. Brad initially resented Stuart because Stuart seemed to be one of the genetic-lottery winners for leanness. Stuart's answer was an eye-opener for Brad:

"Overweight people may look at me and say, 'You've got the right genetics, that's why you're not fat.' I'm not convinced about that. Both my sisters have had weight problems, but different lifestyles and eating habits to mine. And if other people compare their lifestyles and food choices to mine, they will see huge differences in things that they can easily change for the better."

Here's why Stuart consumes more calories than most people and yet doesn't gain weight:

He isn't trying to lose weight—he's lean enough already.

Twice a week, in the morning after breakfast, he lifts weights intensively, and does hard cardio. This may produce the afterburn effect to yield calorie burning for some of the rest of his workout days additional to what he would burn had he not exercised.

He has more muscle mass than he would have if he didn't train with weights, which boosts his caloric needs.

He's very active even when out of the gym, which further boosts his caloric needs.

Although he enjoys his meals—as you must, too—he eats primarily for nourishment, not entertainment.

He never eats crud—no junk food, no fast food, no fried food, and nothing with refined sugar or high-fructose corn syrup in it.

He eats a wide variety of food rich in vitamins, minerals and essential fatty acids; and he takes food supplements.

He eats a fiber-rich diet.

He eats a good breakfast every day.

He rarely eats out.

He never snacks in front of the television.

He eats often but never exceeds his weekly caloric allocation.

He drinks a lot of water, including several mugs of green tea each day.

In many ways, Stuart does what **WEIGHT-LOSS SALVATION** teaches. It's not by chance that he's maintained a lean, steady weight for many years.

Brad now fully understands Stuart's situation because he's now living that type of healthy lifestyle himself.

And now that Brad has maintained his ideal weight for well over three years, many people his age are now saying to *him*, "It must be nice being born with perfect genetics. I wish I could be that lucky."

What an irony. If they could have seen Brad several years ago they would never have made that comment.

How Stuart eats, *and* the value of activity, additional muscle, and healthy eating

Because Stuart doesn't eat meat, and doesn't live in the US, he eats differently to Brad. Furthermore, Stuart has no interest in spending more time in the kitchen than necessary, so he keeps his meals simple and never does any serious cooking. And his wife has the same disinterest in cooking.

His five daily meals are nutritious and healthy, and because he knows the daily quantity of food that keeps him at a stable weight, and his meals are similar in content each day, and his food portions are steady, he controls his caloric intake with ease without counting calories. And you'll be able to do the same, eventually.

Stuart's staples are oatmeal (typically with ginger, and pure honey), almonds, cheese, fresh and dried fruit, vegetables and vegetable juice, salads (with a dressing of extra virgin olive oil, cider vinegar, and herbs), bread, rice, oatcakes, tinned fish, boiled eggs, and olives.

His daily supplements include flaxseed oil, cod liver oil, a multi vitamin-mineral tablet, and additional vitamins C and E.

His daily caloric intake varies between 2,600 and 2,800—an average of about 2,700. This is about 1,000 more than what many inactive men of his height (five-foot ten) need to consume to lose weight.

But if Stuart wasn't so active, didn't train in a gym, and didn't have any muscle additional to what would be natural to him in an untrained state, his current food intake would make him very fat.

Whether you're male or female, and regardless of your age, if *you* become very active in general, build some muscle, train hard and consistently, and eat healthily, then once you've lost your excess weight *you* will be

able to consume many more calories than you may think you can and yet *still maintain a healthy weight.*

"But it's all about your genetics"

Remember that both of Stuart's sisters have struggled with their weights, but they have different lifestyles and eating habits to his.

Most overweight people have different lifestyles and eating habits to Stuart's. If they adopted eating habits similar to his (but with fewer calories), and became much more active, they would lose weight readily.

And they would be able to have a greater food intake than they would otherwise and yet *still lose weight.*

That would satisfy them much more than a lesser food intake, and the extra calories would better enable them to get sufficient nutrients for good health— including healthy fats in foods such as flaxseed oil, extra virgin olive oil, oily fish, and cod liver oil.

Why show a non-dieter's daily fare?

While Stuart's caloric intake is like that of many non-dieters, the food he eats isn't.

He has a 100% healthy, nutrient-rich diet. Among other benefits, this fare keeps his energy level high and steady, which makes it easy for him to be very active. And it prevents food cravings.

But what if Stuart wanted to shed a few pounds? What if he became a dieter?

To lose one pound a week, he would have to create a caloric deficit of about 500 calories or so each day, which could be done by reducing his food intake by that number.

If he wasn't so active, he would need to reduce his caloric intake by another few hundred to compensate for the inactivity.

And if he didn't have any muscle mass additional to what would be natural for him in an untrained state, and didn't train in a gym regularly, he would have to cut his daily caloric intake some more.

So, if he was wanting to lose weight while being inactive and with less muscle mass, he would need to consume at least 1,000 fewer calories, which would take him to about 1,700 (2,700 minus 1,000), which is around what many largely inactive men need to consume in order to lose weight at one pound or so a week.

But if Stuart wanted to lose a pound a week he wouldn't reduce his caloric intake by 500. He would walk briskly for an extra 40 or so minutes a day, and reduce his caloric intake by only 200 or so. And he would distribute his caloric allocation over six or seven small meals, rather than his maintenance format of five.

If Stuart wanted to lose weight he would do *exactly* what WEIGHT-LOSS SALVATION teaches you to do.

She wouldn't let *fat* be her *fate*

As we mentioned earlier, Brad's late mother-in-law was the ultimate food pusher. She pushed her cooking on everyone who crossed her path. Her cooking was terribly unhealthy, overly calorific, and served in huge portions. This was the "life revolves around food" environment that Lisa was raised in.

The environment took its toll on everyone who was exposed to it. The entire family became obese. Lisa was ridiculed at school because of her weight.

Motivated by the cruel teasing, she vowed to make a change. She started swimming because her older brother was heavily involved in the sport. She eventually became a national-level swimmer as a teenager.

The daily swimming, coupled with strength training with the swim team, and regular dance classes, caused her to lose the excess weight. She eventually became one of the leanest and fittest students in her high school.

But the manipulative food pushing at home continued. Because Lisa would never again let herself become "that fat kid," she kept the weight off by keeping her activity levels and exercise at a very high level.

Today, about 30 years later, she continues to be very active, and exercises regularly. But she doesn't have to exercise to the extent she did as a teenager because she now controls what she eats. She strength trains at least three times a week, and enjoys daily jogging or speed walking. And she's very active doing household chores and a great deal of gardening.

But she doesn't *have to* exercise and be very active—she *wants* to. She enjoys these activities, and covets the satisfaction derived from partaking in them. And because of her high energy output she can eat a lot more food than she could if she was a couch potato, and yet not gain weight.

Although occasionally she likes to eat foods that aren't healthy, Lisa keeps her portion sizes in check. Those treats aside, her staples are oatmeal and skim milk for breakfast, a nutritious sandwich for lunch, and usually a Lean Cuisine® low-calorie microwaveable meal for dinner.

Her snacks are typically an all-natural, low-fat cheese stringer, an all-natural meal replacement bar, or a spoonful of peanut butter.

And even though she's never counted calories, she's fully aware of what she eats and drinks. She knows the maximum quantity of food she can eat each day without putting on weight. At 47 years of age, Lisa's the same weight as she was when she graduated from high school.

Since childhood, daily exercise coupled with a very active lifestyle has allowed Lisa to eat pretty much the way she wants yet retain a level of fitness and leanness that people half her age would envy.

How Brad eats now that he's lost his weight

At the end of 2009, Brad was nearly 45 years old, had kept his weight off for over three years, and was well into his maintenance phase.

Once Brad met his goal weight and went into the maintenance phase, he was able to increase his daily caloric intake because he was no longer losing weight. He had previously lost weight at an average of 1.62 pounds of fat a week—which is equivalent to about 5,650 calories each week, or 800 a day.

While Brad still doesn't obsessively count calories or follow specific macronutrient ratios, he's very picky about what he eats and drinks. And although he doesn't eat as perfectly as Stuart and

Mary do, Brad has become accustomed to eating nutrient-rich foods and, like Stuart and Mary, enjoys eating these foods and covets the resulting high, steady energy level, and the absence of food cravings.

Brad is now living his dream, and able to eat like a "normal" person, not as a dieter. He now lives a lifestyle similar to Stuart's. And because Brad is very active from his general daily interests and chores, morning jogging, twice-weekly weight lifting, and daily walking, and because he continues to eat in a very nutritious manner, he can now eat almost as much food as Stuart does. Brad consumes 2,500 to 2,700 daily calories *without gaining weight.*

But remember that these extra nutritious calories Brad is now able to enjoy are earned through a very active lifestyle. When he was fat, most of his calories came from crud, and he had a couch-potato lifestyle.

Brad also knows that exercise doesn't give him a green light to eat anything he wants. He knows that an hour of exercise is easily nullified by five minutes of post-exercise binging.

Follow Brad's example for weight-loss *and* the follow-up maintenance phase. *If he can do it, so can you.*

Everyone in the examples in this chapter used some sort of exercise to help with their weight-loss and/or long-term maintenance.

You have to find at least one activity that works for you. And this has to be something you enjoy, and that's safe for you, whether it's walking outdoors, treadmill walking, spin classes, biking, or hiking, as some of the most common possibilities.

And remember, many people who may have been more obese or elderly than you, lost all of their weight with an exercise program that never evolved past brisk walking. Walking alone, coupled with more daily activity in general (as well as a nutritious, reduced-calorie diet) can still give you the energy imbalance you need to succeed with weight-loss.

Just do something . . . *get moving!*

Maintaining weight is much easier than losing it.

Revel in your lifelong maintenance phase as you enjoy a healthy, active lifestyle as the *new you*.

Part IV

The whole-scoop summary of what you must do for weight-loss success

WEIGHT-LOSS SALVATION has given you a wealth of information to help you lose weight and keep it off. But there's so much guidance that you're unlikely to be able to remember it all.

This section provides a quick-reference summary of the critical preliminaries, and Parts II and III, to remind you of what you must do to stay on track for weight-loss success.

All of the guidance is important, but the items in bold type are of paramount importance.

But please review this section only AFTER you've read the rest of the book in its entirety.

The critical preliminaries 15

> **"Going *on* a diet means someday you're going to go *off* a diet. You can't be on a diet your whole life."**

- ❑ "Diet" and "dieting" are usually associated with bouts of suffering, sacrifice, and deprivation.

- ❑ Restrictive diets and fad diets have a 95% failure rate.

- ❑ There are no quick fixes for long-term weight-loss.

- ❑ Rather than "go on a diet" that's temporary, adopt a fresh outlook on life, nutrition and health over the *long-term*.

- ❑ While some gender-specific issues affect weight and weight-loss, the fundamental ways in which men and women lose weight and keep it off *are the same*.

Successful weight-loss plans must be based on behavior you're comfortable with. If you can't see yourself eating and exercising in the new way for the rest of your life, you'll most likely fail.

- ❑ Nearly two out of three Americans are obese or overweight.

- ❑ People underestimate the number of calories they consume.

- ❑ Get a physical checkup before you begin your weight-loss plan.

- ❑ Your doctor should be an expert on weight-loss and nutrition.

CHAPTER 6

Food addiction 57

Processed foods are *designed* to be irresistible and addictive in order to stimulate the body's inborn emotional responses. *That's* why some foods are so mouth-watering. And that's *also* why many people find it extremely difficult to stop eating some foods.

- ❑ The human body has an innate system that leads you to seek out pleasurable rewards. The pleasure derived from eating is one of these desired rewards.

❐ It's proposed that modern-day processed foods are *chemically designed* to take advantage of this pleasure-seeking programming.

The palatability of food refers to its ability to stimulate your appetite, which in turn prompts you to want more of it. While palatability includes taste, it also comprises the desire to *pursue* the taste further. It's the reason why many people crave certain foods more and more.

Although different people crave different foods, for people with a weight problem the most palatable and the most craved foods are usually the chemically designed ones that contain not just added fat or sugar, but a combination of fat and sugar coupled with salt. And the sensory properties of these chemically designed foods—temperature, texture, color, and aroma—help to stimulate appetite. For many people, these foods provide the most pleasure, and the greatest irresistibility.

But rather than hunger alone, it's the mental stimulation derived from these highly palatable foods that makes so many people crave them. This mental stimulation re-arouses their appetite even after they are done eating.

❐ Food manufacturers discovered that specific combinations of fat, sugar and salt make consumers crave these designer foods even more.

❐ Food manufacturers also discovered that a layer of *additional* fat, sugar and salt can make food *even more* addictive.

❐ People crave these foods to get their fixes of fat, sugar and salt.

❐ These are typically the comfort foods that many people become addicted to.

❐ Foods with higher fat content can "melt in your mouth" easier.

Addictive foods stimulate neurons in your brain because the foods' tastes are hard-wired to the parts of your brain that respond to pleasure. This prompts a strong emotional response to the foods.

- Ads for high-fat, high-sugar and high-salt foods are *designed* to stimulate your senses, and invoke cues to seek and eat the foods.

- This conditioned behavior is similar to that of Pavlov's dogs.

When your senses are exposed to a certain food, bursts of dopamine can be released in your brain, which simulate the pleasure response from the food *without it having been eaten*. Dopamine is a chemical in the brain that contributes to creating the drive to eat. And it's what gives you prominent memories for desirable foods. The more desirable the food, the more attention is directed to it, and the more you're likely to pursue it.

- Dopamine—which is thought to be involved with addiction to alcohol, cocaine, and other drugs—may also play an important role in obesity.

- Obese people may have fewer receptors for dopamine.

- Obese people may eat more to try to stimulate the dopamine pleasure circuits in their brains, like addicts do by taking drugs.

- Eating is a highly reinforcing behavior that induces pleasure.

By capitalizing on their consumers' chemically engineered food addiction, restaurants have slowly upped their portion sizes in an effort to increase their profits. Generally speaking, portion sizes in American restaurants are substantially larger than in other countries.

CHAPTER 7

The psychological aspects of weight-loss   63

- Many weight-loss attempts fail for psychological reasons.

- Many weight battles have an underlying psychological cause.

- Dealing with weight isn't just about self-control and discipline.

- Yo-yo dieting is a major symptom of a compulsive overeater.

Why do you overeat or have a weight problem?

☐ For many people, food is like a drug addiction because it feels good to eat.

☐ Sugary or starchy foods can temporarily boost levels of serotonin.

☐ Food won't solve your problems.

☐ Thinking that it's okay to be obese may indicate living in denial.

☐ Millions of Americans have binge-eating disorder—an *addiction*.

☐ Compulsive overeaters use food for comfort or as "medication."

☐ For compulsive overeaters, restrictive diets must be avoided.

Eating nutritious small meals, or snacks, five or six times a day—while paying attention to the foods' nutritional impact—can eventually eliminate your compulsions for binging and snacking.

☐ Generally speaking, nighttime eating should be avoided.

☐ Be aware of internal and external overeating triggers.

☐ Exercise, or a new passion or hobby, will divert your interest away from food.

☐ Stress can wreak havoc on your waistline and your health.

☐ Alleviate stress through exercise, laughter, or calming activities.

Eliminating comfort food altogether may not be the solution because "If we deny ourselves what we crave, we end up craving it even more." Certain comfort foods in controlled moderation are acceptable.

☐ Many fat-free or sugar-free snacks are still high in calories.

☐ To help curb your cravings, heed the list on pages 86 through 88.

Keep a food journal to foster self-awareness.

☐ Overeating regressions can be triggered by deep-rooted memories.

☐ If temptations or comfort foods aren't there, you can't eat them.

Eating is a basic human function. For those people with a binge-eating disorder, eating should be primarily viewed as a way of acquiring nutrition for sustenance, not as a source of entertainment or comfort.

- ☐ Substitute your bad habits with good habits.

- ☐ Bad habits are acquired behavior that occur automatically and cause you to act in the same harmful ways repeatedly.

- ☐ Eliminate the harmful behavior by creating new patterns of constructive behavior, thus creating good habits.

- ☐ Changing small daily habits can amount to a big change over the long-term.

What bad eating habits can you change? Change isn't as hard as you may think *provided* you approach it *gradually*. Retrain your brain by continually repeating the new satisfaction-generating positive behavior.

- ☐ Watch out for saboteurs and "food pushers."

- ☐ You can only change how you *deal* with stereotypes or criticism.

- ☐ Take responsibility for your own actions regarding your weight.

Everyone has the ability to lose weight. Some people find it harder than others, and some people may need professional help, but if you really want weight-loss success it *will* happen *provided* you know what you're doing.

- ☐ Make a commitment to yourself, and to live in a healthier way.

- ☐ Really appreciate how important good health is.

If you have circumstances in your life that are causing you angst—like a bad relationship, lousy neighbor, or horrible boss—deal with them. You may have to make a major change in your life, and you may need to visit a mental health professional for assistance, but *you must bring an end to the source of your angst*.

❑ Improved physical health will follow improved mental health.

Realize that you're done with traditional dieting, and its temporary measures. You now know that the lifestyle-reform, weight-loss and health plan is the way to success.

❑ Praise yourself for every bit of progress, no matter how small.

❑ Be patient and persistent—move forward *one pound at a time.*

Don't wait to enjoy your new life. Start enjoying it today. Enjoy the ride. Losing weight and keeping it off doesn't have to be boring and tortuous. The lifestyle-reform, weight-loss and health plan may take the weight off slower than crash diets do, *but it works without sacrifice and misery, and the lost weight stays off.* Losing weight is a fun, rewarding journey only if you take your time and allow it to be fun and rewarding.

❑ It may be impractical to eat perfectly all of the time.

❑ Initially, be on track more than you're off track; and then strive to be on track almost all the time.

❑ Caring for yourself and your health will increase your sense of self-pride.

❑ Eventually your inner strength will not let you regress and regain weight.

❑ While you can occasionally cheat, you can't binge.

❑ A binge can negate an entire week's worth of progress.

❑ You must be careful when it comes to your trigger foods.

If you feel like grabbing some comfort food, walk to a mirror, look at your "shiny new self," and ask, "Do I really need to eat this crud?" By remembering the dedication it took to become your "shiny new self," you'll probably end up throwing the crud in the garbage can.

❑ Caring about yourself will help you apply newfound restraint.

❑ You're in charge, not the food.

As Oprah Winfrey says, love yourself and find the inner care you need to make yourself healthy. Make yourself a top priority, and put yourself (and your health) first. Find joy in your everyday life, *but don't let food become that joy.*

And ask yourself these questions: "Why are you overweight? What can you change about yourself? Why have you failed at previous diets? Why do you want to lose weight?" Some deep self-analysis can reveal the underlying issues that are the cause of your weight problem.

❑ No matter how much weight you lose, you'll never be cured.

❑ Your weight must be properly managed for the rest of your life.

❑ You may have to change your mind-set from a *fat person* to a *slim person*.

❑ Adverse life-issues will affect you whether you're fat or slim.

❑ Many people with eating problems suffer from self-esteem issues.

❑ Negative core beliefs can keep you from losing weight, and keep you from enjoying life.

Once you've solved your emotional problems, you'll be more likely to eat for health reasons rather than emotional reasons. And this can help with your self-esteem. The better you feel about yourself emotionally, the better you feel about yourself physically. And the better you feel about yourself physically, the better you feel about yourself emotionally.

❑ The accomplishment from achieving goals will improve your self-esteem.

❑ As you reach your goals, your sense of self-worth will soar.

❑ You'll eventually smile every time you look into the mirror.

❑ You'll enjoy every day and relish the anticipation of tomorrow.

❑ You'll have pride in your appearance.

❑ You'll glow with self-confidence.

Every pound you lose will be another reason to smile, and another reason to take more pride in yourself. You have only one life—start enjoying it!

CHAPTER 8

The physiological aspects of weight-loss   *109*

❑ Losing weight and keeping it off isn't the same for everyone.

❑ Obesity can stem from many medical conditions.

❑ Review the list on page 110.

❑ Most conditions can be corrected with proper treatment.

❑ Health insurance may help cover the cost of these medical bills and procedures.

Obesity should be treated like any other chronic disease, such as hypertension or diabetes. It's a lifelong issue that may need help from a doctor or a psychologist, or both.

❑ The BMI is an inaccurate tool for determining ideal weight.

❑ Consistent fatigue can devastate your ability to lose weight and keep it off.

❑ If you suffer from consistent fatigue, investigate its cause, and seek the appropriate help.

Get enough quantity of good quality sleep so that you're not drowsy during the day. Sleep deprivation can trigger hunger.

❑ If more than two of the symptoms on page 113 apply to you, you probably suffer from a sleep disorder. If so, urgently visit a doctor who specializes in sleep disorders, and deal with the particular disorder or disorders that may afflict you.

❑ There's much at stake—*and not just for weight control.*

❑ If not treated, sleep disorders greatly increase the chance of grave results—heart problems, strokes, and premature death.

Not only will proper treatment boost your energy level and directly help your efforts to lose weight, but it could transform your health in general, which will further help your efforts to lose weight.

☐ The Ad-36 virus may cause weight-gain.

☐ Hypothyroidism can cause the body to store more calories as fat.

☐ Manage perimenopausal and postmenopausal weight with increased activity and reduced calories.

☐ The male menopause, or andropause, can influence the ability to lose weight and keep it off.

☐ Hormonal problems can influence your weight—see pages 116 through 119.

☐ You can still lose weight despite hormonal imbalances.

Do you have a large belly that's hard and not jiggly? If you're a woman, does your waist circumference measure 35 inches or more, and if you're a man, does it measure 40 or more? Do you have high blood pressure? If so, you may have metabolic syndrome.

☐ If you have a medical condition, and get it correctly treated, your life-changing, weight-loss journey can proceed without any medical problem undermining it.

No matter what underlying condition or conditions you may have, everyone can lose weight. Some people may require medical intervention, but everyone can succeed.

☐ You can gain weight because of underconsumption of the right foods as well as overconsumption of the wrong foods.

Most people eat a lot of food that has little nutritional value. Especially when that's coupled with a reduced-calorie diet, malnutrition is inevitable. The lack of key nutrients leads to many problems, including the appetite not being sated properly, which means you may continue

to be hungry even after eating. And when your body is desperate for the nutrients needed for survival, it may still crave food even after a meal.

☐ Eat healthy food rich in nutrients, including phytochemicals.

☐ Take a daily multivitamin-mineral tablet, and additional vitamins C and E.

☐ Take cod liver oil and flaxseed oil, to supply vital essential fatty acids.

☐ But rely on a variety of nutritious foods as your primary source of essential nutrients.

Many people are sedentary because their energy level is so low that they are *incapable of being active and vigorous*. Eating a nutrient-rich diet will boost their energy levels, and add vitality to their lives.

Not eating enough nutrient-rich food is one of the biggest mistakes you can make if you want to lose weight.

☐ Nutrient deficiencies contribute to the obesity epidemic.

☐ Vitamin D deficiency has been linked to obesity.

☐ Get vitamin D from some moderate exposure to the sun.

Your genes can determine how quickly you feel full when you eat, how physically active you're prone to be, and how high your basal metabolic rate may be. And because of this some people may be genetically destined to be more vulnerable to gaining weight, and certain environmental triggers can make these people more susceptible to becoming obese.

☐ Genetics determine your body shape and where fat is stored.

☐ You can lose weight despite a genetic predisposition to obesity.

Obesity tends to run in some families, suggesting a genetic cause. But families also share dietary and lifestyle habits

that contribute to obesity. There seems to be a greater chance that people are heavy because of conditioned behaviors learned from their family, not genetics.

☐ Quitting smoking can cause weight-gain.

☐ It's still possible to exercise and manage weight while pregnant.

☐ Being underweight is dangerous.

☐ Bulimia and anorexia nervosa can be deadly.

☐ Don't follow extreme weight-loss plans used by some celebrities.

Think about the big picture. Being a little more active by burning, say, 300 more calories a day, and reducing your caloric intake by eliminating a daily 300-calorie snack, for example, produces a shift of 600 calories. If that produces a *deficit* of 600 calories—because, previously, you were neither gaining nor losing weight—that change could be equivalent to 62 pounds of fat over a year.

CHAPTER 9

The fundamentals of weight-loss 133

☐ Have confidence in your new weight-loss plan.

☐ You want *fat*-loss, not just *weight*-loss.

☐ Crash diets cause muscle loss and excessive water loss.

☐ Body fat is a long-term store of energy.

The only way to lose body fat naturally is to expend more calories than you take in. You need to establish that energy imbalance via ingesting fewer calories and burning more calories. All successful weight-loss plans have one thing in common: *a marked reduction in calories.*

☐ A calorie is the standard unit for measuring food energy.

☐ One gram of protein has four calories, one gram of carbohydrate also has four calories, but one gram of fat has nine calories.

❑ To lose one pound of fat you must produce a deficit of 3,500 calories. You can do that solely by reducing your caloric intake, solely by increasing your caloric output, or, preferably, by a combination of the two.

The three fundamental ways your body uses calories are through its basal metabolism, from your activities and exercise, and from food digestion. The rate at which your body uses energy at rest (to cover the essential functioning of your organs, muscles, nervous system, and so forth) is called the basal metabolic rate, or BMR, which typically accounts for about two-thirds of an individual's daily caloric requirements.

Active people generally burn more calories—typically 300 to 500 more a day—than sedentary people.

❑ Thin people may burn more calories from a more active lifestyle, not from a faster metabolism.

❑ Heavy people can expend more calories per minute of a given activity because of their bulk, but are less likely to do so because too much effort is required.

❑ Men generally have higher energy expenditures than women because of a higher percentage of muscle mass, and, often, greater overall activity levels.

❑ Additional muscle burns more daily calories, even while at rest.

❑ Most of your weight-loss success will come from a reduction in daily caloric intake.

If you go too long without eating, or if you severely reduce your caloric intake, your body slows its basal metabolic rate as a means of self-preservation. This *starvation effect* causes your body to store fat when you eat.

❑ Don't reduce caloric intake by more than 350 every few days.

A simple way for most people to reduce caloric intake is to gradually eliminate soda, sweets, unhealthy desserts, and excessive dietary fats. Avoid fast food, whole-milk

dairy products, butters, calorie-laden sauces and condiments, and fat-laden meats. And reduce or eliminate nighttime snacking.

❑ No nighttime snacking can produce a loss of 25 to 50 pounds of fat in a year.

❑ Enjoy your food, but eat primarily for nourishment, not entertainment. Choose foods you enjoy *that are also healthy.*

❑ Has your reduction in calories created an energy imbalance?

❑ A daily average energy imbalance of 500 calories—which is 3,500 a week—is equivalent to 52 pounds of fat a year.

❑ Make an energy imbalance a daily rule to live your new life by.

❑ Starving then binging will train your body to store fat.

Find the daily caloric intake that works for you. Many factors, such as your age, weight, height, food intake, body-fat percentage, muscle-mass percentage, overall health, external temperature, and overall activity levels, affect your rate of energy expenditure, and weight-loss. No two people are exactly the same in this regard.

How to determine your daily caloric needs for weight-loss:

For a week, write down everything you normally eat and drink, along with the precise quantities.

Add the total number of calories consumed over the seven days, and then divide the total by seven to produce your current daily average caloric intake.

Then reduce your caloric intake by 250 to 350 every few days. Do this by gradually getting rid of processed food in general, and gradually stopping nighttime eating.

Then, once you're consuming only healthy food, if you still haven't started to lose weight, slowly reduce your calories further.

❑ You can overeat even on exclusively healthy foods.

❑ Monitoring your overall food intake solely through portion sizes can be confusing and ineffective.

❑ Too few daily calories yields deprivation and long-term failure.

❑ Too few daily calories can bring on the *starvation effect,* and slows the basal metabolic rate as a means of self-preservation.

Try a modified version of the "seven-times-bodyweight caloric intake" approach one day, and the higher-calorie approach the next. One day have perhaps 1,400 to 1,600 calories (if you're 200 pounds), but hit the lower end of this range *only* **on your most sedate day each week. And the next day, have a few hundred additional calories for a total of perhaps 1,700 to 1,900. Alternate, day-by-day, between the two approaches. This will average, perhaps, 1,700 daily calories, and keep the starvation effect at bay.**

If the caloric intakes in this illustration are too low for you, choose to lose weight at a slower pace, *or* **increase your activity levels to compensate for the extra few hundred daily calories you need in order to feel satisfied.**

❑ Don't like counting calories? At least know what you're taking in, by reading nutrition labels, and be in the ballpark calories-wise.

❑ For every 10 pounds you lose, reduce your daily calories by about 70.

❑ Permanent weight-loss takes time—*you must be patient.*

❑ The quicker you lose weight, the quicker you're likely to put it back on.

❑ Losing more than two pounds of fat a week is not realistic.

❑ Made-for-TV weight-loss boot camps are unrealistic for dieters in the real world.

❑ Losing more than one pound of fat a week requires greater food reduction, or greater activity level increase, than are practical for most people.

❑ The real-life dieters averaged under one pound of lost fat a week.

Your body is predisposed to be a certain weight, within a range of, perhaps, 20 pounds. Your lowest adult weight—which may be what you weighed in your late

teens, or early twenties, *provided* you were slim at that time—may be a good indication of your lowest achievable target. Getting below that point may not be possible because you can't overcome your bone structure and internal predisposition.

- ❑ Your weight-loss goals must be realistic and obtainable.
- ❑ Trying to look like a supermodel or a ripped athlete isn't a realistic goal.
- ❑ Your ultimate goal must be set in a reasonable time frame.
- ❑ Establish interim goals in small steps—say 10 pounds at a time.
- ❑ Achieving mini goals one at a time makes a long-term goal more attainable.
- ❑ But everyone loses weight *one pound at a time.*

Your first goal should be to get today right, then your next "today" right, then the next, and so on. And further break each new day into one meal and one walk at a time. Anyone can get one day right. And if you can get one day right, you can get the next one right, and then the next, and so on. It soon becomes a habit. Then you'll lose one pound. If you can lose one pound, you can lose another, then another, and so on.

Make *one day at a time*, and *one pound at a time*, your weight-loss creeds.

CHAPTER 10

What's your motivation for losing weight?   *155*

- ❑ The first step is to admit that you need to lose some weight.
- ❑ Are you ready to follow the plan that transformed Brad?
- ❑ Are you ready to commit to eating better, and being more active?
- ❑ Are you ready to change your life for the better?

Just because you said yes to these questions doesn't necessarily mean that you're ready to succeed. To succeed, you'll need strong motivation, because if your heart isn't fully into it, your chances of succeeding are greatly reduced.

☐ 62% of Americans are overweight or obese.

☐ Obesity and an unhealthy lifestyle are leading causes of preventable deaths.

Overweight and obese people are much more likely to develop type II diabetes, have a heart attack, develop heart disease, have a stroke, develop high blood pressure, sustain liver damage, have high cholesterol levels, be more susceptible to cancer, develop sleep apnea, and be vulnerable to many other weight-related ailments. Excess weight can wreak havoc on every part of your body.

☐ Staying alive and healthy should be hugely motivating.

☐ People who follow a healthy lifestyle live an average of 14 years longer.

☐ Make yourself and your health top priorities.

☐ And make it a priority to be healthy for family and loved ones.

Make a commitment to yourself, and follow through. Don't let yourself down. And don't let your friends and family down, either. It's your responsibility and obligation to be around for the people who rely on you and care about you. You have only one life. Don't shorten it by living in an unhealthy body.

☐ For daily inspiration, review your goals and motivating factors.

☐ Look at a photograph of yourself when fat, or slim, as a daily motivational reminder.

☐ Look at a photograph of a child or family member as another daily motivational reminder.

☐ Keep a collage of these photographs by where you store your exercise gear and shoes.

☐ Are you happy with your body and health?

☐ Do you hide from cameras?

☐ Can you look at your naked body and be proud of what you see?

If you aren't satisfied with your body and health, make a conscious decision to do something about it. Each day, visualize yourself as the person you want to be. This will help motivate you to become that person. Losing weight isn't "I'll try," but "I will." Most overweight people make lame excuses for not sticking with their plans.

☐ *Trying* won't produce results, only *doing* will.

☐ And *doing* produces results only if you stick with the plan.

☐ An *epic promise* via short-term goals can yield long-term success.

☐ Don't be pre-defeated or intimidated by your weight-loss plan.

☐ You don't have to be gung-ho to achieve excellent results.

☐ If you upend your life too much, you won't stick with the plan.

There are hundreds of tips in this book to choose from. But you don't have to follow every one of them in order to lose weight. Start by following a handful of tips you think will work best for you, and incorporate more and more of them as you progress. Do what you can for now—getting started is the first step. And good things take time.

CHAPTER 11

Weight-loss scams

163

☐ In 2007, 4.8 million Americans were victims of weight-loss scams.

Snake oil is a derogatory term applied to something that's fraudulent, fake, or ineffective. The term is also applied metaphorically to any product with exaggerated

marketing claims, and questionable or unverifiable quality. In the unregulated, billion-dollar dietary supplement industry, snake-oil peddling is endemic via a huge array of scams that preys on the gullible.

❑ You must be forewarned about this part of the weight-loss industry so that *you* don't fall for any of the scams.

❑ Victims aren't necessarily naïve, but misinformed.

❑ Dietary supplements don't need FDA approval before being marketed, so the potential for scams is huge.

If it sounds too good to be true, it *is* too good to be true.

❑ Many magazines have a vested interest in running deceptive ads.

❑ Some magazines have an editorial bias for certain products.

❑ Most weight-loss products have disclaimers and misleading fine print.

Exaggerated claims of substantial or fast weight-loss are crafted to catch the attention of the gullible. They are supported by fictitious testimonials, bogus "clinical studies," and manipulated before-and-after photos.

❑ Using simple arithmetic can help you determine if a claim is legitimate or not.

❑ Claims of "miraculous benefits" are bogus.

None of the real-life dieters attributed any of their success to a pill, fat burner, or weight-loss supplement. There's no magical weight-loss pill or fat burner that, alone, will cause you to lose 5, 10, 20, or 40 pounds of fat in a month's time. It just doesn't exist. Your doctor will confirm this. Any better-than-average results arise from strict diet and a lot of exercise.

❑ Colon cleansing results in loss of water, and waste, not fat.

❑ Most doctors don't recommend colon cleansing for weight-loss.

- ❐ Excess colon cleansing can result in anemia, malnutrition, and heart failure.

- ❐ Colon cleanse pills bought via the internet or mail order are often part of a credit card scam.

Most of the before-and-after photographs in today's magazines are manipulated, digitally altered, or even completely faked by substituting torsos and other parts of the body from other subjects. They aren't to be trusted.

- ❐ Some of the before-and-after pictures are done on the *same* day.

- ❐ Some models are paid to stage bogus before-and-after photos.

A spokesman for the Federal Trade Commission (FTC) was quoted as saying: "You're not going to find weight-loss in a bottle of pills."

- ❐ Internet snake-oil salesmen are unregulated.

- ❐ The internet is a free-for-all for crooks.

- ❐ Internet "weight-loss pill review sites" are almost always bogus.

- ❐ Internet ads are riddled with fake testimonials and bogus claims.

- ❐ It's foolish to take a weight-loss product bought via the internet.

If you take a pill or potion bought from an enticing internet pop-up ad, you're putting your health at risk. How do you know the product's source is reliable? And how do you know the ingredients are trustworthy? Don't fall for these scams.

- ❐ Many internet weight-loss ads are really credit card scams— don't provide your credit card details to such websites.

- ❐ Don't fall for "free trial" offers—they are often bank-account-draining scams.

Never buy any weight-loss product unless your doctor tells you to. And purchase a doctor-recommended

product from a trustworthy source. Never buy it via the internet because even legitimate-*appearing* products can be counterfeit, and contain hazardous ingredients.

❑ Most fat burners are a dangerous mix of caffeine-type ingredients.

❑ Most fat-burner-type products are terrible for your health.

Most real-life dieters have tried these products, but after a bout of frustration, along with nausea, dizziness, and a racing heart with unnerving skipped beats, the bottles of "magical weight-loss pills" ended up in the garbage can.

❑ The best, legitimate FDA-approved weight-loss pill will, by itself, create a fat-loss of less than one pound a month.

❑ Any snake-oil ad that claims a faster result than this is a lie.

❑ Be watchful of deceptive wording in advertising.

Attention-grabbing headlines such as "Lose 15 pounds a week by following a miracle diet plan" are nonsense. Even legitimate (but highly distorted) claims of huge weight-loss are typically based on rare individual triumphs that are usually a large loss of superfluous water weight, not fat. This is one of the major reasons for the "results not typical" disclaimer.

❑ About 90% of all weight-loss ads are targeted at women.

❑ Women's magazines are known for publishing over-the-top claims for weight-loss.

❑ No matter how far-fetched and misleading they are, catchy covers sell magazines.

❑ Be leery of quirky books or diet fads.

❑ And be especially suspicious of weight-loss plans or products endorsed by celebrities.

Some diet plans have multiple phases, with varying degrees of detoxification practices and procedures.

Almost all weight-loss plans work short-term, but they are usually impractical for the long-term.

❑ The FTC is there for your protection.

❑ Check out the FTC's website: www.ftc.gov

❑ The FTC has several consumer links that offer brochures on weight-loss scams.

❑ Heed the FTC's weight-loss red flags on pages 176 and 177.

The FTC has said, "Claims of anything over three pounds per week can land a company in court. Fast and easy fixes undermine the reality of what it takes to lose weight. People are buying empty promises."

CHAPTER 12

Where your calories should come from   *179*

There are five fundamental constituents of food: the three macronutrients (protein, carbohydrates, and fats), water, and fiber. The macronutrients provide your caloric intake.

❑ Protein is utilized for body tissue repair and growth.

❑ There are two types of protein: *complete* (derived from animal sources, containing all essential amino acids), and *incomplete* (usually plant based).

❑ It takes more energy to digest protein than other macronutrients.

❑ It may take 250% more energy to digest protein than carbs.

❑ The more difficult digestion process increases protein's thermic effect.

By eating more protein on a daily basis—substituting protein for some carbs—your body may burn more calories than it would if less protein but more carbs were eaten (while keeping total calories the same). This is called "diet-induced thermogenesis."

- ❐ Protein also increases your feeling of fullness.

- ❐ A protein-rich diet can help with weight-loss.

- ❐ A protein-rich diet may help muscle-gain and maintenance, and recuperation from exercise.

- ❐ Review the list of protein sources on pages 180 and 181.

- ❐ Be wary of deli meats because some of them are highly processed.

- ❐ Protein shakes aren't necessary. Get your protein from regular food instead.

- ❐ Account for every calorie you eat; and don't waste calories on fast food, junk food, or any other type of processed food.

- ❐ Carbohydrates are the body's primary source of energy.

- ❐ Carbs are divided into two categories: simple, and complex.

- ❐ Simple carbs—essentially sugars—digest quickly and provide a fast but short-lived energy boost.

Complex carbs provide energy for a longer period, and should be a staple of your diet to prevent the highs and lows of the "sugar rush."

- ❐ The glycemic index (GI) is a ranking of carbohydrates on a scale from 0 to 100 by the extent to which they increase blood sugar levels after consumption.

- ❐ Low-glycemic carbs (a GI value of less than 55) may help you lose weight faster.

- ❐ Review the low-glycemic carbohydrate sources on page 182.

- ❐ Visit www.glycemicindex.com for GI ratings of foods.

- ❐ Stay away from high-GI-value carb sources in general, especially those that are processed.

- ❐ Review the list of carbohydrate sources on page 183.

- ❐ Resistant starch may increase fat burning by as much 25%.

- ❐ Foods high in resistant starch include bananas, beans, brown rice, potatoes, pasta, corn, oatmeal, whole-grain bread products.

- ❐ Fruits and vegetables are usually healthier when fresh or frozen, rather than canned.

❑ Canned foods are usually packed in sugary liquids, and contain chemicals—avoid them.

❑ Steaming vegetables helps to preserve their nutritional content.

Some fats, such as margarine, refined vegetable oils, and hydrogenated oil, are harmful and should be avoided.

❑ Not only are some fats not bad, they *are essential for good health.*

❑ Good fats are necessary for the health of your skin and other organs, proper insulin function, red blood cell formation, and the lubrication of your joints, for example.

❑ If you eat a variety of healthy foods, your fat intake should naturally work itself out. About 25% of your total calories should come from healthy fats.

While the weight-loss industry has made almost everyone believe that fat makes people gain weight, it's the *extra* calories, no matter what the source, that are the true culprit. You can lose weight with any diet *as long as* you control your caloric intake. But people who eat a lot of fat-laden foods tend to gain more weight because fat is much more calorific, weight for weight, than protein or carbohydrates.

❑ Essential fatty acids (EFAs) are essential for good health.

❑ Deficiencies in EFAs are linked with cancer, cardiovascular disease, diabetes, arthritis, weakened immune functions, and other health problems.

❑ There are two major families of EFAs: omega-6s, and omega-3s.

❑ Review the EFAs guidance provided on pages 184 through 186.

❑ Extra virgin olive oil is a healthy source of monounsaturated fatty acids that can help enhance fat metabolism. And extra virgin olive oil has many other health benefits.

Monounsaturated fats have numerous health benefits, and can aid in weight-loss. And they may help prevent weight-gain—especially the accumulation of visceral belly fat.

❑ Review the list of monounsaturated fat sources on pages 186 and 187.

❑ Cod liver oil has numerous health benefits.

Regardless of the macronutrient ratios utilized, everyone who lost weight had one thing in common—*a marked reduction in overall calories.* You must keep your calories and portion sizes in check. And regardless of the proportions of macronutrients you eat, you must establish an energy *imbalance* (or caloric *deficit*) to force your body to draw on its energy store—fat.

❑ It's not a prerequisite to adhere to specific macronutrient ratios.

❑ The average macronutrient ratios among the real-life successful dieters were approximately 40% to 50% of calories from protein, 25% to 35% from carbohydrates, and 25% from fats.

❑ The best ratio is the healthy one that you enjoy and can stick with over the long-term.

Most of your meals should have some high-quality protein, complex carbohydrates, and healthy fat. This will stabilize your blood-sugar levels throughout the day because it will slow the rate at which carbs are converted to blood sugar.

❑ Baking, broiling, grilling, frying, steaming, poaching, boiling, and microwaving are the common alternatives for preparing meals.

❑ But the high heat used in baking, broiling, grilling and frying can damage food.

❑ If you stir-fry your food with extra virgin olive oil, a little butter, or non-stick cooking spray, only do it with low to medium heat.

❑ Deep frying should always be avoided.

Because they use the lowest temperature, steaming, poaching and boiling are usually the best methods of cooking—they do the least damage to food, and they preserve its nutritional content.

☐ Buying nutritious foods is an investment in your life.

☐ Look for sales on your favorite healthy foods. Buy in bulk and buy smart.

☐ Don't shop at a supermarket when you're hungry.

The hormone ghrelin improves perception and memory when it comes to food, making food seem tastier; and when you go to the supermarket hungry, every food looks more appealing.

☐ Prepare a shopping list ahead of time, and stick to it.

☐ Purchase no food other than what fulfills your weekly nutritious menu plan.

CHAPTER 13

How to eat for weight-loss 191

☐ Healthy food can be very tasty and enjoyable.

☐ Healthy food builds health, and as your health improves, you'll feel better and function better.

☐ Healthy food makes weight-loss easier to achieve and maintain.

☐ What you eat plays a major role in your weight.

And where you eat plays a major role in your weight. Many social events are centered on or around food. And many of your friends or acquaintances may be poor role models because their poor eating habits can rub off on you. Many people are not obese due to their genetics, *but due to conditioned behavior*.

☐ Many parents pass unhealthy eating habits to their children.

☐ Fast-food eating and junk-food snacking have created many obese families.

Eat often but reduce your portion sizes. Have a 200- to 400-calorie mini-meal every two to four hours.

❑ More frequent mini-meals increase your energy.

❑ More frequent mini-meals increase diet-induced thermogenesis.

❑ Smaller meals help your body fully assimilate what you eat.

❑ More frequent mini-meals help with weight-loss.

Although a given eating pattern won't work the same way for everyone, all successful weight-loss plans have one thing in common—*a marked reduction in overall daily caloric intake.*

❑ Never eat to the point where you're stuffed.

❑ Until you've mastered portion control, always choose a smaller portion size.

❑ Most people greatly underestimate the calories they consume.

❑ Small changes can have an enormous effect over the long-term.

❑ Be aware of the true size of your mini-meals—the difference in effect between 200 and 400 calories per meal is huge.

Be aware of all the food and drink you consume. Make a note of it in a food journal, to track your caloric intake.

❑ Don't overcompensate and overeat just because you exercise.

❑ Don't eat excessive protein just because you may lift weights.

Use a hunger scale to help you gauge when you're full. Formulate a scale from 0 to 10, in which 10 is "stuffed," 0 is "starving," 5 is "comfortably satisfied" and 7.5 is "full." This is based on *your* feelings of hunger. Avoid ever exceeding a feeling of five.

❑ Overeating usually leads to fat storage.

❑ Create a feeling of fullness by eating low-calorie soups and salads.

❑ Eliminate processed food, fat-laden food, and sugars.

❑ Having healthy snacks nearby, or in your purse, can serve as a great diversion.

Processing removes nutrients from food and replaces them with rubbish like hydrogenated fat, sugar, high-fructose corn syrup, and chemicals. Eating processed foods can cause your insulin levels to spike, which triggers your body to store fat. If some food doesn't exist in nature, it's probably a processed food and you should avoid it.

- ❑ "Refined" or "enriched" foods should also be avoided.
- ❑ If a food contains mysterious chemicals, avoid it.
- ❑ Be careful of high-calorie dressings like butter or mayonnaise.
- ❑ Ketchup, steak sauce, barbeque sauce, and other sauces can have high-fructose corn syrup.
- ❑ Ordinary appearing foods can be high in sugar and high-fructose corn syrup.
- ❑ Salad dressings can have hundreds of calories per serving.
- ❑ Watch out for dietary sugars of any kind.

According to the US Department of Agriculture (USDA), the average American ingests 150 pounds of sugar a year, and about a third of it may be converted to body fat.

- ❑ Sugar causes your insulin levels to spike, which triggers your body to store fat.
- ❑ Sugar substitutes, used in moderation, are acceptable.
- ❑ Watch out for "white stuff" — refined foods made from white flour. Eat whole-grain and whole-wheat alternatives instead.

Many studies have shown a compelling link between high-fructose corn syrup (HFCS) and obesity.

- ❑ The average American consumes 63 pounds of HFCS a year.
- ❑ HFCS is in nearly all pre-packaged food.
- ❑ HFCS can impair your liver's ability to break down fat into fuel.
- ❑ The elimination of HFCS can create substantial weight-loss.

Severe caloric reductions can cause your body to store fat when you eat. And severe diets can trigger catabolism, and deplete your muscle tissue.

❑ Starvation can stymie your willpower, and increase cravings.

❑ If you starve then binge, you'll train your body to store fat.

❑ If you're hungry between meals, make time for a "pocket meal" like an all-natural meal replacement bar or drink, some peanuts, a single-serving snack or yogurt, or some skim milk.

People who skip breakfast are four times more likely to be obese than those who eat breakfast.

❑ It's essential to eat a nutritious breakfast.

❑ A well-proportioned, nutritious breakfast helps to control appetite and satisfy cravings.

❑ Skipping breakfast leads to overeating later in the day.

❑ If you're in a rush in the morning, at least have a glass of skim milk, or a granola bar.

Have a cut-off time whereby you stop eating two to three hours before bedtime.

❑ Eliminating nighttime eating can create substantial weight-loss.

❑ Eating larger breakfasts and lunches than dinners may help reduce body fat.

❑ Reduce your carbohydrate intake later in the day.

❑ "Going out to eat after the game" is a sure way to put on weight.

Keep your metabolism revving by varying your caloric intake day-to-day.

❑ By varying your caloric intake you'll outwit your body's innate survival mechanism, and prevent the starvation effect.

❑ But keep your *average* daily caloric intake where it needs to be for weight-loss.

☐ You may have *a little* processed food on one designated treat day a week, if that appeals to you.

☐ Treat days can help to alleviate any perceived dietary boredom.

☐ Over time you'll lose your desire to eat junk food and fast food.

Prevent the "see-food diet" by keeping your home stocked *only* with nutritious, healthy foods. If you don't see irresistible temptations, you won't eat them.

☐ Cook large batches of nutritious foods ahead of time.

☐ Pack your lunch and take it to work.

☐ People who pre-plan their meals are much less likely to cheat on their weight-loss plans.

Pre-packaged meal plans work, at least for the short-term, because they remove human decision-making. But they invariably lead to failure because they are difficult to adhere to over the long-term.

☐ Eating more slowly can help with weight-loss.

☐ It takes about 20 minutes after starting a meal before your brain can signal that you're full.

☐ Eating quickly usually causes you to eat more.

☐ Pretend you're a food critic—savor your food slowly.

When saturated with water, dietary fiber swells in your stomach, and creates a sensation of fullness. Fiber also increases the calories burned as a result of diet-induced thermogenesis because it takes more energy to burn fiber-laden calories. Furthermore, fiber helps to control blood sugar levels and decrease insulin levels.

☐ Having fiber early in the day helps to give you a prolonged sensation of fullness.

☐ Adult women should consume 25 *or more* grams of fiber a day, and adult men 40 *or more*.

- To help the fiber do its job, drink plenty of water.

- Unsalted, dry-roasted peanuts and almonds make a great fiber-rich snack.

- Peanuts and nuts are rich in antioxidants that have health benefits.

- People who snack on peanuts (in moderation) invariably keep weight off.

- Buy dry-roasted peanuts that come in their shells.

- A little vinegar with a meal may help you feel a sense of fullness.

CHAPTER 14

Eating out   *213*

Fast food consumption is a major reason why many people overeat. Read the content in a typical fast-food value meal, and you'll be shocked with how many calories it contains, and how much crud. Eliminating fast food can yield a tremendous loss in body fat.

- Healthy subs are quick-service alternatives to burgers and fries.

- Fast-food wraps, and healthy sandwiches and salads, are good options, too.

- Read labels to make sure that "healthy alternatives" *are* healthy.

When you travel by car, pack a cooler with nutritious foods, to take away any temptation to visit a drive-thru.

- Always be mindful of portion sizes, and caloric intake.

- Even healthy food can be overly calorific if you eat too much of it.

- Don't put high-calorie condiments or fixings on an otherwise healthy sandwich.

Most restaurant food tastes terrific because it's loaded with calorie-laden enhancers that contribute to the mouth-watering taste. Some dishes have multiple sticks of real butter melded into them.

❑ Request that your food is prepared to your liking.

❑ Order smaller portions, or bring half of the meal home.

❑ You should pass on most restaurant appetizers because they add too many calories.

❑ A soup or nutritious salad (or even a whole-wheat bun) can help control hunger.

❑ Heed the salad dressing guidance on pages 186 and 217.

❑ Most desserts are overly calorific and should be avoided.

People tend to overeat when dining in a fun, comfortable social setting among friends, mostly due to spending a longer time in the restaurant than usual, and while paying more attention to the fun atmosphere than to what they are eating.

❑ Avoid "shared food" like wings and nachos.

❑ Sports-themed restaurants or taverns generally have few healthy options.

❑ All-you-can-eat buffets may provide too much temptation.

❑ Cutting down on restaurant dining frees up money for better at-home eating.

❑ It's best not to buy food at entertainment venues like theaters or sports stadiums.

❑ Don't assume that all salads are healthy.

If you're not careful, you can ingest several thousand calories in a single, multi-course meal.

❑ Review the "emergency" fast food choices on pages 219 and 220.

CHAPTER 15

Know what you're eating   *223*

The ingredients listed on a nutrition label are in the order of significance. Pay particular attention to the first few

ingredients, because they are the most predominant. Be especially wary of high-fructose corn syrup, corn syrup, sugar, hydrogenated and partially hydrogenated vegetable oil, chemicals, or anything that says "enriched."

☐ Even accurate food labels can be misleading if you don't fully understand what's on them.

☐ Understand food labels by heeding the FDA-provided definitions on pages 223 and 224.

Be informed and discerning—*read nutrition labels.*

☐ Be careful of deceptive serving sizes in all that you eat and drink.

☐ Be mindful of your sodium intake.

☐ Many people are bloated due to excess water retention because of excess sodium.

While sodium is necessary to help transport vital nutrients around the body, send nerve messages, and contract muscles, many people ingest far more sodium than they need. Excessive sodium intake may contribute to dangerous conditions such as high blood pressure, strokes, osteoporosis, and exercise-induced asthma.

☐ To reduce the negative effects of sodium, load up on healthy, potassium-rich foods. Oats, wheat, potatoes, nuts, legumes, corn, squash, tomatoes, bananas, oranges, and dates are rich in potassium, for example, but with very little (if any) sodium.

☐ Drink more ice-cold water to help reduce bloating.

☐ Heed the bread-buying guidance on pages 226 and 227.

☐ Many cereals are high in sugar, high-fructose corn syrup, and hydrogenated oil.

☐ Opt for cereal of the all-natural variety, or switch to oatmeal.

☐ Review the Nutrition Facts information at www.cfsan.fda.gov/~dms/foodlab.html

CHAPTER 16
Real-life recipes for tasty meals   *231*

These recipes are examples of how you can eat normal foods while on a weight-loss plan. Use any of these easy-to-prepare meals to supplement your favorite nutritious foods and recipes.

❑ Most butters and margarines add excessive calories.

❑ Review the caloric content of any food at www.calorieking.com

❑ Review the list of 200- to 400-calorie mini-meals on pages 232 through 243.

CHAPTER 17
Get moving   *245*

What can you do to be more active? Remember, to lose weight, you *must* use up more calories than you take in. Don't be a couch potato.

❑ Any type of walking is better than lying, or sitting doing nothing.

❑ Obese people are usually less active than lean people.

❑ Sedate obese people burn more than 300 fewer daily calories than lean people.

❑ Periods of four hours or longer of inactivity can cause a near shutdown of an enzyme that controls fat metabolism.

For starters, maintain an activity log to prove that there really is time in the day to do some exercise. Keep track of every minute of every day for a week, and you'll see that there's ample time to be more active no matter how busy you may be.

❑ Even simple activities can burn many calories. For example, a five-mph 30-minute walk can burn as many as 290 calories.

❑ Over time, even small daily activities can amount to huge increases in energy output.

The addition of a three-mph 30-minute daily walk could burn an additional 43,000 or so annual calories (for a 200-pound man illustration), which would be the energy value of about 12 pounds of fat. As he becomes fitter he could increase the pace. A five-mph 30-minute walk would burn more than twice as many calories, which, over 12 months, would be the energy value of about 30 pounds of fat.

Couple this increased energy *output* with a daily *input* reduction of 100, 200, or 300 or more calories, and you'll see how simple it is to lose 50 to 100 pounds in year without upending your life.

❑ Little daily activities—such as tapping your foot, gently swaying in your chair, or twirling your hair—are NEAT (non-exercise activity thermogenesis). If done on and off throughout the day they can have a big impact over time.

❑ Slim people may be slim, at least in part, because they are much more active via daily NEAT.

NEAT activities can burn up to 20 extra calories per hour, or about 350 each day. And that alone could add up to the equivalent of 30 to 40 pounds of fat in a year.

❑ Come up with some fun things to keep yourself more active.

CHAPTER 18

The truth about exercise   *253*

You don't *have to* exercise in order to lose weight, and you don't *have to* exercise in order to keep the weight off. But, when done correctly, exercise *will* help you to lose weight and keep it off, although you don't *have to* go to a gym.

Furthermore, exercise will help you to be healthier, fitter and more robust. *And the healthier, fitter and more robust you are, the better equipped you'll be for everything you do, including losing weight and keeping it off.*

❑ You don't have to exercise fanatically in order to lose weight.

❑ Excessive exercising usually leads to burn-out, injuries, and long-term failure.

Although the ideal exercise regimen includes strength training, cardiorespiratory training, and flexibility work, that's not realistic for most people, especially those starting out on a weight-loss plan.

❑ Leisurely walking is the simplest option for starters.

❑ Many people whose only exercise was walking have lost hundreds of pounds.

❑ Even if you never graduate beyond walking, that's still valuable exercise.

Start with a little exercise, add to it gradually, and as you improve your physical conditioning and see and feel the benefits, you're likely to acquire an increased interest in exercise and take on a bit more of it, and then a bit more still, and so on. *Never start an exercise plan with gung-ho effort.*

Wean yourself onto exercise with this gradual progression:

1. What everyone needs to do for weight-loss

Begin with:
Walking, for weight-loss only, as explained in Chapter 19

Then progress to:
Advanced walking, *and other matters*, for increased weight-loss *and* for fitness, as explained in Chapter 20

2. Optional but highly recommended methods of advanced weight-loss training

Begin with:
Advanced walking, *and other matters* (Chapter 20), *plus* **home strength training** as explained in Chapter 21

Then progress to:
Advanced walking, *and other matters* (Chapter 20), *plus* **home strength training** (Chapter 21), *plus* **home flexibility training** as explained in Chapter 22

The older you are, the more important it is that you exercise. You can add life to your years, and perhaps years to your life, but you must exercise *safely* and *effectively*, or otherwise the results will be injury, frustration, and failure.

❑ The older you are, the greater the need for training consistency.

❑ It's never too late to start exercising. And you're never too old to be fit.

Strength training is the most productive single form of exercise, for men and women. It builds strength, develops muscle, strengthens bones, improves overall fitness, improves posture, slows the effects of aging, increases resistance to injury, and transforms physical appearance. And it can improve blood test results, reduce resting blood pressure, increase resting energy output (because of increased muscle mass), help control body fat, and improve cardiovascular efficiency. No other single type of exercise produces all these benefits.

❑ Safe, progressive, and consistent strength training may offer more health benefits than any other *single* exercise modality.

❑ You'll lose about 1% of your muscle mass a year as you age *unless strength training is employed to prevent it.*

❑ Middle-aged people typically burn hundreds of calories fewer a day because of this loss of muscle mass.

Flexibility training is highly recommended because, without a supple body, movements in general become restricted, dynamic balance is impaired, posture is negatively affected, and aging is accelerated.

Further benefits from exercise:

☐ Strength training, together with cardiovascular exercise, produces further health benefits, including raised levels of high-density lipoprotein (the "good cholesterol"), reduced blood pressure, reduced risk of diabetes, reduced incidence of various cancers, reduced incidence of Alzheimer's disease, and reduced likelihood of depression.

☐ The heart can be trained for greater strength and endurance. The benefits include a healthier cardiovascular system (heart, lungs, and blood vessels), and other internal boons.

☐ Exercise can reduce the mortality rate in seniors.

☐ Via exercise, you'll boost your productivity, usefulness, and enjoyment of life.

☐ If you train properly using activities you like, you'll experience the "exercise high." Your workouts will become an essential part of your life—and they will make you look, function and feel better. Done properly, exercise isn't drudgery. It's a blessing, and a joy.

The combination of strength training, stretching, cardiovascular work, healthy nutrition, and a healthy lifestyle is the closest we can get to the fountain of youth.

Many women are unwilling to strength train because they think it will develop big muscles. This concern is unfounded, and prevents them from obtaining the benefits that strength training produces.

Few women can develop big muscles even if they wanted to. Few women have the genetically determined characteristics required for strength training to yield big muscles. Women are limited in strength and muscular size because of their hormones. They lack the large quantities of testosterone that produce many of the male characteristics.

For the huge majority of women, the development of big muscles is impossible.

❑ Women should train for strength and muscle. Even a little additional muscle can improve appearance greatly, and yield substantial health benefits.

❑ Too much endurance work can break down muscle tissue.

❑ Strength training is great for weight-loss as well as fitness.

❑ Men and women of all ages should strength train.

❑ Serious strength training is needed for serious benefits.

There's no gadget or gizmo that's going to magically speed up fat burning or muscle-gain compared with proper training with conventional equipment.

❑ An exercise gadget alone can't make you ripped.

❑ Most ab training gizmos are rip-offs.

❑ Heed the ab training myths on pages 263 through 265.

Your body has tremendous abilities to adapt to and prosper from exercise *provided* you start out comfortably, and increase the demands *gradually*.

Many people view exercise as boring, and some are intimidated by the word "exercise" because it suggests something unenjoyable. Substitute the word "activity," "sport," or "recreation." And adopt the attitude that you're doing activities you enjoy, to improve your health, and get your heart pumping. You must select exercise or activities that you enjoy if you're to stick with the plan.

❑ Use fitness DVDs or video games like Wii Fit™ and Wii Sport™.

❑ Ultra-fit celebrities exercise their butts off.

❑ Never take good health for granted. It needs to be worked at. Take all possible actions to preserve good health—for your sake *and* those who depend on you.

The health-related benefits that come from exercise should be the primary factors that motivate you to exercise. There must be an investment of time in an exercise program. The potential benefits are so huge that you should *make* the time to exercise. But it's a myth that it's necessary to do a great deal of exercise to achieve good results.

CHAPTER 19

Walk on to weight-loss   *269*

Walking is one of the easiest, most convenient, and cheapest forms of exercise.

☐ Start by walking at a leisurely pace 10 minutes a day, and gradually do more and more until you reach an hour a day.

☐ The one hour of walking can be divided into multiple segments throughout the day.

☐ Build walking into your daily routine.

☐ The one hour of walking every day isn't as difficult as you may think it is if you accumulate a few minutes here and there throughout the day.

Invest in a pair of excellent training shoes appropriate for walking—special shoes for a special activity. Your feet must be properly supported so that you don't develop any problems as you build up your walking workload.

☐ Fix the time or times of day when you walk, and stick to the plan.

☐ Don't let inclement conditions serve as an excuse.

☐ Walk with a companion—human, or canine.

☐ If you walk with company, you may be more likely to stick to it.

☐ If you walk alone, take an iPod or other music player.

☐ Walk with your own thoughts for company, too. Walking can be great thinking or planning time.

At least some of the time, you may prefer bicycling, in-line skating, spinning, aerobics, hiking, dancing, swimming, badminton, active games with your children, in-front-of-television exercise with a DVD for instruction, or other activities.

Do whatever you want provided it's safe, easy to perform, and enjoyable. Walking can satisfy all those requirements, and is also convenient, with zero cost (unless you use a treadmill).

Even if you prefer an activity or activities other than walking, still work up to an hour a day, every day.

Why the big deal about walking for weight-loss?

- ❑ Walking a mile at a leisurely pace can burn approximately 70 calories, and is a great form of exercise for beginners, and *much* better than sitting all day, or lying on a couch. But even at "just" 70 calories a mile, the calories quickly add up.

- ❑ It's much easier to walk a mile at a leisurely pace than it is to run it. Which are you more likely to do on a daily basis, walk at a leisurely pace, or run vigorously?

- ❑ As a pure calorie-burning activity that can be done almost effortlessly on a regular basis, leisurely paced walking is the way to go. When something is almost effortless, you'll not have physical difficulty doing it.

- ❑ If you increase your distance *gradually* (still at a leisurely pace), so that sooner or later you cover four miles more each day than you would from your normal activities, that's about 280 extra calories each day, or about 1,960 each week, or about 102,000 each year.

- ❑ And 102,000 calories is the approximate value of 29 pounds of fat. Over four years, that's equivalent to about 116 pounds of fat—*from just four miles of leisurely walking each day*, which would take about an hour once you've developed a basic level of conditioning..

- ❑ And these calories burned will increase as you gradually pick up your pace in the coming weeks and months. Eventually you may be able to walk at a *sustained brisk pace*, and this may burn around as many calories as running, which is about 100 calories a mile. At that rate, the caloric equivalent of 40 pounds of fat could be burned over a year using the aforementioned four-miles-per-day example.

❑ *But remember that the precise calories burned per mile is affected by your pace, body size and composition, and other factors.*

Now you should see the great value of walking as a part of a weight-loss plan. Make it a mainstay of your weight-loss plan, and then keep it as a mainstay in your keep-the-weight-off plan.

Set a target of eventually doing a *minimum* of 10,000 steps a day—about five miles—from the walking you do from your everyday activities *and* from the additional walking for the primary purpose of burning extra calories. Use a pedometer to track your progress.

❑ Use a pedometer to track your progress.

❑ The awareness of wearing a pedometer is enough to make you walk more.

❑ Have fun pedometer contests to see who can walk the farthest in a day or a week.

❑ Once you hit your goal of 10,000 daily steps, set a new goal of 10,500 daily steps. Once you hit that goal, set a new one for 11,000 daily steps . . . and so on, if you're ambitious.

Walk a few minutes several times during each day—5 or 10 minutes here and there—and take a much longer walk each evening, and at weekends. All the small bursts of walking monitored via a pedometer quickly add up to many miles each day.

❑ Walking indoors on a treadmill is a great option.

❑ You can watch television or talk while walking on a treadmill.

❑ If you buy a treadmill, invest in a quality piece of equipment.

❑ The treadmill should have an adjustable incline.

❑ It should also have a yielding belt, to reduce impact forces.

There are alternatives to a treadmill. An elliptical machine (cross-trainer), has a blend of features from a treadmill, stepper and ski machine. It produces zero impact forces. Stationary cycling, and skiing, climbing and rowing machines produce zero or minimal impact forces.

❑ Before you consider buying a machine, test one or more of them for a few sessions at a local gym or exercise equipment store.

❑ Before a machine can become your staple for home exercising, you must like it. You must enjoy what you're doing if you're to stick with it over the long-term.

No matter whether you're walking or doing an alternative activity, and no matter how you do it or where, build up to a leisurely one hour of it every day. When you've done that for 30 consecutive days, you're ready to progress to *advanced walking, and other matters*—**for increased weight-loss,** *and* **for fitness.**

CHAPTER 20

Advanced walking, *and other matters* 277

To make walking more demanding—for increased fitness benefits, to get more calorie burning in your daily hour of walking, *and* make an even greater contribution to your weight-loss and health plan—*crank up your effort level.* But do so *gradually.*

❑ Never push yourself so hard that you kill your desire to exercise.

❑ Different people have different tolerance levels, and degrees of enthusiasm—*progress at a pace that works for you.*

How to progress to advanced walking:

Over a few weeks—or longer, if required—*gradually* increase your pace from leisurely, to brisk but not exhausting.

Move at a brisk but not exhausting pace for a minute, then return to your normal leisurely pace for a few minutes, then again move at the brisk clip for a minute, and so on.

Gradually increase the length of the brisk stretches, and reduce the length of the leisurely stretches. Eventually, perform the entire hour at a brisk but not exhausting pace.

But you don't have to do the one hour continuously. If you prefer to break it up into two or more short stints rather than one long one, that's fine.

As you increase your conditioning, and reduce your weight, you'll find it easier to maintain a brisk pace, and you may be able to make the pace brisker without any apparent increase in required effort.

Again, your body is wonderfully adaptive *provided* you increase the demands on it *gradually*, and you're *patient*.

Many middle-aged, women dieters eventually worked up to an hour or even 90 minutes of low- to moderate-intensity exercise several times a week, if not six or seven times a week.

- ❑ How much exercise is best for weight-loss? As much as you can perform *consistently*, which means it must be safe, and you must enjoy it. Our minimum recommendation is one hour a day of walking.

- ❑ Doing too much, and then burning out and giving it all up, is a classic error of exercising.

- ❑ Start off with just *a little* exercise, then add to it as your enthusiasm and physical conditioning increase.

An hour a day of walking—spread over one, two or more bouts—but done every day, year after year, is much better than an initial burst of enthusiasm that manifests in a two-hour gym workout on four days a week, and two hours of vigorous walking on each of the other three days, *but then after two months the gym is given up, and walks happen only rarely.*

- ❑ Feedback from dieters confirms that an hour a day of exercise isn't difficult to achieve *if you make it part of your daily lifestyle.*

- ❑ *Advanced* walking can produce a terrific workout.

The bottom line for weight-loss:

❐ No matter how much you exercise, in order to lose fat *you still have to expend more calories than you consume.*

❐ **There are two huge benefits from exercising. First, you can eat more food and yet still lose weight, which produces more satisfaction from eating, and a greater supply of nutrients. Second, the exercise, provided it's safe and you enjoy it, is good for your physical and mental well-being.**

❐ It's possible to do no exercise whatsoever and yet still lose weight *provided you eat very little.* It's also possible to lose weight while consuming lots of food *provided you burn lots of calories through a great deal of activity and exercise.*

❐ It's also possible to be hugely active and burn lots of calories and yet still *gain* weight *if you consume more calories than you need to maintain your bodyweight.*

❐ Find the right balance for you. For most people, it's moderate caloric intake, and moderate activity and exercise levels. If you want to eat a lot more, and yet still lose weight, you would have to be far more active in order to burn more calories, which isn't practical for most people.

Once you can readily walk at a brisk but not exhausting pace for an hour or so, increase its intensity some of the time by, for example, including a hill in the walk, or some undulating terrain. You may even wear a weighted vest, or a backpack, to add resistance so that even walking on level terrain can be made more demanding.

❐ Eventually, walk up flights of stairs as a supplementary activity.

❐ And then *gradually* build up to a couple of minutes of climbing flights of stairs *two* steps at a time. — but without rushing the pace.

An excellent method of increasing walking intensity is "interval walking." After walking at a slow-to-moderate pace to warm up, walk at a brisk but not exhausting pace and interject 30- to 60-second periods of fast, exhausting

walking throughout your workout. After each 30- to 60-second higher-intensity interval, walk at your normal, comfortable level for a few minutes—this is the recovery interval. Allow your breathing to return to normal, and then crank up the effort level for another 30 to 60 seconds. Repeat this pattern as often as you can.

As your conditioning improves, your recovery period will shorten, and the frequency of the exhausting bursts can be increased. Progress *gradually.*

☐ Using a treadmill, you may increase the incline for the higher-intensity bursts.

☐ Brisk walking, and interval walking, can produce sufficient cardiovascular exercise.

☐ Cardio is short for cardiovascular exercise, and is any activity that elevates your heart rate sufficiently to produce breathlessness.

☐ Cardio will strengthen your heart, and boost your health.

These higher-intensity variations of walking can produce the same effect on your heart as running, but without the same risk of injury. Many people, especially heavy people, shouldn't run, or even jog, because the stress on their joints and backs is excessive.

Many of the heavier or more elderly real-life dieters achieved their weight-loss success, *and* dramatically improved levels of fitness, while never graduating past higher-intensity walking. Anything more demanding than vigorous walking put too much stress on their joints.

☐ Be inspired by the real-life interval training success story on page 282.

☐ Even very heavy people can gradually progress to cardio training *provided* the exercise is low impact.

☐ Exercise can be performed on a variety of machines—spin cycles, ellipticals, ski machines, or rowers, for example—in addition to, or instead of, walking.

Higher-intensity exercise is *not* for everybody. Nor is it imperative for weight-loss. And for many people it's not fun. *But*, for many people, high-intensity exercise *is fun*. And it can accelerate fat-loss once you've progressed to the level of fitness required.

❑ Do the best that you can do, even if you feel your level of fitness is embarrassing, or subpar. Personal competition makes the journey more fun—and increasing your fitness is satisfying.

❑ Don't rush into high-intensity exercise—*build up gradually.*

Do some exercise first thing each day. Get up earlier, to exercise. When you exercise in a fasted or semi-fasted state—before you eat breakfast—your body may derive more of its fuel from your stored body fat.

❑ But it's best not to do intensive exercise—weight-lifting, or hard cardio—on an empty stomach first thing in the morning. Do it an hour or longer after a meal.

❑ Go to bed an hour earlier to wake up an hour earlier to exercise.

High-intensity interval training, or HIIT, is popular among exercise enthusiasts. HIIT is an upgrading of interval training, to make it more rigorous, formal, and effective for weight-loss, and for increased fitness benefits. This is a form of hard cardio work, where breathlessness and a greatly elevated heart rate are produced. HIIT can accelerate fat-loss substantially.

❑ If you want to progress to running, do it gradually, and be sure that you're suited to running.

❑ For running, wear proper shoes, and, perhaps, do it *only* on a treadmill (like in Stuart's example).

But jogging and running aren't for everyone. For many people they result in injury. Rather than jog or run, with their higher impact forces and risk of injury than from walking, you're probably better off to walk very briskly

(perhaps with a bag on your back for additional resistance), or walk at a slight incline on a treadmill. This especially applies to people who are overweight. The larger your mass, the greater the impact forces.

☐ Workout logs can help keep you organized, and motivated.

The "afterburn effect"—excess post-exercise oxygen consumption, or EPOC—is when an *intensive* workout may burn calories for a period of time after your workout *additional* to what you'd burn had you not exercised. It does this by elevating your metabolism above its normal resting state.

☐ To take advantage of this possible afterburn effect, do at least some of your hardest workouts in the morning, but after you've eaten.

☐ Place your treadmill, stationary cycle, or any other exercise gear in a room with natural light, and pleasant surroundings.

Build up, as described, to the one hour of higher-intensity walking (or other exercise) every day. When you've done that for 30 consecutive days, and if you want to further improve your fitness and your ability to lose weight and keep it lost, add *home strength training*.

CHAPTER 21

Home strength training   *293*

Once again . . . strength training is the most productive *single* form of exercise, for men and women.

☐ Gut-busting workouts at a gym aren't necessary.

☐ Review the five calisthenic exercises starting on page 296.

☐ Make slow, incremental progress.

☐ Some muscular soreness is fine, but you should *never* experience exercise-related pain.

❑ Have no time for the foolish maxim "No pain, no gain."

❑ Don't overtrain. You must recuperate fully between workouts. For your muscles to build the *overcompensation* tissue, and grow, you need adequate recovery time and sleep, and proper nutrition.

❑ Use correct exercise technique.

❑ Determine the weekly routine that best fits your schedule, according to the guidelines on page 309.

❑ Record your progress in a training logbook.

CHAPTER 22

Home stretching routine   *313*

By being supple you'll stay young for your years, and you'll be better equipped for being an active, vigorous person. And that will directly help you to lose weight and keep it lost.

Furthermore, if done properly, stretching is enjoyable and invigorating.

❑ Combine stretching with advanced walking, and home strength training.

❑ Stretch twice a week, immediately after your strength training.

❑ Make slow, incremental progress.

Many dieters stretch in front of the television while watching a specific program, such as the evening news.

❑ Do three reps of each stretch (or three reps for e*ach side* for two of the stretches). Hold each rep for at least 20 seconds.

❑ Review the five stretches starting on page 317.

❑ Never force yourself to feel pain, but you must feel tension during each stretch. Never have anyone force you into a stretch.

❑ Have no time for the foolish maxim "No pain, no gain."

CHAPTER 23

Additional weight-loss tips and tidbits   *327*

If you cheat on occasion, or give in to cravings, don't fret. Just get back on track tomorrow. There's no need to be a party pooper because you think that you aren't allowed to have fun on a weight-loss plan.

☐ You're still supposed to enjoy life while losing weight.

☐ Cheating "on occasion" doesn't mean weekly.

☐ A few days of splurging out of *a year* is okay, but weekly splurging isn't.

☐ If you stuff yourself with food, what's your plan to burn it off?

☐ Weight-loss plateaus are to be expected—your body always tries to adapt to what you do to it.

☐ You won't lose weight every week.

☐ A plateau can be the result of muscle-gain, or water-weight-gain.

☐ A plateau can be caused by not periodically reducing your caloric intake.

☐ A plateau can be the result of underexercising.

☐ A plateau can be the result of medication.

☐ Heed the plateau-busting tricks on pages 328 through 330.

A plateau is often the result of overeating. Perhaps some of your 200- to 400-calorie mini-meals have crept up to 500 or 600 calories. Get your food journal back out, and monitor what you're truly eating.

☐ To monitor progress, consider how your clothes fit, and keep tabs on fat pinch-points.

☐ When using the scale, weigh yourself under the same conditions.

☐ Most successful dieters weigh themselves regularly.

☐ But inadvertent water retention can skew your scale readings.

❑ Only body fat composition tests can determine if you're truly losing fat.

Variety keeps you fresh. Vary the exercises you enjoy doing. Come up with a list of nutritious foods that you enjoy eating, and vary them.

❑ Vary your entertainment while exercising.

❑ It's easier to succeed when you have a support group.

❑ Ask friends and family for their support.

❑ Find a weight-loss buddy to go through this with you.

❑ People who joined weight-loss support groups lost three times as much weight as people who had no support groups.

❑ Try an exercise group, or form one yourself if it doesn't exist.

❑ Perhaps, periodically, employ the services of a registered dietician, personal trainer, or psychologist.

❑ Use smaller plates, bowls and glasses when you prepare meals.

❑ A meal appears larger when heaped over a small plate.

❑ Blue plates and bowls are the least likely to stimulate appetite.

Brush your teeth after every meal—this may keep you from snacking between meals. If you get the urge to snack, you can also gargle with mouthwash, or put a breath strip into your mouth.

❑ Most obese people don't necessarily have more fat cells than slim people.

❑ Your body can replace fat cells over time.

❑ When you lose weight, you don't get rid of fat cells, you merely shrink them.

❑ Liposuction is a procedure for localized fat removal for normal-weight people. It's not a solution for overall weight-loss.

❑ Bariatric surgery—of which gastric-bypass surgery is the most common form—is only for the super obese, morbidly obese or clinically obese who are also suffering from serious obesity-related health problems. It requires a lifelong commitment.

❑ You must be thoroughly educated by a doctor to see if bariatric surgery is for you.

❑ Gastric-bypass surgery has serious risks and complications.

❑ Most gastric-bypass patients gradually regain 20% to 25% of what they lose.

❑ Gastric band surgery and obesity implants are alternatives to gastric-bypass surgery.

❑ Bariatric surgery is very expensive, and it may not be covered by insurance.

Gastric-bypass surgery can lead to a serious, post-surgery complication called "addiction transfer." Former patients eventually transfer their addiction from food (which they can no longer overeat on) to another addiction such as alcohol, shopping, compulsive spending, compulsive gambling, smoking, or even promiscuity.

CHAPTER 24
Drink up   *343*

Drink plenty of water and other fluids, preferably ice-cold. Being properly hydrated is essential for your health, and sufficient fluids can also produce the sensation of fullness that can help reduce food consumption.

❑ Drink enough water over the course of the day to produce at least four *clear* urinations a day (in addition to colored ones). The quantity will vary relative to your activity level, and the climate you live in.

❑ Don't consume calorie-laden drinks like soda, coffee drinks, fruit-juice drinks, or even 100%-pure fruit juices.

❑ While sugar-free soda is low in calories, it's still processed, usually contains chemicals, and should be avoided.

❑ Many vitamin-enhanced drinks or sports drinks are high-calorie, sugared water.

❑ Watch your portion sizes when drinking nutritious drinks like skim milk.

Liquid calories don't satisfy your body in the way that solid-food calories can, but can easily add up to many low-nutrient calories. Watch out for excessive calories, dietary sugars, or high-fructose corn syrup in anything you drink. By eliminating a few sugar-laden sodas each day you can lose 10 to 30 pounds in a year.

❑ 86% of adult Americans responsibly enjoy alcoholic drinks.

❑ In moderation, alcoholic drinks can be healthy.

"Moderation" for Americans means no more than one drink a day for women or lighter-weight men, and no more than two drinks a day for other men. A drink is a 12-ounce can or bottle of beer (or wine cooler), a 5-ounce glass of wine, or 1.5 ounces of 80-proof liquor.

❑ Excessive drinking of alcoholic beverages yields many consumed calories, and often causes excessive eating because of reduced inhibitions.

❑ Alcohol can suppress your body's ability to burn fat.

❑ Your body will burn the alcohol first, and store your food calories as fat.

❑ Be more active when you drink at social events—by standing and walking around.

❑ Eat a balanced meal and drink plenty of water before you begin drinking any alcohol.

❑ Beer drinking doesn't directly create a beer belly.

❑ A beer belly accrues when caloric intake regularly exceeds caloric expenditure.

❑ If you've overdone drinking, work off the calories with exercise.

Heavy alcohol consumption is associated with reduced longevity and increased risk of a diversity of diseases.

CHAPTER 25

Weight-loss aids   *353*

While there are many dietary supplements that claim to provide weight-loss benefits, most are *not* backed by legitimate, unbiased scientific research conducted on human beings. And because of this, most of these products can't be trusted.

❑ Even the best legitimate weight-loss aids may help only a few percent at best.

If you were to lose 100 pounds, about 98 of it would be from your exercise and diet, and only two or so would be from the contribution of a weight-loss aid.

The only proven means to substantial, sustainable fat-loss that experts agree on, is *proper diet and exercise*.

❑ Omega-3 fatty acids can trigger enzymes that can help to lower body fat.

❑ Vitamin C plays a critical role in the fat oxidation process.

❑ Take a daily RDA-level multivitamin-mineral tablet that has the USP symbol.

❑ Caffeine is a central nervous system stimulant and mild diuretic.

❑ Caffeine may prompt you to exercise harder, and you may burn more calories as a result.

❑ Studies show that caffeine *alone* may not have fat-burning effects.

❑ Coffee drinks and energy drinks can be very high in calories and sugar.

❑ Use caffeine in moderation because too much can be dangerous.

Green tea, or green tea extract capsules with EGCG, are a good source of caffeine, and have been shown to accelerate fat-breakdown, and increase endurance.

❑ Green tea also serves as a powerful antioxidant, which helps to protect cells.

- Certain micronutrients (including some phytochemicals) may help weight-loss.

- The best legitimate FDA-approved weight-loss pill will, by itself, create a fat-loss of less than one pound a month.

If you're considering trying a food supplement, or a weight-loss aid, first review it with your doctor to see if it's appropriate for you. And if it is appropriate, discuss the dosage that's right for you.

CHAPTER 26

How to succeed when you have children   *361*

If you eat healthily but while everyone else in your family eats processed food, you'll most likely fail with weight-loss over the long-term. To succeed, it usually requires a support group. Make your support group within your own family. If you can get your family on the same page, you can all live a healthier lifestyle, and help each other.

- Allow children to adapt to healthier eating *electively*.

- During the interim, give them their own personal zone where they can store their processed food.

- Have your own personal zone for your healthy, nutritious foods.

Set a great example with your own healthy eating, weight-loss, and much improved fitness, and you may win your children over to the better lifestyle *provided* it's not forced upon them. If you eat healthily, they may eventually learn to enjoy eating healthily, too.

- Just because you're on a weight-loss plan doesn't mean your children also want to be on one.

- If you eat junk food and fast food, your children will probably emulate you and eat junk food and fast food, too.

- If you become more active, so may your children.

Perhaps the most effective way to lose weight and get healthy is for your entire family to do it together, as a team. But it has to be a long-term, lifestyle-reform, weight-loss and health plan, not a temporary diet.

CHAPTER 27

Excuses are no excuse   *367*

☐ Everyone has time to exercise—if President Obama can find time, so can you.

On a blog written by a middle-aged lady who lost 200 pounds, Brad found this exchange:

"How do you find time to do so much walking and exercise?"

"I make the time by not watching so much television."

☐ Combine indoor, low-intensity exercise—such as treadmill walking—with TV watching, telephone calls, or social interaction.

☐ Find time to eat healthily by planning better, or pre-preparing meals in advance.

☐ If you make exercise fun and rewarding, you won't hate it.

☐ Very heavy people can still do a variety of low-impact exercises.

☐ You're never too old to exercise or improve your health.

If dieting is too hard, don't make it so hard. At least initially, eat correctly just 80% to 90% of the time. Enjoy your favorite foods, and enjoy some occasional cheating. If you don't enjoy working your plan, and don't adopt a strategy you can readily stick with for the rest of your life, you'll never succeed over the long-term.

But eventually you'll find that healthy food tastes better than processed food, you'll lose desire for crud, and then you may not want to eat any of it.

☐ Don't blame others for your weight problem.

❑ Take responsibility for your actions, and you'll have a good chance of losing weight, and changing your life for the better.

Does obesity run in your family via genetics, or via conditioned behaviors? Many generations of families are obese because that's all they know — and it's got nothing to do with genetics.

But you can still lose weight and keep it off *even if your obesity has a genetic component.*

❑ It's your responsibility to be healthy for yourself, and for people who rely on you.

❑ Take excellent care of your health.

You won't succeed with weight-loss unless you give up excuses, get some motivation, and get into a healthy lifestyle with commitment.

In just three or four weeks, a healthy lifestyle will become second nature. *Just give it a chance.*

Most people who succeed at weight-loss say the same thing — *once you get over the initial hump, you're almost home-free.*

CHAPTER 28

What you can learn from the new Brad   *373*

Brad's story is similar to the stories of many other real-life dieters who struggle with their weight.

Are any of these symptoms similar to yours?

Brad's weight problems really began when he went to college, away from the realm of parental control.

He became addicted to processed food.

Eating also became a form of entertainment and social interaction.

He equated eating with comfort and happiness, much like how it was during his childhood.

Healthy eating was off his radar as a young adult.

He couldn't control his eating.

A lack of patience spawned a decades-long cycle of crash diets.

He was forever searching for the weight-loss holy grail.

He was gullible, and trusted the ads for weight-loss products.

Here's what New Brad advised Young Brad:

- ❑ "Fast results" weight-loss pills are a sham.

- ❑ It's unrealistic to lose more than two pounds a week.

- ❑ Restrictive diets and extreme exercise can't be maintained over the long-term because they take you too far from your normal comfort zone.

- ❑ Don't go on a temporary diet, but have a fresh outlook on life, nutrition and health over the *long-term*.

- ❑ Your plan must be based on behaviors you're comfortable with. The best diet is the one you don't know you're on.

- ❑ It's okay to cheat *a little* every now and then. You can't be perfect all the time.

- ❑ Keep yourself active, and stop being a couch potato. Even little daily activities like standing and moving around can amount to several pounds lost over time.

- ❑ Stop late-night and weekend binges. Where do you think the thousands of late-night calories end up if you do nothing to burn them off?

- ❑ Don't eat anything two to three hours before bedtime.

- ❑ Eat a nutritious mini-meal or snack every two to four hours. You can still enjoy burgers and sandwiches—just prepare them in a nutritious manner, and don't make them so big.

- ❑ As you eat, remind yourself that what you eat provides nourishment for your body. Eat primarily for nourishment, not entertainment. *Get pleasure from your food, of course, but get it from food that's also nourishing and healthy.*

❏ Be patient. Stop trying to rush your weight-loss. You've failed every time with crash diets. Just take it one step at a time—day-by-day, week-by-week, pound-by-pound.

❏ Stop being gullible—gimmicks, shortcuts, and pills and potions that claim to have "miraculous benefits" aren't the answer for weight-loss. Not a single person I interviewed attributed their weight-loss to any of these fallacies.

❏ Take pleasure in the process because it will eventually become your new, permanent lifestyle. People who succeed with weight-loss, and keeping it off, exercise and eat well because they *want* to, not because they feel they *have* to.

❏ Find new hobbies and interests to divert energy away from food and eating.

❏ To lose body fat you *must* expend more calories than you take in, to create an energy imbalance in your body. Consume fewer calories, and burn more calories.

❏ *Every day*, produce the required energy imbalance. Then you'll make progress *every day*.

Brad followed a model based on real-life success. *It's now time for you to do the same.*

CHAPTER 29

You've lost the weight . . . now what? *381*

❏ Get rid of the "fat clothes." Indulge in new and fashionable "thin clothes."

❏ Treat yourself to a spa treatment, massage, manicure, and a fabulous haircut.

❏ Spoil yourself with fun things like these, *not food*.

It's imperative that you continue to follow the basic principles that created your weight-loss in the first place. The biggest mistake that dieters who have lost a lot of weight make is to think that they've "crossed the finish line," and assume that they are done.

They mistakenly believe that they no longer have to eat sensibly and exercise once they are "done" with the program. The right approach has no finish line.

☐ Adjust your calories and exercise to a level that allows you to comfortably maintain your ideal weight for the rest of your life.

☐ Don't forget about the hundreds of hours of dedication it took you to succeed.

☐ Don't fall off the weight-loss plan wagon and let yourself down.

☐ Stick with the program, and enjoy it for the rest of your life.

If you keep your activity levels somewhat high, and continue to eat in a nutritious manner, you can enjoy a relatively normal lifestyle and yet still break even bodyweight wise.

Maintaining your weight is much easier than losing weight. The maintenance phase—which will be the rest of your life—is a breeze, comparatively speaking. Just don't stray from the general principles and guidelines that you utilized to realize your fabulous results.

Make changes that you can live with forever, and follow through day after day, month after month, year after year.

Although it may seem like a pipe dream now, the healthy lifestyle you'll live will eventually become second nature. And you'll wonder how you could have lived an unhealthy lifestyle in the first place.

☐ For long-term maintenance you must stay active via exercise.

☐ If you stray from the principles that created your weight-loss, you'll regain your weight.

☐ It's acceptable to fluctuate a few pounds throughout the year.

☐ Make your goal a range within, perhaps, three to five pounds.

☐ You can still enjoy holidays and special occasions. If you're overly strict and don't enjoy your life, you'll fail to lose weight and keep it off.

❑ It's okay to make occasional mistakes. Focus on the big picture.

Everyone is capable of achieving lasting weight-loss.

Never forget these fundamental principles of weight-loss:

To lose weight you must establish an energy imbalance in your body. So, the next time you overeat, what's your plan for burning the extra calories off? And what will happen to the extra calories if you don't burn them off— *they will be stored as body fat.*

When you're in maintenance mode you can vary your daily caloric intake and output somewhat, *but be consistent with your weekly figures*. Then, provided you match your input and output figures every week, you'll effortlessly maintain your weight.

CHAPTER 30

How real people ate to *lose* weight, and how real people eat to *maintain* their healthy weights *387*

❑ The typical day in Brad's life during his transformation, shown on pages 388 and 389, provides ideas for when you design your own daily schedule.

❑ And also review the account on pages 390 through 392 of how Mary lost 80 pounds and kept it off.

❑ If you want to consume more calories than Brad or Mary did, you can, but you'll lose weight at a slower pace. Of course, you must still produce an average daily caloric deficit, although not necessarily to the same extent as Brad did.

For most of his life Brad resented slim people. He would look at a lean person and think to himself, "It must be nice being born with perfect genetics. I wish I could have been that lucky."

But as Brad researched why people are slim, he came to another conclusion. A very few people are winners of

life's genetic lottery for leanness, *but most lean people are that way because of their lifestyle and eating habits.*

Why Stuart can eat more than many people and yet not gain weight:

- ❑ He isn't trying to lose weight—he's lean enough already.

- ❑ Twice a week, in the morning after breakfast, he lifts weights intensively, and does hard cardio. This may produce the afterburn effect to yield calorie burning for some of the rest of his workout days additional to what he would burn had he not exercised.

- ❑. He has more muscle mass than he would have if he didn't train with weights, which boosts his caloric needs.

- ❑ He's very active even when out of the gym, which further boosts his caloric needs.

- ❑ Although he enjoys his meals—*as you must, too*—he eats primarily for nourishment, not entertainment.

- ❑ He never eats crud—no junk food, no fast food, no fried food, and nothing with refined sugar or high-fructose corn syrup in it.

- ❑ He eats a wide variety of food rich in vitamins, minerals and essential fatty acids; and he takes food supplements.

- ❑ He eats a fiber-rich diet.

- ❑ He eats a good breakfast every day.

- ❑ He rarely eats out.

- ❑ He never snacks in front of the television.

- ❑ He eats often but never exceeds his weekly caloric allocation.

- ❑ He drinks a lot of water, including several mugs of green tea each day.

In many ways, Stuart does what **WEIGHT-LOSS SALVATION** teaches. It's not by chance that he's maintained a lean, steady weight for many years.

Most overweight people have different lifestyles and eating habits to Stuart's. If they adopted eating habits

similar to his (but with fewer calories), and become much more active, they would lose weight readily.

❑ That Brad's 47-year-old wife, Lisa, has a very active lifestyle, and exercises regularly, allows her to eat as she pleases yet maintain a healthy weight. Although occasionally she still eats food that isn't healthy, she always keeps her portion sizes in check. But treats aside, she eats nutritiously.

❑ Lisa is also fully aware of what she eats and drinks. She knows the maximum amount of sustenance she can have each day without putting on weight, and she doesn't exceed that quantity.

How Brad eats now that he's lost his weight:

❑ Once Brad met his goal weight and went into the maintenance phase, he was able to increase his daily calories because he was no longer losing weight.

❑ Brad had previously lost weight at an average of 1.62 pounds of fat a week (the equivalent of 5,670 weekly calories, which amounts to about 800 daily calories).

❑ Brad has become accustomed to eating more nutrient-rich foods and, like Stuart, enjoys eating these foods, and covets the resulting high, steady energy level.

❑ These extra nutritious calories Brad is now able to enjoy are earned through a very active lifestyle as part of his lifelong maintenance phase.

Brad now fully understands Stuart's situation because he's now living that type of healthy lifestyle himself. And now that Brad has maintained his ideal weight for well over three years, many people his age are now saying to him, "It must be nice being born with perfect genetics. I wish I could be that lucky."

What an irony. If they could have seen Brad several years ago they would never have made that comment.

Follow Brad's example for weight-loss *and* the follow-up maintenance phase. *If he can do it, so can you.*

Maintaining weight is much easier than losing weight. Revel in your lifelong maintenance phase as you enjoy a healthy, active lifestyle as the new you!

Good luck with *your* weight-loss. *And cheers to the new you!*

Help spread the word

The purpose of this book is to change lives, and save lives.

Everyone hears stories about people as young as 35 to 45 suddenly dying of a heart attack, and invariably those people were overweight and unhealthy.

Weight-related issues have become the second leading cause of preventable death in the United States—second only to smoking. And the same issues occur in many other countries. We can prevent many of these annual deaths, *one person at a time*. It has become one of our passions to do something about this global epidemic. But we can't do it alone. *We need your help.*

Once you begin to get healthy by utilizing the guidance offered in **WEIGHT-LOSS SALVATION**, help everyone you care about to get healthy, too. Urge them to read their own copies of this book

We've helped many people get healthy and turn their lives around. Get healthy yourself, turn your life around, and spread the word about this book so that others can achieve the same great results themselves.

Help spread the word!

Let's stay in touch

We want to hear from you. We want to see photographs of your progress, and read accounts of it.

Please e-mail your information to *brad@weightlosssalvation.com* or *stuart@weightlosssalvation.com*

We're all in this together, and we want you to be part of our ongoing support group. You can be part of our posse of successful real-life dieters

Visit our website at www.weightlosssalvation.com

About the authors

Bradley Cailor

Brad was born in 1965 in Youngstown, Ohio. He is a recovering compulsive overeater. He had a 30-year battle with binge-eating disorder and its associated yo-yo dieting. He tried every diet and weight-loss pill, and lost over 600 pounds of fat during that period.

At age 40, haunted by thoughts of dying from a heart attack, Brad needed a permanent change. Armed with over 25 years of research, and input from hundreds of successful, long-term dieters, he achieved a net fat-loss of 114 pounds over one continuous stretch. And he has maintained his current weight for over three years.

Brad was a personal trainer for seven years, coach of national- and world-caliber powerlifters, president of Kent State University's Weightlifting and Exercise Association, a competitive powerlifter, and a school-record athlete in high school. He has a college degree in health education, post-graduate schooling in nutrition, and was a certified health teacher for almost a decade.

He currently lives with his wife and numerous pets outside of Columbus, Ohio.

Stuart McRobert

Stuart was born in 1958 in Stockton-on-Tees, England. At age 14 he started a lifelong fascination with exercise, nutrition, and health.

In 1981 he started writing instructional articles, and has subsequently had over 500 published in newsstand magazines in the US and the UK.

He graduated from college in 1982 but was unable to find a teaching post in England. In 1983 he started teaching at an international school on the Mediterranean island of Cyprus.

In 1989 he founded CS Publishing, and started *Hardgainer* magazine. Shortly afterwards he retired as a school teacher. Over the next 15 years he wrote five books on exercise instruction and related topics: *Brawn, Beyond Brawn, Further Brawn, The Insider's Tell-All Handbook on Weight-Training Technique,* and *Build Muscle, Lose Fat, Look Great.* He has guided countless people on how to transform their bodies. He retired *Hardgainer* in 2004, and then diversified his writing and publishing.

He continues to live in Cyprus, with his wife and two daughters.

Index

See directs you from a term not used in the index to the synonym where the information will be found. *See also* indicates that additional information is available under a related subject.

The Whole-Scoop Summary has not been indexed.

Referenced publications

Dement, William C., M.D., Ph.D., *The Promise of Sleep*, 115, 350
Hirschmann, Jane R., and Munter, Carol H., *Overcoming Overeating*, 64, 80
Johnson, Richard J., M.D., and Gower, Timothy, *The Sugar Fix*, 119
Kessler, David A., M.D., *The End of Overeating*, 57, 59
Peters, Lulu Hunt, *Diet and Health: With Key to the Calories*, 135
Schuler, Lou, et al, *Testosterone Advantage Plan*, 180
Thayer, Robert E., Ph.D., *Calm Energy: How People Regulate Mood with Food
                and Exercise*, 84
Guinness Book of World Records, 15

Documentaries

Referenced institutions and bodies